# OVARIAN FUNCTION
# AND ITS DISORDERS

# DEVELOPMENTS IN OBSTETRICS
# AND GYNECOLOGY

VOLUME 3

1. J. E. Jirásek, Human fetal endocrines, 1980. ISBN 90–247–2325–6.
2. P. M. Motta, E. S. E. Hafez, eds., Biology of the ovary, 1980. ISBN 90–247–2316–7.
3. J. Horský, J. Presl, Ovarian function and its disorders, 1980. ISBN 90–247–2326–4.
4. D. W. Richardson, D. Joyce, E. M. Symonds, eds., Frozen human semen, 1980. ISBN 90–247–2370–1.
5. E. S. E. Hafez, W. A. A. van Os, eds., Medicated intrauterine devices, 1980. ISBN 90–247–2371–X.

Series ISBN 90–247–2334–5

# Ovarian Function and its Disorders

JAN HORSKÝ, M.D., D.Sc.
JIŘÍ PRESL, M.D., D.Sc.

*Institute for the Care of Mother and Child, Prague*

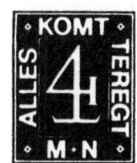

1981
MARTINUS NIJHOFF PUBLISHERS
THE HAGUE / BOSTON / LONDON

*Distributors:*

*for the United States and Canada*

Kluwer Boston, Inc.
190 Old Derby Street
Hingham, MA 02043
USA

*for all other countries*

Kluwer Academic Publishers Group
Distribution Center
P.O. Box 322
3300 AH Dordrecht
The Netherlands

*for Hungary, Albania,*
*Bulgaria, China,*
*Cuba, Czechoslovakia,*
*German Democratic Republic,*
*Democratic People's Republic*
*of Korea, Mongolia, Poland,*
*Roumania, Soviet Union,*
*Democratic Republic of Vietnam,*
*and Yugoslavia*

AVICENUM,
Czechoslovak Medical Press,
Prague

ISBN-13:978-94-009-8197-3     e-ISBN-13:978-94-009-8195-9
DOI: 10.1007/978-94-009-8195-9

© *Translation: K. Ošancová, Ph.D.*

*Copyright* © *1981 by Martinus Nijhoff Publishers bv, The Hague.*
*Softcover reprint of the hardcover 1st edition 1981*

# Contents

# ABBREVIATIONS USED IN THE TEXT

| | |
|---|---|
| ACTH | adrenocorticotropic hormone |
| BM | basal metabolic rate |
| BSA | bovine serum albumin |
| BT, BBT | basal body temperature |
| cAMP | cyclic adenosine-3′, 5′-monophosphate |
| CBG | corticoid-binding globulin (transcortin) |
| cGMP | cyclic guanosine-3′, 5′-monophosphate |
| Chr | chromatography |
| CL | confidence limits |
| CoA | coenzyme A |
| CPB | competitive protein binding |
| CRF | corticotropin-releasing factor |
| DA | dopamine |
| DHEA | dehydroepiandrosterone |
| DHT | dihydrotestosterone |
| DID | double isotope dilution |
| DNA | deoxyribonucleic acid |
| E | oestrogens ($E_1$-oestron, $E_2$-oestradiol, $E_3$-oestriol, $E_t$-total oestrogens) |
| EE | ethinyloestradiol |
| FSH | follicle-stimulating hormone |
| GABA | $\gamma$-aminobutyric acid |
| GH | growth hormone (synonym: STH) |
| GLC | gas liquid chromatography |
| Gn | gonadotropic hormone |
| h | human (before abbreviation of the hormone) |
| hCG | human chorionic gonadotropin |
| hCS | human chorionic somatotropin (synonym: hPL) |
| HMG | human menopausal gonadotropin |
| HMG-IRP-2 | 2nd International Reference Preparation of HMG |
| HPG | human pituitary gonadotropin |

| | |
|---|---|
| hPL | human placental lactogen (synonym: hCS) |
| 3β-HSD | 3β-hydroxysteroid dehydrogenase |
| HSG | hysterosalpingography |
| KI | kymoinsufflation |
| LH | luteinizing hormone |
| LTH | luteotropic (luteomammotropic) hormone (synonym: PRL) |
| ME | mestranol, ethinyloestradiol methylether |
| IU | international unit |
| MCR | metabolic clearance rate |
| MSH | melanostimulating hormone |
| NAD | nicotinamide adenine dinucleotide |
| NADH | NAD in reduced form |
| NADP | nicotinamide adenine dinucleotide phosphate |
| NADPH | NADP in reduced form |
| NE | norepinephrine |
| o | ovine (before abbreviation of the hormone) |
| OAAD | ovarian ascorbic acid depletion |
| p | porcine (before abbreviation of the hormone) |
| PBI | protein-bound iodine |
| PG | prostaglandin |
| PIF, PIH | prolactin inhibiting factor or hormone |
| PMSG | pregnant mare serum gonadotropin |
| PPG | pneumopelvigraphy |
| PRH | prolactin releasing hormone |
| PRL | prolactin |
| RF | hypothalamic releasing factor |
| RH | hypothalamic releasing hormone |
| RIA | radioimmunoassay |
| RNA | ribonucleic acid |
| SBP | sex steroid-binding protein (synonyms: SBβG, SHBG, TeBG, TEBG) |
| SBβG | sex steroid-binding β-globulin (synonyms: SBP, SHBG, TeBG, TEBG) |
| SD | standard deviation |
| SE | standard error |
| SHBG | sex hormone-binding globulin (synonyms: SBP, SBβG, TeBG, TEBG) |
| STH | somatotropic hormone (synonym: GH) |
| T | testosterone ($T_T$ total, $T_F$ free) |
| $T_4$ | thyroxin |

XVI

| | |
|---|---|
| TeBG | testosterone-binding globulin (synonyms: SBP, SBβG, SHBG, TEBG) |
| TEBG | testosterone and oestradiol binding globulin (synonyms: SBP, SBβG, SHBG, TeBG) |
| TGA | total gonadotropin activity |
| TRH | TSH releasing hormone |
| TSH | thyrotropic hormone |

# CONVERSION INTO SI UNITS

1 pg of oestradiol/ml    = 3.67 pmol/l
1 ng of progesterone/ml = 3.12 nmol/l
1 pg of testosterone/ml  = 3.45 pmol/l

# Development of Ovarian Activity and its Control

## SEX DETERMINATION

Gonadal sex in the human is determined at the moment when after fertilization of the ovum, impregnation, karyogamy occurs, i.e. fusion of the haploid female and male pronucleus. The human fertilized ovum, zygote, contains a diploid set of chromosomes 2n = 46. This number comprises 44 autosomes and 2 hetero-chromosomes (gonosomes), XX in the female zygote and XY in the male zygote.

In mammals gonosome Y determines the male sex, gonosome X carries certain factors which determine the female sex. Without gonosome Y the testis does not develop. Not even the simultaneous presence of two or more X gonosomes in the chromosomal complement will prevent differentiation of the indifferent embryonic bipotential gonad into the testis. For the normal differentiation of the ovary in humans two X gonosomes without a Y gonosome are needed. In the presence of gonosome Y the ovary does not develop, regardless of the number of X gonosomes. One X gonosome, when the other is lacking or abnormal, does not suffice for the normal development of the ovary. Gonosome X carries moreover a number of sex-linked Mendelian genes which are vital for the organism and thus the chromo-somal constitution of 44,00 (i.e. absence of the two X gonosomes) is lethal. Thus we can never find out whether differentiation of the embryonic bipotential gonad into the ovary would also start in the absence of both X gonosomes.

During the very earliest embryonic period both X gonosomes ($X^m$ of maternal and $X^p$ of paternal origin) are fully active; in primates during the period of the implanted blastocyst [in humans between the 12th day (in the trophoblast) and 16th day (in the embryo) after fertilization] one of them undergoes heteropyknosis, and practically already genetically inactive, is pushed out towards the nuclear membrane as so-called sex chromatin (Barr's body), which can be detected in normal women in 36–76% of cellular nuclei in smears from the buccal mucosa (199); its incidence varies in relation to the menstrual cycle. The inactivation of this heterochromosome is, however, neither complete nor permanent; evidence of this is the phenotypic difference between a normal woman 46,XX, and an individual with gonadal dysgenesis 45,X0. In some somatic cells a heteropycnotic change of chromosome $X^m$ occurs, in others of $X^p$. Mammalian females are in this respect carriers of the mosaic $X^m X^p$.

Sexual differentiation of the indifferent embryonic bipotential gonad depends obviously on gonosomal factors which determine sex in the earliest phase of intrauterine life, probably before the

1

heteropycnosis of one of the X gonosomes, i.e. before the formation of the gonadal primordium (primordial germ cells in the genital fold already have sex chromatin).

Recent observations make this assumption more definite. Ovulating women with Turner's phenotype and 45,X0 leucocytic karyotype were described who had also the ovarian karyotype 45,X0. Since an ovarian karyotype is obtained from a cell culture of fibroblastic tissue and only reflects the status of the primitive gonadal ridge, it can be concluded, that the limiting factor in normal ovarian differentiation is not heterochromatic X of the gonadal ridge tissue but the integrity of germ cells. The occurrence of a specific "reverse" non-disjunction during the mitotic phase of germ cell proliferation has been postulated with formation of a large number of 46,XX daughter cells, thus explaining the observed differentiation of functioning ovarian tissue (260).

From the genetic determination of gonadal sex, which is determined by the gonosomal sex, it is essential to differentiate the postgenetic determination of subsequent stages of sexual differentiation of the individual. Their hierarchy can be summarized as follows (119):

    I. gonosomal (genotypic) sex
   II. gonadal sex
  III. somatopsychic sex: a) genital and somatic (phenotypic) sex
                                 b) hypothalamic and psychic sex
  IV. gender identity

# DEVELOPMENT OF THE REPRODUCTIVE SYSTEM, ITS FUNCTION AND CONTROL

## DEVELOPMENT OF THE OVARY

At present the view is generally accepted that in all vertebrates incl. humans *primordial germ cells* (*primary gonocytes*) develop outside the gonads. In man they were identified first in the entodermal epithelium of the yolk sac in the vicinity of the diverticulum of the allantois during the third week after fertilization. From there they move by active migration, shifts caused by the uneven growth of tissues and perhaps also due to lytic activity into the entoderm of the cloaca and then through the mesenterial mesenchyma into the indifferent gonads. This primordium (Anlage) of the gonad develops by hypertrophy of the primitive coelomic (meso-blastic) epithelium which covers the transient embryonic developmental stage of the kidney, mesonephros, before migration of the primordial germ cells. The condition of its further growth is the presence of a certain number of these cells. The migration of the primordial germ cells is terminated about 40 days after fertilization; the cells are deposited in the epithelium and underlying mesenchyma and begin to divide mitotically (division may have started during migration).

For the subsequent development the direction of differentiation of the somatic blastema in the root of the **indifferent gonad** which is determined by the gono-

2

somal complement is decisive. The somatic blastema of the indifferent gonad communicates with the blastema located cranially to the indifferent gonad from which the adrenal cortex differentiates. It seems that ovarian, testicular and adrenal steroid-producing cells have a common origin. This is also suggested by the common metabolic pathway of steroid biosynthesis where gestagens, androgens and oestrogens are only individual steps (for review see 375).

Primordial germ cells and oogonia respectively which develop from them by mitotic division are incorporated at the periphery of the gonad into cellular cords of the blastema and there they divide further and differentiate into oocytes. In deeper layers around oocytes in meiosis a sheath of follicular cells is formed, aggregations of primordial follicles not separated by connective tissue develop, the first at the menstrual age of 4.5–5 months. During the subsequent differentiation of the ovary the mesonephros disappears. At the site of the original contact the mesoovarium and the ovarian hilus develop. The remnants of the cranial portion of the mesonephros persist in the mesoovarium as the epoophoron (homologue of the epididymis of the testis), the caudal portion of the mesonephros in the broad ligament as the paroophoron (homologue of the paradidymis of the testis) and in the hilus as the rete ovarii. At the age of 7–8 weeks after fertilization we may already identify reliably in a human female embryo the gonad as the so-called **embryonic ovary** (240, 241)).

The first follicular structures in the ovary are described as primordial and formed at some sites by an irregular, incomplete layer of flat follicular cells. The follicles are not yet separated by reticular fibres. About one month later isolated primary follicles appear which at first are completely surrounded by a layer of cubic granulosa cells. Vesicular follicles with cavitation in the multiple layer of granulosa cells and the formation of an antrum with follicular liquid are found in the ovary within a very variable range of 21–36 weeks of menstrual age. The formation of the antrum is associated or preceded by the differentiation of the theca and its epitheloid cells. Rarely, in the last trimester of pregnancy in the ovary of the foetus large cavitated follicles are also described resembling preovulatory Graafian follicles. It seems that the human foetal ovary is relatively inactive despite the high concentration of circulating gonadotropins, endogenous hypophyseal FSH and LH and placental hCG (for review see 254, 429). Therefore the idea is feasible that the action of gonadotropins on the foetal ovary is blocked or inhibited. In this connection the existence of an gonadotropin-inhibiting factor in the pineal gland of the human foetus is of interest (see p. 22).

The **postnatal ovary** is from the age of 2 months to 11 years (397) an actively growing ovary in most instances which contains in addition to preantral also cavitated follicles. A "*quiescent ovary*" which contains mainly quiescent primordial and primary follicles was not found; it seems that in those instances a developmental disorder is obviously involved, observed e.g. in children with Down's syndrome. The gradually increasing number and size of cavitated follicles is evident after the age of six years in coincidence with the rise of urinary excretion of total oestrogens. After the age of seven the latter for the first time exceed values recorded in adult ovariectomized women, along with the first manifestations of oestrogenic stimulation in vaginal smears, the subsequent colonization of the vagina with Döderlein's lactobacillus and the onset of the growth of mammary glands (409).

## OOGENESIS

The *primordial germ cells* (*primary gonocytes*) divide in the early developmental stage of the ovary and oogonia develop which divide further by mitotic division. The first oogonia enter meiotic division already during the 8th–9th week following fertilization and change into *primary oocytes*. The presence of meiosis and the absence of isolated primary follicles characterize the so-called **early foetal ovary.** The stimulus for the onset of meiosis (and perhaps also for the formation of follicular cells) comes most probably from the rete ovarii. The first meiotic maturation division (reductional) reaches in the prophase the diplotene, i.e. the period of the terminated crossing over when genes are exchanged between homologous chromosomes; during the subsequent late period of the diplotene [in the dictyotene (dictyate)] in a sort of resting stage meiosis stops. In this stage which is reached by the first oocytes about the 90th day after fertilization and by the last shortly after delivery, the primary oocytes persist in the human ovary for 10 to 50 years unless they degenerate. Only shortly before ovulation this resting stage is interrupted and meiosis proceeds. It seems that the arrest of meiosis coincides with the formation of a sheath of follicular cells; a causal relationship (inhibition on the part of the follicle) seems probable. The presence of isolated primary follicles with oocytes in the diplotenic resting stage of meiosis and with primary stroma in the cells of which for the first time the activity of 3β-hydroxysteroid dehydrogenase can be detected characterizes the so-called **late foetal ovary.** For the transformation of the early into the late foetal ovary, for the formation of a complete sheath of follicular cells two X chromosomes in the gonosomal complement are essential. (In 45,X0 foetuses the oocytes degenerate shortly after the formation of primary follicles, because the sheath of follicular cells is incomplete.)

The number of oogonia and primary oocytes in the foetus reaches its peak approximately during the fifth month after fertilization (according to estimates there are about two million oogonia and five million primary oocytes) and then the number declines rapidly — by termination of mitosis of oogonia and as a result of degeneration of oogonia and primary oocytes. The ovary of the newborn infant, the so-called **perinatal ovary,** contains about one million oocytes. Its typical feature is the presence of growing follicles with a multi-layer granulosa and differen-

4

tiated theca with 3β-hydroxysteroid dehydrogenase activity in the epitheloid cells, and cavitated follicles. With the above "stock" of oocytes the individual enters postnatal life. The majority of contemporary authors agree that postfoetal or postnatal oogenesis in humans does not exist (for review see 148, 149). The majority of oocytes disappears during life-time, during the fertile period of females some 400–500 mature to the stage of ovulation, i.e. approximately 1 of 5,000 in the ovaries of newborn infants.

Shortly before ovulation the follicle increases rapidly in size to a diameter of 15–20 mm in particular at the expense of the antrum and a Graafian follicle develops. Its primary oocyte proceeds in the interrupted prophase of the first maturation division (reductional) of meiosis and a haploid secondary oocyte is formed and the first polar body. The impulse of reactivation of meiosis is not known; it is probably associated with the preovulation release of gonadotropins from the pituitary. The second maturation division (equational, i.e. mitotic) of meiosis begins several minutes before ovulation proper and fertilization is the prerequisite of its termination. After penetration of the sperm cell (fertilization usually takes place in the outer third of the oviduct and the sperm cell penetrates as a whole through the zona pellucida, deprived of 3,000–4,000 cells of the corona radiata) in the oocyte the second polar body is separated and the remaining nucleus of the secondary oocyte changes into the female pronucleus. Although several sperm cells can penetrate into the oocyte, only one participates in fertilization. By the fusion of haploid pronuclei (karyogamy) the new diploid set of chromosomes of the zygote is formed.

The first division of the zygote takes place about 30 hours after fertilization. The morula migrates through the oviduct and after four days the developing blastula reaches the uterus where 6–6.5 days after fertilization the blastocyst begins to be implanted. If fertilization does not take place, the oocyte perishes 12–24 hours after ovulation, and is destroyed in the uterine cavity.

It is obvious that the exact equivalent of the spermatozoon, the ovum, i.e. the cell which develops after termination of the second maturation division of meiosis, does not exist. Either it is fertilized as the secondary oocyte and changes into a zygote or, if fertilization does not occur — it perishes as a secondary oocyte at the onset of the second meiotic maturation division.


## DEVELOPMENT OF THE GENITAL APPARATUS

The genital organs develop in close association with the urinary system. The first primitive foetal kidney, *pronephros*, appears at the end of the 3rd week after fertilization high in the cervical region and disappears after one week. Its duct leading into the cloaca persists and combines secondarily as the *Wolffian duct* with the second foetal kidney, the *mesonephros* (corpus Wolffi) which is formed during the 4th week caudally from the pronephros in the thoracic and upper lumbar region and disappears after the 7th week (while the definitive kidney, the *metanephros*, differentiates caudally from the mesonephros during the 5th week).

On the median surface of the mesonephros coelomic epithelium hypertrophies to form the earlier mentioned genital fold, it becomes invaginated on the lateral surface and the paramesonephric *Müllerian duct* is formed which during the 9th week reaches the urogenital part of the original cloaca, the urogenital sinus. In female foetuses (where testicular testosterone and "factor X" are lacking, which in the male foetus induce proliferation of the Wolffian system and degeneration of the Müllerian) about 10 weeks after fertilization the Wolffian duct disappears. Its residuum is Gärtner's duct which runs parallel with the Fallopian tube, uterus and vagina. From the cranial portion of Müller's ducts Fallopian tubes are differentiated and from their caudal fused part the uterovaginal canal. From the cranial portion of the uterovaginal canal the uterus is formed, and from the caudal part the vagina. The indifferent external genitalia develop in a female way and in a three-month-old foetus it has already a definite female character (for review see 240, 241).

*What is the biological meaning of this autonomous differentiation of the female genital apparatus?* Natural selection favoured viviparity in mammals with a prolonged development of the new individual which is relatively safe inside the maternal organism. Therefore evolution has substituted the phylogenetically lower prototype of autonomous development of male and the induction of female sex organs by oestrogens (in reptiles and birds) by the reverse in mammals. In the mammalian embryo, regardless of its genetic sex, the female pattern of development of the genital apparatus (and of secretion of pituitary gonadotropins) is inherent. Therefore the development of the female sex is relatively autonomous; the development of the male genital apparatus, on the other hand, is induced, i.e. the differentiation into the testis takes place only as a result of the action of testicular androgens — this mechanism protects against the action of maternal oestrogens. If this radical evolutional change did not occur, male foetuses would run the danger of feminization by maternal oestrogens (68).


# DEVELOPMENT OF THE ADENOHYPOPHYSIS


The adenohypophysis, i.e. the glandular, epithelial part of the pituitary, develops according to the classical concept from invagination of the entoderm of the primitive oral cavity apparent during the 4th week after fertilization (adjacent secondarily to the primordium of the neurohypophysis which is formed from the ectoderm of the base of the diencephalon). The present concept, however, postulates that the adenohypophysis shares with the hypothalamus the same ventral neural ridge of the neuroectoderm for its origin. Thus, all peptide hormone-producing cells are derived from the neural ectoderm, as are all neurons. The whole hypothalamo--hypophyseal complex appears to be a neuroendocrine derivative of the ventral neural ridge.

As early as from the 8th week after fertilization a common glycoprotein $\alpha$-sub--unit can be detected in the pituitary by immunocytochemical methods; during the 15th week — probably due to the action of hypothalamic regulatory peptides — the synthesis of FSH$\beta$ and LH$\beta$ begins, as in adult life, both sub-units in the same cell (191). This observation is consistent with the findings that about at the age of 16 weeks the human foetal pituitary begins to respond to hypothalamic trigger hormones by gonadotropin secretion *in vitro* (465; 505). The secretion of the α-sub-unit persists into adult life; peripheral breakdown of intact glycoprotein hormones is not involved (129). Immunoreactive FSH in plasma was demonstrated from the 84th day after fertilization, LH from the 99th day (254). The concentration of circulating gonadotropins is highest at the end of the first half of pregnancy when it reaches values found in women after castration or the menopause.

During the first six months after birth the plasma gonadotropin levels decline; their secretion then remains relatively stable up to the onset of puberty.

## DEVELOPMENT OF THE HYPOTHALAMUS

In the third lunar month of pregnancy the hypothalamic morpho-functional areas associated with the regulation of the gonadotropin secretion by the pituitary are defined. During the fourth month their shape and structure resemble the adult state and cell differentiation begins (development also proceeds postnatally, in particular during the first 2–4 years after birth) (51). The original multilayer cell matrix in the preoptic area and anterior hypothalamus is used up, and between the 25th and 28th week of pregnancy it has the appearance of a single-layer ependyma. This stage corresponds to the degree of morphological development of the hypothalamus of the female rat at the end of the critical postnatal period of neuronal competence where it is possible to alter the future cyclic release of pituitary gonadotropins by exogenous androgens or oestrogens and thus to induce anovulatory sterility (120).

By means of immunocytochemical detection of LH-RH in the hypothalamus of the human foetus the first immunoreactive neurons are revealed during the 13th week after fertilization (in rare instances even earlier); their number increases and reaches a peak about the 20th week. They are dispersed in certain preferential areas, in the anterior, mediobasal and posterior hypothalamus (64). In the extract of the foetal hypothalamus LH-RH can be detected by radioimmunological methods, from the 6th week after fertilization; its concentration rises up to the 20th week (8). Starting at the 16th week some LH-RH immunoreactive fibres end on the capillary loops of the primary portal plexus which is found approximately during the 14th week. The continuity of the primary and secondary plexus of the portal system is, however, formed only after 18–21 weeks of intrauterine life (64, 361).

# DEVELOPMENT OF THE PINEAL ORGAN

The pineal is formed later than the pituitary and has a double origin. About 7 weeks after fertilization the caudal part of the roof of the diencephalon becomes invaginated; the anterior lobe is a derivative of the ependymal lining, the posterior develops most probably from specialized subcommissural ependyma. The pineal loses all nervous and vascular connections with the brain; from this aspect we cannot compare the epithalamo-epiphyseal system with the hypothalamo-pituitary system. Typical cells of the epiphyseal parenchyma, pinealocytes, are derivatives of the neuroepithelial basis of the gland; they are specialized ectodermal elements of the neuroglial series, like pituicytes of the neurohypophysis (for review see 255).

The involution of parenchymal cells begins in humans during childhood; in autopsy findings calcifications were detected even in the first year of life and their incidence is steadily increasing (previous X-ray studies usually detected pineal calcifications only after puberty). It was not possible to detect any morphological changes linked with a definite postnatal period (for review see 543).


# SEXUAL DIFFERENTIATION OF THE HYPOTHALAMUS

In the rat, the adult sexual pattern of pituitary gonadotropin secretion depends on the presence or absence of testicular androgens during the postnatal critical period of neuronal competence of the hypothalamus. The presence of androgens will decide on the future male tonic character of gonadotropin secretion. Lack of androgens means that the original, to both gonosomal and gonadal sexes common and inherent pattern of the future cyclic, i.e. female secretion of gonadotropins, persists and becomes fixed. Early castration "feminizes" the hypothalamic regulating areas in the male and conversely early administration of androgen to the female causes "masculinization" of the appropriate areas of the hypothalamus. In the first case the ovary transplanted to a male will start its cyclic function in adult life, in the second case the female will develop anovulatory sterility (for review see 178). [Similarly, the metabolic pattern of steroid transformation in the rat liver differentiates sexually, depending on neonatal testosterone (105).]

A similar effect as that caused by androgens in the critical period is exerted also by oestrogens. It seems that androgens do not act directly but only after conversion into oestrogens in the target tissue. Inhibitors of aromatization block the action of testosterone. Antioestrogens block not only the effect of oestrogens but also that of androgens. Dihydrotestosterone which cannot be aromatized and which is also formed in the hypothalamus after administration of testosterone therefore does not have a local masculinizing effect on gonadotropin secretion. Endogenous oestrogens do not play a part in female rats because at that time the ovary has not yet started the biosynthesis of oestrogens (for review see 404) and the rat brain seems to be temporarily protected against the effect of relatively high concentration of circulating oestrogens of adrenal origin (327a).

The developmental stage of the human foetal hypothalamus which corresponds

8

to the termination of the critical postnatal period of neuronal competence of the hypothalamus in the rat is attained between the 25th and 28th week of pregnancy (120). In the second trimester in the median basal hypothalamus the first mono-aminergic neurons are also found (324). If the conditions revealed in laboratory rodents apply also to primates, the critical period of neuronal competence of the hypothalamus in man would start by the differentiation of hypothalamic nuclei (between the 14th and 16th week of intrauterine life) and terminate at the end of the 2nd and beginning of the 3rd trimester of pregnancy respectively.

Because in the human female foetuses a high circulating oestradiol concentration (equal or higher than in the mother — 428) does not interfere with the development of the future cyclic secretion of pituitary gonadotropins, it is obvious that it is protected against the action of oestradiol. The brain of human and subhuman primate foetuses is protected so effectively against the masculinizing action of placental oestradiol (and testicular testosterone in foetuses with male gonadal sex) that even in male foetuses masculinization of the hypothalamus does not occur. In castrated men and male monkeys after suppression of increased gonadotropin secretion a functioning stimulatory (positive) feedback of oestrogens can be found, similarly as in women and female monkeys (256, 284, 494). Female monkeys with an external genital masculinized after administration of testosterone to pregnant mothers also have the mechanism of the stimulatory oestrogen feedback preserved (494). "Pseudomasculinization" of the hypothalamus in male primates with tonic secretion of gonadotropins is only the manifestation of masking the ability of cyclic secretion by postnatal testicular hormone (of non-steroid but peptide character), as proved by the appearance of the stimulatory feedback of oestrogens after orchidectomy (495).

We assume that a prenatal disorder of protective mechanisms can cause masculinization of the hypothalamic pattern of pituitary gonadotropin secretion by placental oestrogens; the clinical manifestation would be a) primary or b) secondary (delayed) anovulatory disorders of the menstrual cycle and sterility (p. 197).

# Sexual Maturation

**Menarche,** the first menstruation, the typical manifestation of the genital cycle in higher primates is in the life of women a period which — although it is not identical with sexual maturity — is a certain culmination of the previous development of the genital apparatus and its regulatory mechanisms. It is preceded by growth acceleration and the development of secondary sex characteristics.

*Table 1* Onset and termination of the development of clinical characteristics of sexual maturation of an urban (Prague) group of 1,300 girls (311)

| Clinical Sign | Onset | Termination |
|---|---|---|
| | age (years) | |
| Oestrogen stimulation of the vaginal epithelium | 7.1 | 13.6 |
| Breast growth | 7.6 | 19.0 |
| Döderlein's lactobacillus vaginal colonization | 7.7 | 13.8 |
| Pubic hair | 8.3 | 15.5 |
| Axillary hair | 9.1 | 17.5 |
| Uterine growth | 9.1 | 19.6 |
| Menarche | 9.8 | 17.2 |

(For statistical evaluation of clinical data see p. 166)

The sequence of the development of sex characteristics is described generally as follows:

(1) first manifestations of oestrogenic stimulation of the vaginal epithelium, colonization of the vagina with Döderlein's lactobacillus and change of the pH of the vaginal secretion, (2) development of the breasts (thelarche) (preceded by enlargement of the pelvis and rounding of the hips), (3) development of pubic hair (pubarche), (4) development of axillary hair, (5) development of the uterus and (6) menarche (311). The onset and termination of the development of clinical signs of sexual maturation in the urban population of Prague is summarized in Table 1.

The practical *clinical classification of sexual maturation* (238) differentiates between the following stages:

11

P1 — absence of clinical characteristics of sexual maturation;

P2 — beginning of growth of breasts, sparse pubic or axillary hair or both — early puberty;

P3 — further development of the breasts (the areola is above the outline of the breast), more abundant pubic and axillary hair — mid-puberty;

P4 — breasts developed (the areola fuses with the outline of the breast), pubic and axillary hair, but still without menarche — late puberty;

P5 — postmenarcheal girls.

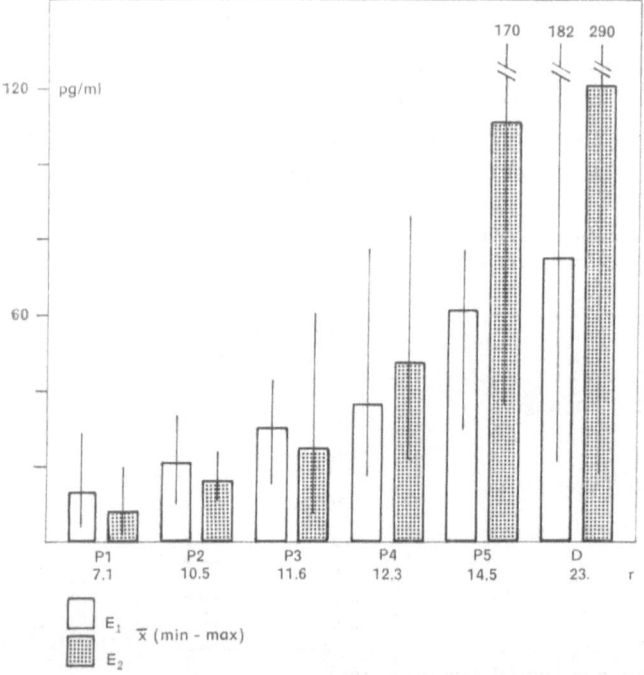

*Fig. 1.* Mean concentrations of plasma oestrone ($E_1$) and oestradiol ($E_2$) in relation to sexual maturation. (P1–P5 — stages of puberty, D — adult women and mean age in different groups) (41).

This clinical classification correlates markedly with the rising concentration of plasma oestradiol and oestrone (Fig. 1) (41). In clinical practice, we prefer this classification to a more simplified one differentiating only two pubertal stages, the early and the late.

There is considerable terminological confusion in the interpretation of the concepts of puberty and adolescence. In our opinion **puberty** in girls can be defined as the interval between the first clinical manifestations of sexual maturation and the attainment of menarche, i.e. the interval which in the above five-grade classification comprises stages P2, P3 and P4.

During the period of menarche, or shortly afterwards the rapid phase of pubertal acceleration of somatic growth culminates; the degree of bone maturation, characterized among others by the state of ossification of the metacarpus of the thumb, correlates significantly with menarche (46).

We consider menarche as the onset of **adolescence.** This term is used for the period when the slow phase of pubertal acceleration takes place and which ends by the stabilization of the menstrual cycle with a predominance of ovulatory cycles and adequate function of the corpus luteum. The termination of adolescence corre-

*Fig. 2.* Variability of length of menstrual cycle in relation to menstrual age (calculated from menarche), calendar age and premenopausal age (related to menopause). (On x-axis interval after menarche; calendar age and interval before menopause in years; on y-axis on left — mean length of cycle in days, on right — intervals of selected mean m) (513).

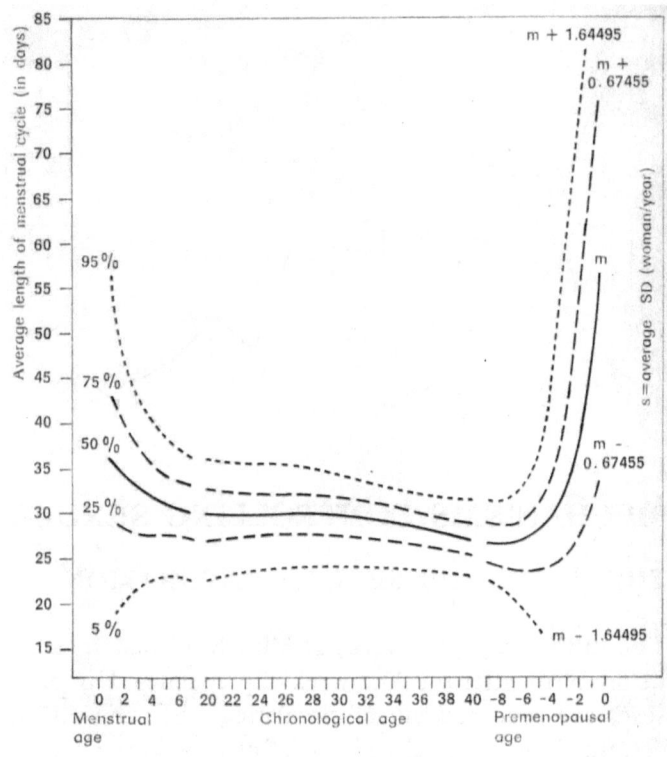

sponds to the disappearance of epiphyseal plates of the long bones of the arm, radius and ulna (not earlier than two years after menarche, as a rule after 24–36 months) (46).

The variability of the first menstrual cycles after menarche is considerable (276) (Fig. 2). At first anovulatory cycles predominate and luteal phase inadequacy is frequent. With increasing "menstrual experience" the incidence of anovulatory cycles declines, while that of ovulatory cycles increases (Fig. 3). After the first 24 cycles an obvious tendency towards regularity is observed. It is maintained that irregularity of menstrual cycles during the first two years after menarche is no reason for fears (106). Irregularity persisting for longer than two years is considered, however, a primary menstrual dysfunction (405). The prognosis of this disorder is poor. The probability that the cycles will remain dysfunctional is greater than in adolescent girls and women where the pattern of a normal menstrual cycle is stabilized and disorders of the cycle develop only secondarily (486). Further, the future fertility of women with primary menstrual dysfunction is markedly impaired (486).

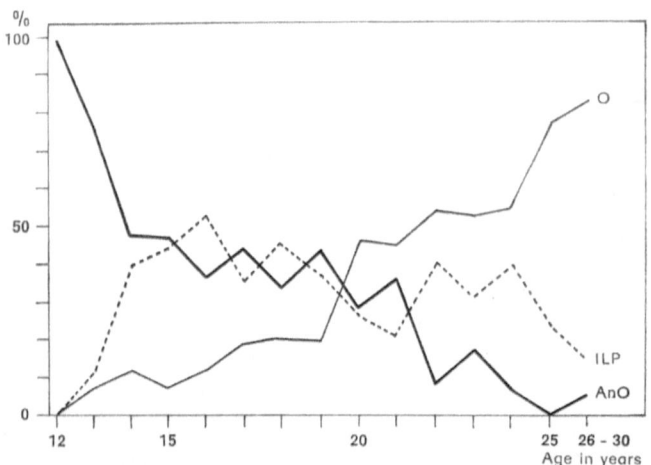

*Fig. 3.* Stabilization of ovulation mechanism in women after menarche (1471 cycles in 303 women). (O — incidence of ovulatory cycles, AnO — incidence of anovulatory cycles, ILP — inadequate luteal phase (115).

# MECHANISMS CONTROLLING SEXUAL MATURATION

## THE BRAIN AND SEXUAL MATURATION

**The inhibitory (negative) feedback of oestrogens** (p. 38) operates probably before birth, after the 20th week of pregnancy. Up to that time in foetuses of both sexes the concentration of circulating FSH and LH increases despite the high oestradiol plasma level which is of placental origin, and only then the secretion of foetal pituitary gonadotropins declines briskly (see review by 186, 254, 429). At that time apparently in the brain and pituitary of human foetuses a specific cytoplasmic oestrogen receptor develops (101).

The responsiveness of oestrogen-sensitive areas of the brain which are decisive for the inhibitory feedback declines gradually during ontogeny. Hohlweg's and Junkmann's hypothesis of 1932, derived from experiments on rats, was also confirmed in humans and the dose of oestrogens needed to reduce the urinary FSH secretion in prepubertal girls increases in the course of puberty (259, 282). According to this concept the pubertal rise of tonic gonadotropin secretion is a manifestation of disinhibition of the release of hypothalamic regulatory peptides. The position is, no doubt, more complicated. The pubertal rise of gonadotropin secretion also occurs when normal ovaries and or ovarian oestrogens are lacking (e.g. in gonadal dysgenesis — 88, 422), probably as a result of an autonomously programmed change in the setting of the hypothalamic gonadostat. The participation of this central mechanism is also suggested by the substantially slower rise and lower plateau of secretion of both gonadotropins after ovariectomy in prepubertal female monkeys — the distinct rise occurs only during the period corresponding to puberty (112). An alternative explanation is the possible interference of adrenal androgens during adrenarche.

**The stimulatory (positive) oestrogen feedback** (p. 39) potentially operates in girls during late puberty (P4), i.e. during premenarche (412); in monkeys this mechanism matures only several months after menarche. Contrary to the typical ovulatory cycle, in girls before menarche only LH is released. The feedback cyclic secretion of both gonadotropins in females thus matures in a different way, that of FSH only after menarche. It is assumed that there is also an increase in the responsiveness of the appropriate oestrogen-sensitive target areas of the hypothalamus — contrary to the inhibitory feedback the level of circulating oestrogens exceeds its threshold and thus the first release of ovulatory hormone takes place (404).

From the facts mentioned it ensues that the increase of tonic, and later the onset of cyclic secretion of pituitary gonadotropins depends on the appropriately changed release of hypothalamic trigger hormones which is controlled by monoaminoergic neurons. Therefore there is no doubt that the key factor in the onset of puberty is the functional maturity of certain central catecholaminergic neurons. The hypothesis on the growth of terminal arborization of their synapses on peptidergic neurons with subsequent enlargement of the hypothalamic impulse for activation of the pituitary ovarian axis (442) creates for the first time the idea of a mutual relationship between nutritional and metabolic factors and puberty. Cerebral catecholaminergic neurons respond to the neuronal growth factor (NGF) which is as to its structure and function close to pancreatic proinsulin secreted into the peripheral circulation. Pancreatic secretion depends, as known, on food supply and body mass — proinsulin could stimulate the appropriate central neurons and act thus as a messenger between the metabolism and hypothalamus during sexual maturation. In juvenile diabetes delayed menarche is actually described (40, 87, 541).

## INFLUENCE OF AGE, BODY-WEIGHT, BODY COMPOSITION AND METABOLISM ON SEXUAL MATURATION

The **age** when humans reach sexual maturity is probably genetically programmed. There is evidence on the striking coincidence of menarche in monozygotic twins and on the similarity between mothers and daughters or siblings. It seems that the expression of this prototype of menarcheal age in the human species can be influenced by the conditions of the external environment. The observed secular trend of acceleration of menarche is explained by the conditions of the external environment and their improvement: during the last century the age of menarche gradually declined (Fig. 4). While it was relatively constant from classical times to the beginning of the modern era, round the year 1500 it began to delay in Europe and this

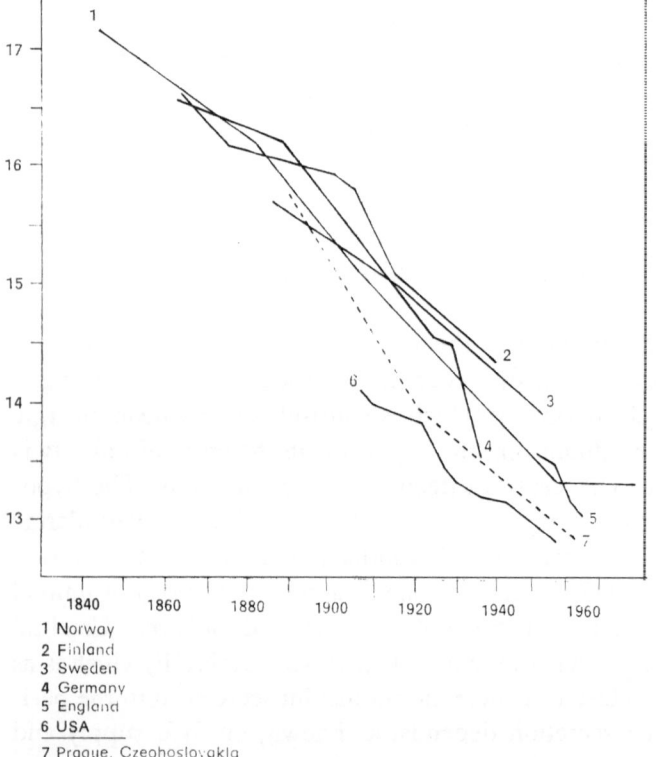

*Fig. 4.* Gradual reduction of menarcheal age in different countries (16).

1 Norway
2 Finland
3 Sweden
4 Germany
5 England
6 USA
7 Prague, Czechoslovakia

trend reached its peak at the end of the 18th century. At the beginning of the 19th century the menarcheal age began to decline, obviously due to advancing industrialization and improvement of socioeconomic conditions of the population (16). The age of menarche is thus a certain indicator of the living standard of the population. It seems that in recent years in some countries (e.g. Norway and USA) the acceleration of menarche has already stopped.

Extensive literature suggests that formerly overrated racial and climatic influences on menarcheal age are not as important as formerly assumed. Much more important is the comprehensive action of social and economic conditions, in particular in conjunction with the urban environment. No doubt, an important

16

part is played by economic prosperity with a high nutritional standard. Acceleration of menarche seems to be only part of the general acceleration of somatic development which is manifested by the attainment of a higher average height and body weight.

Recent investigation revealed that the age at menarche is more closely related to **body weight** than to chronological age. The correlation with body weight is so significant, that some authors speak of a "critical body weight" associated with the attainment of menarche (158, 159). It has been known that in monkeys there exists a close relationship between body weight and menarche: the scatter of body weight at menarche is smaller than the scatter of chronological age. By growth acceleration and by earlier attainment of average menarcheal weight with anabolic drugs in female monkeys it proved possible to reduce the age of menarche. In humans earlier menarche is also associated with accelerated skeletal maturation. In the US population the critical body weight at menarche is reported to be $47.8 \pm 0.5$ kg (the 25th percentile is 43.0 and the 75th percentile 51.5 kg) (158). Comparable data for the Czech population are lacking so far.

The level of **basal metabolism** is even more closely related with menarche; again for the US population the critical value is a decline to 28 cal/kg/h (117.2 J/kg/h). In keeping with this are observations that in juvenile thyrotoxicosis menarche is usually delayed (423), while in hypothyroidism the reverse is true (237, 540a). The raised metabolism during treatment of hypothyroidism leads to regression of manifestations of early sexual maturation (445, 522). Based on experimental results it is assumed at present that there exists a pituitary factor which reduces the response of peripheral tissues to thyroid hormones. It seems that its formation starts during puberty; subsequently its production increases further (104).

The condition when menarche is reached is characterized better by the critical **body fat ratio** than by the critical body weight, the same body fat ratio being attained by individuals with a very different height and body weight. During menarche the body fat ratio is about $23.5\%$, i.e. about 11 kg (these data pertain again to the US population). From menarche to the period of stabilized body composition, i.e. to the age of 16–18 years, there is an average increment of 4.5 kg body fat. This interval corresponds to the described adolescent sterility with a predominance of anovulatory cycles. The resulting total amout is about 16–17 kg fat, a reserve of readily mobilizable energy for future pregnancy and lactation. An interaction between energy homeostasis and the reproductive function of the female is assumed (160). In obese girls earlier menarche is observed (121). In this connection we would like to recall the already mentioned idea that proinsulin acts as a possible factor of neuron growth and that it plays a part in the maturation of catecholaminergic neurons of the CNS in areas controlling the secretion of pituitary gonadotropins (p. 29).

Human adipose tissue contains some enzyme systems participating in steroid biosynthesis; it is able to aromatize androgens and is thus an important extragonadal source of oestrogens (see p. 86). An increase in body weight with an increase of body fat is moreover associated with a change of the oestrogen metabolism: 2-hydroxylation of oestradiol (formation of 2-hydroxyoestrone) is reduced and its 16α-hydroxylation (oestriol formation) increases. (The reverse trend is observed when the body weight declines in anorexia nervosa.) 2-hydroxyoestrone is biologically less active than oestriol and it cannot be ruled out that it acts as an endogenous antioestrogen.

## PITUITARY AND SEXUAL MATURATION

**Gonadarche,** the onset of ovarian oestrogen secretion and the subsequent beginning of puberty is logically associated with increased secretion of pituitary gonadotropins. This secretion does not change substantially during the first years (391). During the prepubertal period significantly lower concentrations of circulating gonadotropins are reported than in adult women (for review see 283). Although most frequently a rise of both plasma gonadotropin levels is described and a more rapid rise of FSH than of LH, depending on the stage of sexual maturation, so far unequivocal evidence has not been provided whether gonadarche is due to the concomitant rise of secretion of one or both gonadotropins.

The reactivity of the adenohypophysis in relation to LH-RH markedly changes during postnatal ontogeny. Before puberty there is a greater response of FSH than of LH, from the onset of puberty, however, the response of LH rises progressively (152, 186), obviously as a result of stimulated synthesis and storage of LH and gradually it acquires the adult pattern. This striking change of pituitary response to exogenous LH-RH appears to be associated rather with adrenal androgens than with pubertal changes of ovarian steroid secretion. In preteenage girls with gonadal dysgenesis the reaction of gonadotropic secretion to LH-RH resembles the reaction in prepubertal girls and although the steroid production in their gonads does not change through the teenage years, the secretory response of the pituitary changes similarly as in pubertal girls (422). These observations suggest at the same time that changes in the secretion of two pituitary gonadotropins do not necessarily imply the existence of two independent hypothalamic releasing hormones. The different action of exogenous LH-RH, depending on sexual maturation, indicates that a single releasing hormone on the background of the changing steroid spectrum is sufficient.

The urinary gonadotropin excretion acquires in the course of puberty a dominant rhythm, at first with a two-day frequency; the rising oestrogen excretion, however, does not display the corresponding variations (212). At a certain time before menarche a gradual change towards a longer cycle takes place (31, 203).

# PINEAL GLAND AND SEXUAL MATURATION

b Although it is tempting to assume that in the mechanism of sexual maturation a part is played
y pineal antigonadotropic factors (p. 22), no unequivocal conclusions can be drawn from hitherto
accomplished investigations.


# ADRENALS AND SEXUAL MATURATION

A prerequisite among others of normal sexual maturation is a normal function
of other endocrine glands, in particular the adrenals — especially in conjunction
with the development of pubic and axillary hair (**pubarche**). At the time of incipient puberty the excretion of 17-oxosteroids rises (**adrenarche**), and for the first
time dehydroepiandrosterone appears in the urine; it was not detected in girls
before the age of 8 years, not even after stimulation with exogenous ACTH (390).

The level of plasma androstenedione rises in girls already at the age of about
8 years, i.e. in coincidence with the first clinical manifestations of sexual maturation
and the rise of circulating oestrone. The plasma testosterone level rises later, about
at the age of 10 years, during the period of pubarche, along with a brisk increase
in the circulating oestradiol concentration. The correlation with pubertal stages
P1–P5 is in both androgens (and oestradiol) highly significant (85, 539).

The finding that there is a better correlation between the maximum plasma LH
increment during a LH-RH test and androstenedione or testosterone than with
oestradiol in girls is remarkable (85). Assembled data seem to indicate that the
adrenal gland is the first to be activated in the process of sexual maturation
(57a, 90c).

Androstenedione serves, moreover, as an extragonadal precursor for the peripheral oestrogen formation; by aromatization in the growing adipose tissue which
typically increases in girls during puberty the oestrogenization of the organism
increases. The urinary excretion of total oestrogens rises during the 7th and 8th
year of life and at that time it exceeds for the first time values recorded in adult
ovariectomized women (409).


# QUALITATIVE CHANGES IN STEROIDOGENESIS
# AND SEXUAL MATURATION

The oestrogen metabolism in humans changes markedly during ontogeny. During the second
trimester of pregnancy it is already more active in the foetus than in adult life, but oestriol is not
the final metabolite. The product of excessive hydroxylation of oestradiol is 15α-hydroxyoestriol,
oestetrol, which passes into the maternal circulation and is excreted in the urine as oestetrol-
glucuronate. In the foetus at term its plasma concentration is twelve times higher than in the

mother. Oestetrol which acts as a physiological antioestrogen (516) helps to protect the foetal hypothalamus against biologically active placental oestrogens (p. 9). Only during the 2nd–4th year after birth the oestrogen metabolism acquires an adult pattern.

The decline of the relatively high plasma FSH persisting several months after delivery in girls during early childhood, i.e. during the period of minimum production of ovarian oestrogens and their low concentration in the peripheral blood and urine tempts us to assume that the infantile human ovary secretes a non-identified factor(s) which is(are) active in the inhibitory feedback (539). In fact pathological conditions associated with the absence of potentially functioning gonads in childhood are associated with hypersecretion of gonadotropins (538).

# Control of Ovarian Activity

## EXTRAHYPOTHALAMIC STRUCTURES AND THE CEREBRAL CORTEX

### LIMBIC SYSTEM

The limbic system is a phylogenetically old part of the brain comprising the limbic lobe and various subcortical areas which are bilaterally connected with the hypothalamus, with areas of peptidergic neurons producing GnRH (for review see 537). The original idea that this part of the brain serves in particular the sense of smell (rhinencephalon) has been abandoned. Two main functional systems are differentiated, the so-called amygdaloid circle and the septal circle with the hippocampus. Both systems participate in the control of gonadotropic pituitary function.

The limbic system is considered a mediator between sensory impulses of the external environment and the hypothalamus. In humans, however, the determining influences of the external environment were replaced by psychosocial factors and the analysis and integration of sensory information from the external environment shifted to phylogenetically younger structures, in particular to the neocortex. This does not reduce in any way the role of the limbic system in putting into effect instinctive, genetically fixed patterns of behaviour, although in humans they frequently lost their original stereotypically programmed character. In this connection it is apt to remember the frequent coincidence of disorders of the menstrual cycle and ovulation and disorders of food intake.

### THE PINEAL GLAND

During phylogeny the pineal gland has gone through an interesting development from the original photosensory organ to a secretory glandular organ. Pinealocytes are the product of evolutional transformation of sensory cells, not a modification of nerve cells. It is not known whether their secretory products are transmitted to the capillaries of the glandular parenchyma or into the cerebrospinal fluid. However, in the latter the melatonin concentration is higher than in the peripheral blood (for review see 425).

The original direct nervous connection with the epithalamus is interrupted; the main innervation are postganglionic adrenergic sympathetic fibres from the perivascular plexuses which originate in the superior cervical ganglion. In monkeys, also preganglionic parasympathetic fibres enter the pineal gland and these fibres terminate on cholinergic autonomic nerve cells which are typical for the pineal gland of primates.

The pineal gland contains various biogenic amines; histamine, norepinephrine, dopamine and in primates in particular serotonin (5-hydroxytryptamine). It is found in pinealocytes, but is synthesized also in autonomic nerve fibres. Serotonin is a precursor of *melatonin* (N-acetyl-5-methoxytryptamine) — the best known pineal hormone — which is formed by the action of hydroxyindole-O-methyltransferase (HIOMT), an enzyme which is typical for the pineal gland. The HIOMT activity in the human pineal body does not change during postnatal ontogeny. In monkeys it is also present in the epithalamic habenula and in rats also in the retina; melatonin thus can also be formed extrapineally.

In mammals the pineal also remains an indirect photosensory organ the photic impulses being transmitted by sympathetic fibres. There also exist direct retinohypothalamic pathways; some of them end in the suprachiasmatic nucleus which is considered to be the site of the endogenous circadian rhythm. The synthesis of secretory products in pinealocytes is photo-dependent. Light reduces the HIOMT activity, while darkness promotes it. Therefore also in humans the melatonin concentration in the pineal body and its urinary excretion during the night and during sleep is higher than in day-time. Also the plasma melatonin concentration in the peripheral blood during the night is four to five times higher than during the day.

The pineal is not an endocrine gland in the true sense of the word, it is a neuroendocrine transducer (similar to the adrenal medulla) which converts the neural input into an endocrine output, i.e. it secretes hormones in response to the neurotransmitter — norepinephrine stimulates melatonin synthesis. The pineal responds, however, in a similar way also to adrenal epinephrine, liberated from the adrenal medulla during stress (for review see 544).

The majority of authors nowadays inclines to the view that the mammalian pineal is an antigonadotropic organ. $^3$H-melatonin is preferentially accumulated in the hypothalamus and ovary. The concentration of circulating melatonin in women displays an obvious relationship with the menstrual cycle; it is maximal during menstruation and lowest near ovulation. Its participation and that of the pineal respectively in the control of the axis hypothalamus — pituitary — ovary is suggested by preferential accumulation of $^3$H-oestradiol, $^3$H-progesterone and $^3$H-testosterone (and its 5α-reduction and aromatization) (for review see 413). Ovarian steroids perhaps modulate the melatonin synthesis by direct action on the pineal body.

In addition to melatonin other hormones the pineal produces are: (1) other methoxyindoles (e.g. 5-methoxytryptophol, in many respects more effective than melatonin) and (2) peptides (for review see 434). In particular arginine–vasotocin, a phylogenetically very old nonapeptide, which during the evolution of mammals differentiated into two specialized hormones, vasopressin and oxytocin, is produced. It was identified as a gonadotropin-inhibiting principle in the pineal gland of human foetuses. Moreover, in the pineal other antigonadotropic peptides with a so far not identified structure are formed, and finally LH-RH is accumulated and possibly also formed there. Nothing is known so far about factors which control the synthesis and secretion of pineal peptides. It is assumed that the site of their antigonadotropic action might be the adenohypophysis, while pineal indoles might influence the metabolism of cerebral monoamines and/or catecholamines (with the resulting reduction of LH secretion due to the action of melatonin, and FSH secretion due to the action of 5-methoxytryptophol) in addition to the direct action on the ovary (perhaps by inhibition of the gonadotropic effect).

The pineal is probably particularly involved in the slow seasonal adaptation of the reproductive system to conditions of the external environment, but certainly it is not essential for reproductive function. Pinealectomy, denervation of the pineal or permanent light or darkness usually do not have substantial and permanent consequences on the reproductive activity of lower mammals. In primates, and in particular in man, the importance of diurnal photic stimulation of the gonadotropic function of the pituitary — mediated probably by the pineal — has receded further. Artificial periodicity of alternating light and darkness does not influence the menstrual cycle of monkeys, in contrast to its effect on the genital cycle of rats; and the known infertility and irregular menstrual cycle of monkeys in summer cannot be explained by this mechanism (133). Consistent with the fact that in primates the preovulatory release of gonadotropins does not depend on the time of day is also a recent finding, that — in contrast to laboratory rodents — the preoptic suprachiasmatic area of the hypothalamus in monkeys is not essential for the development and transmission of the signal for cyclic LH release respectively (279).

## CEREBRAL CORTEX

The cerebral cortex (neocortex) is the phylogenetically youngest part of the brain which developed immensely during the process of hominization. Its volume in humans accounts for approximately $44\%$ of the volume of the hemisphere and the corticalization of functions is maximal. It is the supreme analyzing and integrating organ of information from the external and internal environment. The neocortex has also in primates direct efferent cortico-hypothalamic connections from the frontal and temporal lobe. Impulses from the neocortex can also penetrate indirectly into the hypothalamus after switching over on the thalamic nuclei.

Removal of the neopallium shortly after birth does not interfere with future fertility in female rats and the disorder of the ovarian cycle after decortication in adult female rats is only temporary. In monkeys after bilateral frontal lobotomy the menstrual cycle is not affected. Bilateral temporal lobectomy, however, severely influenced the menstrual cycle (it was irregular and prolonged and there were ovulatory disorders) and bilateral amygdalectomy alone had a similar effect. Direct cortico-hypothalamic pathways from the temporal lobes appear indispensable for the reproductive function of primates.

On the other hand, experimental neurosis causes a disorder of the oestrous cycle either without or with ovulatory disorders even in rats. In monkeys experimental neurosis is also associated with different disorders of the menstrual cycle (oligomenorrhoea or amenorrhoea or irregular bleeding). It seems thus that although the neocortex is not essential for reproductive functions, alteration of its corrective function according to Bykov's classical concept on corticovisceral pathology (for review see 285) may cause severe damage of the normal function of mechanisms regulating the gonadotropic function of the pituitary. It is of interest that experimental neuroses in animals lead to similarly varied disorders of ovarian activity as it is the case in psychosomatic menstrual dysfunction in human females (see p. 249). It cannot be ruled out that the central nervous system may influence ovarian activity also by parahypophyseal routes, i.e. via the autonomic innervation of the ovary. Similarly it cannot be entirely ruled out that the autonomic innervation influences the sensitivity of peripheral target tissues to ovarian steroids.

Starting with the classical experiments of Pavlov's school with castration neurosis, the reverse effect of gonadal steroids on the cerebral cortex was also confirmed (for review see 17).


PHEROMONES

In the evolution of primates to man olfaction became subordinated to vision and hearing, and even somaesthesis. However, in the control of the reproductive function also in some microsmatic mammals, such as subhuman primates, olfaction participates. The main terminal point of the olfactory tract is the piriform cortex, a primitive cerebral cortex (archicortex). Connection with the primary receiving area of the neocortex (the orbito-frontal area) is established only after several relays in the limbic system. Thus the olfactory connections are quite different from the visual, auditory and somaesthetic systems, where there are connections first with the neocortex which after several relays reach the limbic system. The olfactory sense organ has connections not only with the amygdala and hippocampus but also with the septal complex, the preoptic area and the hypothalamus.

24

The chemical messengers of information during interindividual sexual communication of mammals are specific signal factors acting through smell, *pheromones* (for review see 86). In subhuman primates they have the nature of signalling pheromones with a trigger effect, i.e. they act directly on sexual behaviour. Detailed investigations in women provided evidence of an individually very variable composition of the organic volatile (odorous) constituents of vaginal secretions (acids, alcohols, hydroxyketones and aromatic compounds) the origin of which is fairly complex. As to short-chain aliphatic acids ("copulins") that have sex-attractant properties in subhuman primates, in women only acetic acid is present; lactic acid is the major acidic compound consistently found near the time of ovulation, along with acetic acid and urea (223). Women on oral steroid contraceptives had lower amounts of volatile fatty acids and did not show any rhythmic changes in acid content during the menstrual cycle (332).

We have only indirect evidence on the role of sexual pheromones in humans. Hormone-dependent pheromonal signalization of women, i.e. non-behavioural cue to the partner explains the variable rate of coituses, observed by some and denied by others, in relation to the menstrual cycle with a maximum during the period of ovulation and a marked drop during the luteal phase. Moreover the tendency of synchronization of the menstrual cycle in women living in a close community and dormitories and relatively frequent oro-genital contacts during sexual activity in primitive as well as highly civilized societies is interpreted by olfactory communication. In the treatment of sexual dysfunctions of married couples olfactory perceptions are also emphasized and preferred odours are recommended as an adjuvant. Residual olfactory communication in humans need not always be apparent, as olfactory mechanisms may act at a sub-threshold level of consciousness. The idea of previously unsuspected influences of specific, naturally occurring body odours on social and sexual behaviour of man may, however, be due to an unsuitable experimental set-up with subhuman primates. The effect of associative learning in the monkeys rather than a pheromonic phenomenon appears to be an alternate interpretation of the evidence assembled to date.


## INNERVATION OF THE OVARY

The ovary of subhuman primates and man is innervated by the sympathetic (adrenergic) and parasympathetic (cholinergic) component of the autonomic nervous system. Because the indifferent embryonic gonad develops at the thoracic level, it is assumed that the *sympathetic innervation of the ovary* originates in the lower thoracic part of the spinal cord (probably Th 9-11). The fibres pass via the plexus coeliacus (long postganglionic fibres) and the ovarian plexus (short postganglionic fibres) and subsequently enter the hilus of the ovary along with blood vessels; the afferent fibres take a similar course. The *parasympathetic innervation of the ovary* which is less abundant is probably of vagal origin. A sensitive cerebrospinal innervation is also described, the fibres of which enter the posterior spinal roots via the plexus coeliacus (for review see 19, 526).

Adrenergic fibres are most abundant near the blood vessels and in the stroma in fibromuscular tissue. Nervous fibres also run in the close vicinity of follicles regardless of their developmental stage, they are relatively abundant in the external theca (probably vascular fibres are involved), they do not pass through the granulosa but they enter the corpus luteum along with blood vessels. The findings of sympathetic ganglionic cells in the ovary are controversial. There are fewer cholinergic fibres, which are found along the blood vessels and in the stroma. Contemporary histochemical investigations of sympathetic and parasympathetic fibres by means of detection of norepinephrine and acetylcholine esterase do not confirm older findings of nervous fibres (using impregnation of neurofibrils) which in the ovary of the monkey and human penetrate through the granulosa to the close vicinity of the oocyte already in the foetus in the third trimester of pregnancy.

Although experiments with the denervation of the ovary gave negative results, i.e. they did not interfere with the menstrual cycle and did not affect the fertility of females, they do not rule out the role of vegetative innervation in the control of ovarian function. Complete and permanent denervation of the ovary is impossible. Even heterotopic transplantation of the ovary does not eliminate nervous influences; revascularization which is the condition of restored function is associated with regeneration of adrenergic fibres (for review see 19).

The physiological role of the vegetative innervation of the ovary is only now being elucidated. A vasomotor and perhaps also a secretory function (nerve endings on steroid producing cells) is assumed. A permissive or synergistic action with that of gonadotropins cannot be completely ruled out either. Soviet authors consider the sensitive innervation of the ovary important for interoceptive signalization (for review see 526).

At present innervation of the smooth muscles of the human ovary is most probable, the muscle cells being abundant in the theca externa and stroma. The ovary of the monkey and human display spontaneous contractility *in vivo* and *in vitro* which is more marked when the ovary does not contain the corpus luteum. Contractions, in particular of smooth muscle fibres, may influence adjacent collagen fibrils and thus help to open the apex of the follicle impaired by collagenolytic enzymes (see p. 75).

## HYPOTHALAMUS

The hypothalamus is a small portion of the diencephalon with a diameter of only 2.5 cm between the optic chiasma and the mammillary bodies. It is an organ which coordinates and controls the majority of vitally important processes in the organism incl. reproduction. Anatomically it is divided into the anterior, medial and posterior hypothalamus. While in lower animals a swelling can be observed on the base of the hypothalamus, described as median eminence (of the tuber cinereum), in humans and monkeys due to phylogenetic and ontogenetic changes the swelling has disappeared and the appropriate area is part of the pituitary stalk which connects the hypothalamus and the pituitary. The blood supply of the hypothalamus is ensured by the anterior cerebral artery and the posterior communicating artery.

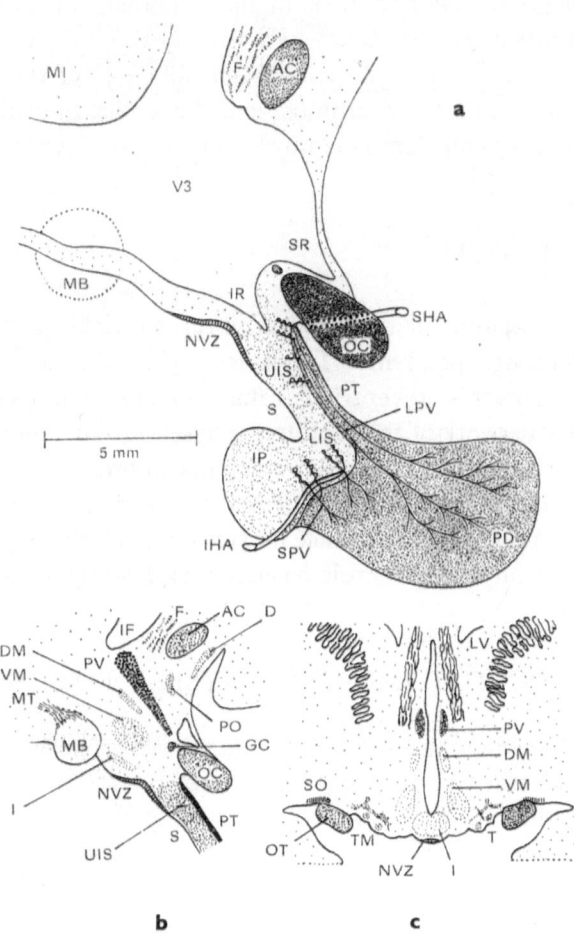

*Fig. 5.* Human hypothalamus, adjacent parts and hypophysis. a) Midline sagittal section. b) Lateral sagittal section. c) Coronal section. (AC — anterior commissure, D — nucleus of diagonal band, DM — dorsomedial nucleus, F — anterior column of fornix, GC — Gudden's commissure, I — infundibular nucleus, ventricle, IF — intraventricular foramen, IP — infundibular process, IR — infundibular recess of third ventricle, LV — lateral ventricle, LIS — lower infundibular stem, LPV — long portal vessel, MB — mamillary body, MI — massa intermedia, MT — mammillothalamic tract, NVZ — neurovascular zone, OC — optic chiasma, OT — optic tract, PD — pars distalis, PO — preoptic nucleus, PT — pars tuberalis, PV — paraventricular nucleus, S — pituitary stalk, SHA — superior hypophyseal artery, SO — supraoptic nucleus, SPV — short portal vessel, SR — supraoptic recess of third ventricle, T — lateral tuberal nucleus, TM — tuberomammillary cells, VM — ventromedial nucleus, UIS — upper infundibular stem, V3 — third ventricle) (98).

## HYPOTHALAMIC NUCLEI AND THEIR NERVOUS PATHWAYS

The hypothalamus contains a major number of clearly and vaguely defined groups of neurons described as nuclei (Fig. 5). The most readily visible are the supraoptic nucleus and the paraventricular nucleus made up of magnocellular neuro-endocrine cells. Their unmyelinated fibres form the supraopticohypophyseal tract which conveys neurohormones for the posterior lobe of the pituitary. The preoptic, infundibular (arcuate nucleus in animals) and the ventromedial hypothalamic nuclei are made up of parvicellular neuroendocrine cells and their unmyelinated fibres end in the median eminence as the so-called tubero-infundibular tract (not confirmed so far in humans), and convey releasing hormones to the portal system for the adenohypophysis (for review see 98, 204). From experiments in rats two areas of the hypothalamus appeared important: the preoptic--suprachiasmatic area where the signal for the cyclic preovulation release of LH is generated, and the hypophysiotropic area of the medial basal hypothalamus, the centre of the tonic output of gonadotropins. In primates the structures of the median basal hypothalamus control both, i.e. the cyclic and tonic gonadotropin release.

## EPENDYMA

On the base of the third cerebral ventricle in the hypothalamus is the so-called tanycyte ependyma. Tanycytes are special ependymal cells which are centrally in contact with ventricular fluid and their end feet terminate in the primary capillary network of the portohypophyseal circulation in the median eminence. In these cells structural changes develop in conjunction with the ovarian cycle. The assumption was expressed that it could be a transport link between the cerebrospinal fluid and the median eminence for steroids and releasing hormones resp. So far, however, their physiological role has not been assessed conclusively.

## HYPOTHALAMO-HYPOPHYSEAL PORTAL SYSTEM

The hypothalamo-hypophyseal portal system is a vascular link between the hypothalamus and the adenohypophysis. It starts as the primary capillary network in the median eminence. The capillary network is made up of loops which form complex structures, described by various terms, which join up into several vessels in the stalk of the pituitary. The blood supply is ensured by the branches of the a. hypophysea superior. The portal vessels in the adenohypophysis divide again to form a network of sinusoids which are in close contact with strands of glandular cells which produce gonadotropins. First they were described only from the anatomical aspect, later the centrifugal trend of the circulation was revealed. The physiological explanation of this system as a humoral link between the hypothalamus and pituitary was presented by Green and Harris (1947). Numerous experiments provided evidence that through the portal vessels neurosecretory factors are conveyed which are essential for the function of the adenohypophysis. The neurosecretion of hypothalamic cells and the portal circulation became the basic links in the neurohumoral concept of the hypothalamo–hypophyseal–ovarian regulatory mechanisms of the genital cycle. The final confirmation of the concept was the discovery of releasing hormones and this term replaced the term neurosecretion.

## BIOGENIC AMINES

Numerous papers revealed that in the regulation of gonadotropic secretion a major number of biogenic amines participate which act as neurotransmitters in addition to releasing hormones in the hypothalamus. The latter include catecholamines (norepinephrine and dopamine), indolamines (histamine) and acetylcholine (for review see 377).

Nowadays the adrenergic mechanism seems most important and **norepinephrine** (NE) at the synapses in the hypothalamus stimulates via LH-RH release the output of LH. Intraventricular administration of NE in oestrogen--primed ovariectomized rats causes release of LH (280), in rats with persistent oestrus it induces ovulation (511) and in oestrogen-primed rabbits it causes a pre-ovulation rise of LH (447), while direct NE stimulation of the pituitary is without effect. Using immunohistochemical methods and the punch technique NE was revealed in large amounts and was found to be evenly distributed in nuclei of the hypothalamus (15, 384). In the morning and afternoon during prooestrus in rats a treble increase of NE was detected in the nucleus suprachiasmaticus (463).

**Dopamine** (DA) inhibits the control of LH-RH secretion and thus LH and inhibits prolactin secretion. Apart from other cerebral systems which produce dopamine, for the gonadotropic function the tuberoinfundibular dopaminergic system is important. The bodies of neurons are located in the arcuate nucleus and in the periventricular hypothalamic areas. The nerve endings project into the lateral palisade zone of the median eminence and inhibit by axo-axonic action the secretion of LH-RH into primary capillary plexuses. DA neurons for prolactin inhibition are projected into the median palisade zone of the median eminence. A dopamine infusion in females and males reduces the blood level of LH with a subsequent rebound effect, while the FSH level is not affected. It also significantly reduces the prolactin blood level (292). The effect is either via PIH, or directly on the adenohypophysis, as dopamine receptors were also detected in the pituitary. Various authors are steadily more inclined to think that PIH is a dopamine (321). Catecholamines thus play a part in the gonadotropic regulation and the hypothesis was expressed that the negative (inhibitory) feedback action of oestrogens is leading to an increase in the DA/NA ratio in the median eminence, whereas the positive (facilitatory) feedback action causes a marked reduction of this ratio (161).

**Serotonin** is another biogenic amine which was found not only in the epiphysis but also in major amounts in the arcuate nucleus and numerous data provide evidence of its inhibitory effect on the episodic output of LH under experimental conditions or its stimulating action on ovulation after pinealectomy.

In the control of gonadotropin release some part is also played by **histamine.** Its highest concentration in the CNS is in the hypothalamus and experimentally, after its intraventricular administration in rats, a rise of serum prolactin was found and a small but significant LH output in serum, while the FSH level remained unaltered (301).

A cholinergic mechanism is probably also involved in the gonadotropin output, and has been demonstrated *in vitro* as well as *in vivo*. **Acetylcholine** enhances the LH and FSH output in incubation medium *in vitro* or serum *in vivo* (144), in other instances anticholinergic substances (BL 14) reduced serum LH and FSH and raised the serum level of prolactin (162).

Among transmitters acting at the level of the hypothalamus **GABA** (γ-amino-butyric acid) also is included. Nowadays it is assumed that GABA neurons directly or indirectly play an important part in the control of hypothalamic function (127). Intraventricular administration in rats increased serum LH (379) and the GABA-ergic substance, ibotenic acid reduces the dopamine turnover in the median eminence of the rat and is thus involved in the control of LH-RH and prolactin secretion (162).

## HYPOTHALAMIC RELEASING HORMONES

Releasing hormones control the function of the anterior lobe of the pituitary. Today we recognize six hormones stimulating and three hormones inhibiting pituitary hormones: TRH, LH-RH, CRH, PRH, SRH, MRH; PIH, SIH, MIH. The abbreviations have many synonyms and often the term factors is still used although there exists an official terminology which differentiates between stimulating liberins and inhibiting statins. Their function is more pertinently covered by the term regulatory hypothalamic peptides. There also exist other regulatory hypothalamic or extrahypothalamic peptides such as α-endorphine, β-lipoprotein, substance P, fibroblast growth factor and others. Neurosecretion first shown by E. and B. Scharrer, and demonstrated for a long time only for oxytocin and vasopressin, has a wider significance as peptide secretion interferes with many sections of physiology and medicine (for review see 188, 377, 451).

## LH-RH (GnRH, LH/FSH-RH, LRF)

LH-RH (according to the new terminology luliberin) was isolated first from pig and sheep hypothalamic tissue in 1971 and in the same year its structure was assessed and the substance was synthesized. As to its chemical nature it is a deca-peptide: pGlu-His-Trp-Ser-Tyr-Gly-Leu-Arg-Pro-Gly-$NH_2$. LH-RH stimulates the release of LH and FSH into the blood stream, in addition it also stimulates the formation of both hormones. Its action is probably species-non-specific as it was detected in humans and in many species of lower mammals, subhuman primates, birds, amphibians and fish.

The problem of two or one gonadotropin releasing agents seems to be resolved in favour of a single one, LH-RH, as separate FSH-RH was not detected. The synthetic decapeptide has the same effect as the natural one, it is equally effective when administered by the i.v., i.m. and s.c. route. The nasal route is 50 times less effective, while administered orally it is almost ineffective ($1000 \times$ less).

LH-RH is found above all in the hypothalamus but also outside it. By RIA estimation in rats it was found that most of the LH-RH detectable in the medial basal hypothalamus is in the arcuate nucleus (385). Investigations of the human hypothalamus revealed a maximum LH-RH concentration in the preoptic area which is probably the site of synthesis and in the pituitary stalk which is probably the site of release (378). By immunohistochemical methods in monkeys and humans (28) neurons containing LH-RH in the highest concentration were found in the medial basal hypothalamus and in the lamina terminalis and the neighbouring preoptic area. They give rise to the tuberoinfundibular LH-RH tract which could control the tonic secretion of gonadotropins, and to the preopticoterminal tract, perhaps for the acute release of LH-RH (cyclic gonadotropin release). Some LH-RH neurons are also in the septal, pericommissural and retromammilary area and in the rostral mesencephalon. They give rise to the extrahypophyseal tract which can modulate the activity of certain telencephalic or mesencephalic structures (for review see 28). Because of this extrahypothalamic occurrence of LH-RH neurons, of the participation of LH-RH in sexual behaviour and stress, and of its postnidation inhibitory action, it seems that the control of LH and FSH output may be only one part of its biological importance. Ovarian LH-RH receptors discovered recently can explain the inhibition of ovarian steroidogenesis by direct action of LH-RH (202a). It is assumed that LH-RH may play a wider role as a neu-rotransmitter or synaptic mediator (320). LH-RH is also formed in the placenta and could control both the output and secretion of hCG.

The initial findings pertaining to LH-RH circulation indicate that LH-RH does not bind with plasma proteins and is not inactivated by them. It disappears rapidly from the circulation, biological half-life $t_{1/2}$ (disappearance rate) = 2.9 min during the first five minutes after administration, after 5–20 min $t_{1/2}$ = 10 min and after

20 min it can no longer be detected by biological methods. By means of the RIA method a biexponential curve is found with $t_{1/2} = 5.3$ min in the first phase and $t_{1/2} = 27.4$ min in the second phase (236). The value of MCR is $1,640 \pm 59.7$ ml/min (399). Hypothalamic peptidases inactivate LH-RH and may play a part in its regulation. This degradation system contains L-cystine aryl amidase and is found not only in the hypothalamus but also in the adenohypophysis and is activated by high LH levels. It is probably an important factor in the mechanism of the gonado-tropin feedback (281). Inactivation of LH-RH results from breakdown between the 6th and 7th amino acid. The main metabolite is probably des-pGlu-His-LH-RH. The stimulus for the formation and release of LH-RH passes via biogenic amines (see p. 29). Prostaglandin $E_2$ and in particular sexual steroids also participate in the release. LH-RH accumulates in the eminentia mediana (135), and as has been proved in monkeys, is released in pulse-like waves into portal hypophyseal vessels (74). In the adenohypophysis it is bound to a specific receptor (for review see 251). In the subcellular mechanism of the effect of LH-RH on LH and FSH release according to the majority of authors the system adenyl cyclase – cAMP acts as mediator. There is also evidence that LH output is preceded by a raised cGMP level (431). The action of LH-RH requires the presence of $Ca^{2+}$ ions.

**LH-RH and its action under physiological conditions.** Immunoreactive LH-RH was identified in the human foetal brain from the age of 4.5 weeks *intra utero* and this is consistent with the first occurrence of LH and FSH in foetuses in the 5th week of gestation. The effect on the output of LH and FSH, however, is still lacking with this LH-RH between the 15th and 22nd week of gestation in experiments *in vivo*, while *in vitro* in the mid-term human foetus LH-RH is already able to release LH (167). After birth and in the quiet stage of sexual development the response in LH and FSH to LH-RH is about treble compared with basal values and increases significantly at the onset of puberty, gradually in different stages according to Tanner (P2–P5), i.e. the threshold of pituitary responsiveness changes (107). The maximum response of FSH before and at the onset of puberty in girls, which declines in the course of puberty, is striking.

In adult women LH-RH doses of 10–200 µg by the i.v. route significantly increase the plasma level of LH with a maximum after 30 minutes. The increase is 3–16 times the original level, after one hour it declines rapidly and after 8 hours it reaches the normal level. The effect on plasma FSH is substantially less, the increase is 2–5 times the original level with a maximum after 45 minutes. The decline to normal is delayed, compared with LH and occurs on average after 13 hours. There is an obvious and direct dose-response relationship for LH as well as FSH (for review see 152, 450, 451, 547).

In the course of the normal menstrual cycle the sensitivity of gonadotrophs in the anterior lobe of the pituitary to LH-RH changes. The response after a single dose of LH-RH is least during the early proliferative stage after which it rises, and is highest during the period of preovulatory rise of LH and somewhat lower, but higher than during proliferation, in the secretory stage (356, 364, 546). In women after the menopause there is after LH-RH an increased response of LH, with high basal values, compared with a normal cycle, the response of FSH being small (151). In women using oral contraceptives the response of both gonado-tropins, according to some only of LH, is reduced or suppressed. The sensitivity of the adenohypophysis is reduced more in combined and sequential preparations, only slightly in depot gestagens (Depo-Provera) or does not change at all, e.g. after minipills (393, 529).

During pregnancy the response of LH and FSH after LH-RH declines rapidly and from the third day there is a relative insensitivity of the adenohypophysis which persists up to ten days during the puerperium and only 3–4 weeks after delivery the responses to LH-RH return to normal. The position is similar after abortions — however, the reduction of response in the second trimester is greater than in the first. The reduced sensitivity of the adenohypophysis thus depends on the period of gestation (336, 519). The conclusion was drawn from some physio-logical changes that the effect of LH-RH on LH and FSH formation and output depends directly on the plasma oestradiol level. The relationship is, however, not simple and therefore much attention was devoted to investigations into the action of steroids on the sensitivity and responsiveness of the adenohypophysis and its capacity.

*Effect of sexual steroids on the gonadotropin response after LH-RH (sensitivity of the anterior lobe of the pituitary).* Sexual steroids administered exogenously reduce in the majority of subjects the release of LH and FSH after LH-RH, but sometimes they induce a rise. This modulating action depends on the dose, time, way of administration and hormonal milieu (152, 508). *Oestrogens* exert both a stimulatory and inhibitory effect. Small amounts (2.5 µg/kg body weight) enhance, while large doses (50 µg/kg body weight) reduce the response to LH-RH. LH responds rather to the stimulatory action of oestro-gens, and FSH more to the inhibitory action. The response of FSH after LH-RH declines proportionately to the increasing dose of oestrogens. There exists, however, also a biphasic action of oestrogens in time: following one dose of oestrogens after 24 hours the response to LH-RH declines and after 48 hours it increases. Biphasic action was demonstrated in amenorrhoic women (219), in a normal cycle (469) and in different animal species *in vivo* and *in vitro*. It may also have the physiological impact on primary cumulation of gonadotropins in the adenohypo-physis in the first inhibitory phase of sensitivity and their subsequent output in the second stimulatory phase. For clinical practice it is important to consider the reduced sensitivity of the adenohypophysis after large and repeated doses of oestrogens. The direct action on the sensitivity of the pituitary is the second route by which oestrogens may influence the regulation of ovarian activity, in addition to the action via the output and synthesis of hypothalamic LH-RH.

The modulating action of *gestagens* on the response after LH-RH depends on the dose and previous oestrogen treatment. Large doses of progesterone (3–5 mg/kg) reduce the response after LH-RH, smaller doses do not alter the response (470). After pretreatment with oestradiol (1 mg oestradiol benzoate) even a dose of 25 mg progesterone can increase the response of the two gonadotropins after LH-RH in amenorrhoic women, although the dose of oestrogens alone suppressed the response after LH-RH. It is therefore assumed that the preovulatory increase of progesterone contributes towards the increased sensitivity of the adenohypophysis during the preovulatory peak of LH secretion in the cycle (365).

*Testosterone* in small amounts does not alter the response after LH-RH but its 5α reduced metabolites (androstandiols) enhance the response. Large doses of testosterone either have no effect or reduce the response, metabolites (DHT and androstandiols) always reduce the response after LH-RH (132). Results both *in vitro* and *in vivo* are similar. Results *in vitro* confirm only that the adenohypophysis is influenced by androgens at least partly by a direct route.

Repeated administration of LH-RH in 2-hour pulses and in a 4–6 hour i.v. infusion gave new results and led to the idea of two gonadotropin pools in the function of the pituitary (547). The first immediately releasable pool of LH corresponds to the sensitivity of the adenohypophysis and the second reserve pool plus rate of synthesis of new LH corresponds to the capacity and the reserve of the adenohypophysis resp. In keeping with this concept, after the long-term infusion of LH-RH a biphasic response of LH after LH-RH was demonstrated with one peak after 15–45 minutes and a second higher peak after two hours. FSH did not display a biphasic character and rose steadily. The magnitude of response of the two pools is modulated by a feedback of oestradiol and progesterone and by the self-priming effect of LH-RH and changes in the course of the menstrual cycle (103, 213). In long-term infusion of LH-RH (48 hours) in monkeys gonadotropin release declined 4–28 hours after initial stimulation (141).

The determining factor for the sensitivity of the adenohypophysis to LH-RH is the content of cellular and nuclear oestrogen receptors, which at least in the cycle of the rat changes parallel with the sensitivity of the adenohypophysis to LH-RH (464).

**Anti-fertile action of LH-RH.** Pharmacological doses of LH-RH or of super-active analogues block implantation and terminate pregnancy in rats. Chronic administration of these high doses causes temporary and reversible disorders of ovarian function with a reduction of the LH and FSH levels in both animals and humans (91, 446). Investigations are in progress attempting to make use of the anti-fertile action of these substances for a new contraceptive method.

**LH-RH serum levels.** Several methods were suggested for the assessment of LH-RH levels in biological fluids. The first was biological, but the more recent methods are radioimmunological. So far, depending on the antiserum used, the method of iodidation and the extraction methods, the values differ and it will be necessary to improve the sensitivity of the methods. The serum levels during the cycle are usually lower than the sensitivity of the method. In mid-cycle some authors did not find raised values, while others found a maximum consistent with the preovulation peak of LH (0.2–1.5, 2–17 and 30–100 pg/ml resp.). The serum levels of women after the menopause are raised. The LH-RH levels in portohypophyseal circulation in monkeys are reported to be 10–150 pg/ml. The LH-RH content of the hypothalamus in rats rises after ovariectomy.


## LH-RH ANALOGUES

Investigations of the structure and function of different amino acids in the LH-RH molecules revealed two series of many new analogues: superactive or conversely inhibitory (for review see 93).

The substitution of glycine at the 6th position by another D-amino acid as well as substitution of glycinamide at the 10th position by alkylamide led to a striking increase of biological activity. There are several very strong and clinically used *superactive analogues*, i.e. super releasers. (D-Ala$^6$, des Gly-NH$_2^{10}$) LH-RH ethylamide and (D-Leu$^6$, des Gly-NH$_2^{10}$) LH-RH ethylamide cause a 9 or 5 fold greater LH and FSH release resp. than LH-RH (221, 485). They have moreover a protracted action and the maximum is reached only after three hours, the raised levels decline after 6 hours, and reach normal levels after 24 hours. D-Trp$^6$ LH-RH and D-Ser(TBU)$^6$(EA$^{10}$) LH-RH$^{1-9}$ (buserelin) raise LH and FSH in women in the follicular phase 40 times and 21 times resp. more than the appropriate amounts of LH-RH alone (156, 233). The response in women is always higher than in men. Due to the mediated action via gonadotropins after administration of analogues the oestradiol plasma level rises significantly, the maximum being after 8–9 hours. The high potency and prolonged duration of action of these analogues may be useful for stimulating ovulation in women.

*Inhibitory analogues* were obtained by the removal of histidine in position 2 and its substitution by D-phenylalanine, by substitution of glycine in position 6 by D-alanine, D-leucine or preferably D-phenylalanine and finally by substitution of L-tryptophan in position 3 by L-phenylalanine. Highly effective inhibiting analogues are nowadays (D-Phe$^2$, D-Leu$^6$)LH-RH, (D-Phe$^2$, D-Phe$^6$)LH-RH, they have, however, also a small stimulatory activity of LH-RH. A minimum LH-RH activity is possessed by (D-Phe$^2$, Phe$^3$, D-Phe$^6$)LH-RH and (D-Phe$^2$, Phe$^5$, D-Phe$^6$)LR-RH which have a protracted action for a period of eight hours and inhibit the action of LH and FSH to an extent of 75–95%. Artificially induced ovulation was inhibited by these analogues in experiments on rats, hamsters and rabbits. In monkeys in the luteal stage of the cycle the action of subsequently administered LH-RH was suppressed (192). In humans the nowadays most effective inhibiting analogue (D-Phe$^2$, D-Trp$^3$, D-Phe$^6$)LH-RH was administered in males; after one dose of 90 mg by the i.m. route it reduced significantly the response after 25 $\mu$g LH-RH for a period of 1–24 hours (174). This same analogue inhibits gonadotropin release in the chimpanzee (211). The mechanism of action is at the level of hypophyseal receptors. The results suggest the possibility of establishing a new method of birth control.

**Clinical value of synthetic LH-RH.** (1) The LH-RH test serves for the differentiation of hypothalamic and hypophyseal causes of disorders of the menstrual cycle. In hypophyseal disorders only a minor or no increase of the LH and FSH serum level is found after an i.v. injection of LH-RH.

For diagnostic purposes also the mediated release of oestradiol after LH-RH is used for the assessment of the sensitivity of the ovary (see p. 228).

(2) Therapeutically LH-RH can stimulate the maturation of the follicle and induce ovulation. In animals it induces ovulation easily, in women the results are not regular, not even after pretreatment with HMG or clomiphene. Perhaps superactive analogues will give better results (see p. 330).

(3) The application for contraceptive methods is in the experimental stage. Inhibitory analogues were prepared which by competition at the level of hypophyseal receptors prevent the physiological action of LH-RH and ovulation in rodents. The results in monkeys and humans are also promising (see p. 374). The newly confirmed antifertile action of chronic doses of superactive analogues seems to be another pathway to a method of birth control.

Antisera against LH-RH were also prepared which in rats and hamsters block the preovulatory release of LH and ovulation. However, in intact and ovariectomized monkeys it did not prove possible to block a positive feedback, i.e. oestradiol--induced LH release, while tonic release of LH and FSH was reduced to 40%, compared with controls (327).


PRH

The trigger of prolactin secretion was isolated from extracts of bovine pituitaries and from the median eminence. In males it was detected in serum after methanol extraction (190). The existence of a special trigger, however, has not been established conclusively. It is considered possible that the action of PRH is produced indirectly by TRH or other peptides or biogenic amines which are known to promote prolactin release *in vivo* but not *in vitro* (serotonin) (for review see 518).

# HYPOTHALAMIC INHIBITORY HORMONES

## PIH

In contradistinction to other hormones of the hypothalamus, PIH has an inhibiting effect on prolactin secretion which was experimentally proved in both female and male animals. The presence of PIH was detected in hypothalamic extracts of many mammalian species. By appropriate processes it proved possible to separate it from hypothalamic releasing hormones. So far it has not been detected in plasma and its chemical structure was not assessed. Many factors have an inhibitory action on PIH and thus stimulate prolactin release. The latter include in particular gonadal steroids: oestrogens, progesterone, testosterone, cortisone and also the sucking stimulus during lactation, some psychopharmaceutical substances (reserpine and other tranquillizers) and stress. A stimulating action on PIH and inhibitory action on prolactin secretion is exerted by prolactin itself in the feedback, as well as by L-DOPA, monoaminoxidase inhibitors and ergot preparations. The action on PIH is mediated, as has been mentioned before, by the dopaminergic route.

Some evidence suggests that most of the inhibitory effect of PIH on prolactin secretion is produced by dopamine by direct action on the adenohypophysis (for review see 321).

# FEEDBACKS IN THE HYPOTHALAMO-HYPOPHYSO-OVARIAN RELATIONS

The feedback principle is an important constituent of every cybernetic system in general and an important component in the control of biological processes in the organism. It is a reverse flow of information in the system of control where the controlling link receives information on the controlled link. A negative or inhibitory feedback ensures the release of such instructions between the controlling and controlled link that compensate deviations in the activity of the system. In our case the increased secretion of ovarian steroid hormones leads to a reduced release of gonadotropic hormones and vice versa. A positive or stimulatory feedback does not eliminate but promotes deviations. In our context the rise of steroid levels in the periphery induces an increased release of gonadotropins in the centre. It is not a question of simple linear feedback as in technical spheres or in the control of other endocrine glands. The complexity of the relationship between the hypothalamus and ovary is due to the fact that in addition to the quantitative aspect in the course of the cycle also the chronological aspect is involved and that the secretion of two gonadotropic (FSH and LH) and two ovarian hormones (17β--oestradiol and progesterone) is involved.

The mechanism is even more complicated, as in addition to gonadotropins of the anterior lobe of the pituitary further factors interfere with the feedback: hypothalamic releasing hormones, biogenic amines at the synapses and the sensitivity of the adenohypophysis which all respond to 17β-oestradiol.

## LONG (EXTERNAL) FEEDBACK OF OVARIAN STEROIDS

A long feedback exists between the ovary and hypothalamus; it is negative or positive and is found in all three sexual steroids.

**Negative (inhibitory) feedback of oestrogens.** A negative feedback of oestrogens and gonadotropins between gonads and the pituitary was demonstrated for the first time by Moore and Price and between gonads and the superior centre in the hypothalamus it was postulated by Hohlweg and Junkmann 1932. Further investigations in rodents, using different methods (castration, lesions and subsequent administration of exogenous oestrogens) confirmed this feedback (for review see 347). Numerous investigations in humans revealed a rise of FSH and LH level after castration and a reduction to suppression of both levels after administration of oestrogens. Extensive experiments in ovariectomized monkeys imitated by administration of minor amounts of oestradiol its normal level (70 pg/ml) as in the early follicular stage, and reduced the LH level to that corresponding to common tonic secretion (257). Other results obtained by quantification of steroids and proteohormones in monkeys revealed (271) that 17β-oestradiol acted in a negative as well as a positive feedback, depending on the height of its blood level and its persistence. The decisive threshold for the change of a negative into a positive feedback was 100 pg/ml persisting for 36–42 hours. It was thus found that in primates the long negative feedback of oestrogens is the main physiological regulator of tonic LH secretion.

**Negative feedback of progesterone.** Animal experiments had already long shown a block of ovulation after large doses of progesterone administered by the systemic route or implanted into the hypothalamus or adenohypophysis (for review see 25). Doses of 5–10 mg/d progesterone or 0.3 mg/d norethisterone acetate suppress the preovulatory peak of LH and FSH and ovulation in the normal cycle of women. Progesterone also reduces the duration of the preovulatory peak of LH by blocking the response of the adenohypophysis to LH-RH in rats (24).

**Negative feedback of testosterone.** The effect of castration in animal experiments and in men leads to a rise of the LH level and slight rise of FSH. To reduce the LH level in men one dose of 50–100 mg testosterone propionate is sufficient; FSH declined only slightly (for review see 66). In women the LH level also declines after testosterone propionate, but not the FSH level (218). Dihydrotestosterone and

5α-androstan-3α,17β diol cause an even greater decline of LH than testosterone (for review see 322).

**Positive (stimulatory) feedback of oestrogens.** For the first time a positive feedback was described many years ago by Hohlweg (1932) and Bradbury (1946). In subsequent animal experiments it was found after systemic administration as well as after implantation into the hypothalamus. In experiments on castrated monkeys but also on monkeys with an intact cycle it proved possible by single doses of oestradiol benzoate (50 µg/kg) to induce release of LH resembling the preovulatory peak in the cycle. In women exogenous oestradiol benzoate (1–5 mg i.m.) causes such regular LH release that this phenomenon has been used as a clinical test (468, 532). It is generally accepted that this positive feedback of oestrogens to LH release is also the physiological basis of the preovulatory release of LH in women (271), i.e. a regulator of cyclic LH secretion.

**Positive feedback of progesterone.** Progesterone induces a rise of the LH and FSH plasma level by a feedback mechanism in castrated women and women after the menopause pretreated with oestrogen (296, 373). The greatest increase was observed in women who were pretreated in the early follicular phase with oestradiol benzoate (2.5 µg/kg/12 h) and then were given progesterone (1.25–5 mg/ /12 h). It is assumed that also a normal preovulatory rise of LH stimulates progesterone production and that the latter not only causes an increase of LH but together with oestradiol causes a mid-cycle rise of FSH (79).

The feedback mechanism is implemented by cytosol and nuclear receptors which as regards oestradiol were found in the highest concentration in the preoptic area and in the eminentia mediana of the hypothalamus, and also in the adenohypophysis and further dispersed in different concentrations elsewhere in the brain. In women no specific nuclear receptors for progesterone were detected in the hypothalamus and hypophysis, although according to some work they exist in animals. The effect of progesterone is mediated by an increase in oestradiol receptors in these tissues or the increase in oestradiol receptor is caused by a progesterone-mediated block of a later step in the oestradiol – receptor – genome interaction (426). The positive feedback of progesterone is implemented probably after conversion of progesterone to 5α reduced metabolites. The negative feedback is probably a property of progesterone itself (322).

So far, however, it remains obscure at what site the feedback circle closes. From animal experiments it was concluded, based on surgical disconnection by means of Halasz' knife which blocked ovulation in rodents, that the site of the positive feedback was in the anterior hypothalamus. More recently by quantification of steroids and proteohormones it was demonstrated that by the same method in monkeys different results were obtained and therefore the positive feedback was postulated as being in the medial basal hypothalamus (279). More recent work provides evidence that the site of positive and negative feedback of oestradiol in primates is the adenohypophysis (354). Even today experimental evidence and advocates are found for all three sites.

In the first group of studies, based on surgical disconnection of MBH in rats, the assumed site of the positive oestradiol feedback is the limbic-preoptic-hypothalamic system, while the site for progesterone is the preoptic suprachiasmatic area and the anterior hypothalamic area (258) and the medial basal hypothalamus is ruled out as the site of a positive feedback of oestradiol (176). Based on stimulatory and separation methods, the medial preoptic area was considered as primary for FSH/LH ovulatory release and the dorsal anterior hypothalamic area for tonic FSH release (82). In monkeys bilateral destruction of the preoptic and anterior hypothalamic area also blocked spontaneous ovulation (369), contrary to results reported by Krey.

The latter group of studies (279) also confirmed the importance of the medial basal hypothalamus for the release of LH and FSH after oestradiol benzoate in monkeys deprived of the preoptic-anterior hypothalamic area (207) and by selective lesions they established that the area of the arcuate nucleus is the primary structure mediating the hypothalamic control of gonadotropin secretion in monkeys (402).

The same group elaborated the third view that oestradiol can produce a negative as well as positive feedback effect on gonadotropins at the level of the adenohypophysis (354), based on experiments with ovariectomized monkeys with hypothalamic lesions where the endogenous LH-RH production was eliminated and replaced by chronic intermittent infusion of synthetic LH-RH. Direct evidence was even provided in castrated rats with pharmacological destruction that the arcuate nucleus, the eminentia mediana and the tuberoinfundibular system play no part in the tonic feedback regulation of LH and FSH (181).

When applying the concept of a simple feedback of steroids and gonadotropins, considering only the quantitative aspect, a clear relationship is found between steroids and LH, while the relationship with FSH is less clear. One explanation is the hypothesis of the pleiomorphism of FSH and thus a qualitative feedback for FSH. According to it the adenohypophysis secretes three types of FSH: neuter-FSH, andro-FSH, gyno-FSH, with a different index of discrimination, molecular weight and capacity to survive in the circulation, depending on the absence of hormones or under the influence of androgens or ovarian steroids (50). Another explanation is that in the control of FSH secretion ovarian inhibin is involved (see p. 44).

## SHORT (INTERNAL) FEEDBACK OF HYPOPHYSEAL GONADOTROPINS

Evidence was provided that the eminentia mediana in addition to receptors for feedback for steroids also possesses receptors sensitive to LH. This is a negative feedback where excess *LH* released by the anterior lobe into the blood stream reaches receptors in the hypothalamus, where it inhibits further production of hormone via LH-RH. In castrated rats LH implanted into the eminentia mediana led to a reduction of LH reserves in the pituitary and to a decline of plasma LH (100). For *FSH* this relationship was demonstrated later. This feedback was also proved in rats with an oestrous cycle. In women after castration this negative short feedback was found in some cases after administration of Pergonal, when the total gonadotropin level declined significantly, compared with the original level (501). It could be assumed that in women under physiological conditions this feedback could terminate the release of LH required for ovulation. A similar short feedback is also found in prolactin which at the hypothalamic level inhibits its own secretion (6).

## "ULTRASHORT" FEEDBACK OF HYPOTHALAMIC RELEASING HORMONES

The synthesis, accumulation and release of hypothalamic releasing hormones are controlled by the plasma level of sex steroids (long feedback) and the LH and FSH level (short feedback). Experiments on rats revealed that the subcutaneous administration of crude extract from the rat hypothalamus considerably reduced FSH-RH output from the hypothalamus in castrated and hypophysectomized rats. It is therefore concluded that hypothalamic releasing hormones also regulate their own release (227).

Other investigations, however, did not reveal this ultrashort feedback and in castrated rats administration of an LH-RH analogue did not alter the LH-RH content in the hypothalamus (446).

## CONTROL OF FSH AND LH SECRETION

### TONIC AND CYCLIC MECHANISM OF GONADOTROPIC SECRETION

By investigating the anterior lobe of the pituitary which was transplanted into various parts of the hypothalamus, a group of Hungarian workers defined in animal experiments a semicircular space in the anterior basal hypothalamus where the transplanted lobe preserved its normal cytological and functional character. This space comprising in particular the anterior hypothalamic region of the ventro-median nucleus and arcuate nucleus is described as the hypophysotropic area and is the site of the mechanism of tonic release of plasmatic FSH and LH. After severing of afferent nervous pathways it was revealed that in males the gonadotropic activity was not altered, while in females there was a permanent oestrus without corpus luteum formation. These findings gave rise to the idea that the male type is characterized by tonic, i.e. basal or even slightly varying secretion of FSH and LH induced by releasing hormones produced in the neurons of this hypophysotropic area. For the female type of control in addition to the tonic secretion also cyclic secretion is typical. A higher centre in the preoptic area of the hypothalamus emits nervous impulses into the hypophysotropic area for the cyclic release of LH-RH and thus for the cyclic release of plasmatic LH needed for ovulation. Other nervous impulses modulating (i.e. stimulating or inhibiting) the function of the hypophysotropic area originate from the adjacent anterior and lateral hypothalamic area, from the limbic system and epithalamo-epiphyseal complex, as discussed elsewhere. Neurons of the parvicellular system from the hypophysotropic area, in particular the nucleus arcuatus, conduct the releasing hormones through the tuberoinfundibular tract to the vicinity of capillaries of the portal system.

This idea which developed on the basis of animal experiments seems very simplified today. In primates, and thus also in humans, the tonic as well as the cyclic mechanism of gonadotropic secretion is closed in the medial basal hypothalamus and can also close in the anterior lobe of the pituitary (see feedbacks). In the anterior lobe of the pituitary steroids can directly control the sensitivity of gonadotrophs. In the control thus a hypothalamic as well as direct hypophyseal mechanism may participate and it is not clear which is primary or whether they run parallel. The hypothesis of a direct hypophyseal mechanism is reinforced by the new evidence that intermittent release of LH-RH is only a permissive, however necessary component of the control of menstrual cycle in the rhesus monkey (271a).

## MUTUAL RELATIONSHIP BETWEEN GONADOTROPINS AND STEROIDS DURING THE MENSTRUAL CYCLE AND OVULATION

The original idea of a time signal in the hypothalamus which controlled ovulation and rhythmic processes during the menstrual cycle has been abandoned. The basis of the processes is the ovarian signal in the shape of a positive feedback of oestrogens (Fig. 6). In the first stage of the menstrual cycle the growth of follicles begins as a result of the rise of FSH in plasma during menstruation. This secretion rise of FSH is the result of a negative feedback after the drop of oestradiol at the end of the previous cycle. Six to twelve follicles begin to grow but as the local concentration of ovarian oestrogen rises one follicle continues to grow while the remainder undergo atresia. It seems that after the beginning of follicular growth the raised FSH level is no longer needed and during the subsequent follicular phase it is on a low level. Along with the preovulation development of the follicle the plasma oestradiol level and the 17α-hydroxyprogesterone and progesterone level resp. rise. Oestradiol (a level of at least 150 pg/ml) acts as an ovarian signal either alone or together with the rise of progesterone (first, stimulatory part of its effect) on the preovulatory rise of LH and FSH. This rise of LH then causes ovulation. The difference between the two peaks is 24 hours. This sequence of processes was proved in lower mammals as well as in primates. It seems that an important part is played by the time factor and the rise of oestrogens must persist for at least 12 hours. The interval between the peak of LH and ovulation is different in different species, from several hours to 24 hours, in women 9 hours (389). For luteinization and the development of the corpus luteum, the function of which persists for 12–14 days, the presence of a small amount of LH is essential. This was demon-

Fig. 6. Regulatory mechanisms of ovarian function. (Gr —granulosa cells, Th—theca cells, CL —corpus luteum, C-E — catecholoestrogens, GnRH — gonadotropin releasing hormone, R — hormone receptor, $E_2$ — oestradiol, Andro — androgens, P — progesterone, (+) positive and (—) negative feedback) (314)

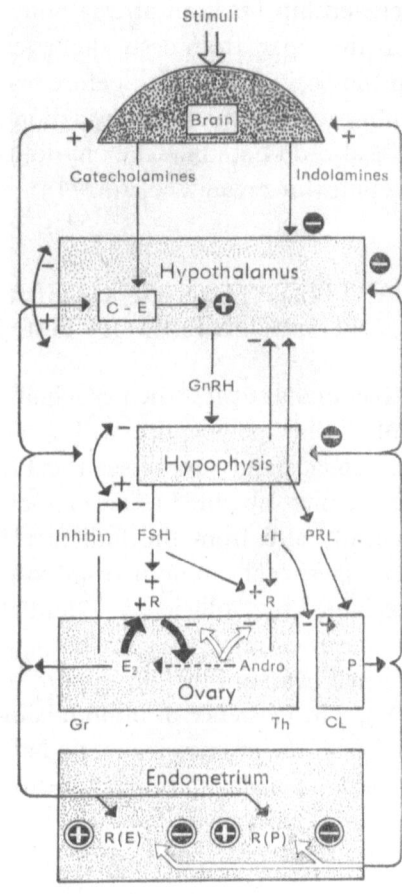

strated during treatment of sterile women where after induced ovulation a small amount of LH or hCG ensures the function of the corpus luteum for 12–18 days. As during the luteal phase the oestradiol and progesterone levels rise, those of LH and FSH decline to levels lower than during the follicular phase. Progesterone displays here the second inhibitory part of its biphasic action on the LH level. The decline of the plasma level of oestradiol and progesterone occurs at the end of the cycle when the function of the corpus luteum terminates. The termination is at

43

least partly an intrinsic property. The luteotropic action of prolactin for the maintenance of the function of the corpus luteum in women is important as high and very low levels of prolactin reduce ovarian steroidogenesis (progesterone).

In processes of the menstrual cycle there are many obscure or controversial facts. It is not known to what extent further hypothalamic factors, other than GnRH, or extrahypothalamic factors (sensitivity of the adenohypophysis, inhibin, neurophysin) modify LH and FSH secretion. It is not known what controls the relationship between atresia and the development of the follicle. It is not clear whether apart from oestradiol a stimulatory action is also exerted by progesterone in the positive feedback before ovulation and what causes the change of its stimulatory action into inhibitory action on LH and FSH in the luteal phase of the cycle. We also do not know the physiological importance of short feedbacks of gonadotropins (for review see 26, 374).

## PARTICIPATION OF OTHER SUBSTANCES IN THE CONTROL OF THE MENSTRUAL CYCLE

Recent data suggest the participation of *inhibin* in the control of the ovarian cycle. Inhibin is a polypeptide with a molecular weight of 23,000 which is produced by the gonads and suppresses the FSH serum level much more than the LH level. It was first obtained as an extract from testes and the seminal plasma, but more recently also from the follicular fluid of cows, sows and from human ovaries. In experiments inhibin from sow follicles suppressed resumption of meiosis in explanted sow follicles (515) and also suppressed the secondary rise of FSH in the prooestrous rats (461). In human ovaries there is more inhibin in women with normal ovarian function than in ovaries with cystic follicles in the premenopause (99). The existence of inhibin could explain changes in the LH-FSH ratio during puberty, the premenopause and after castration. In addition to lowering spermatogenesis in males it could, by direct action on hypophyseal FSH, prevent maturation of the primordial follicle and thus interfere with fertility.

Another substance of this type is the *oestrogen-neurophysin*, a protein produced by the hypothalamus which rises in plasma parallel with LH, or even several hours earlier after injection of oestradiol benzoate to ovariectomized monkeys and is perhaps related to the positive feedback of oestrogens on LH release (462).

# PULSATILE RELEASE OF GONADOTROPINS

The blood level of hormones is proportional to their production and metabolic clearance which in turn is influenced by episodic, diurnal or seasonal factors and other factors of the external environment. The level of circulating gonadotropins thus does not persist in a steady state, not even during tonic secretion. It was revealed that it is made up of pulses or oscillations which occur repeatedly at about hourly intervals (therefore the term "circhoral" or episodic release is used). They were first observed in ovariectomized monkeys, but not in regularly menstruating animals, and later in castrated rats of both sexes, intact bulls, rams, men and women. In women the pulsatile waves occur during the cycle, in particular in LH, during the menopause in LH as well as FSH and they coincide. The length and height of the waves change in the course of the cycle: during the early follicular and early luteal phase the frequency is 1–2 hours, during the mid-cycle and late luteal phase about four hours. The height of LH waves is 5–15 m/IU/ml during tonic secretion and 10–30 mIU ml during the preovulatory peak of the cycle. The pulsatile release is the determining factor of basal tonic secretion of LH and is responsible for the range of variation of values. The mean rise of LH in the wave in menopausal women is 18 mIU ml, in FSH 14 mIU/ml. From this a greater variation of gonadotropin values in menopausal women ensues. The episodic secretion of LH and FSH was also confirmed in pathological agonadal and hypogonadal conditions; it is lacking, however, in children before puberty, after hypophysectomy, after administration of oestradiol and cyproterone acetate. It reflects thus the normal function of the hypothalamo-hypophyso-gonadal axis. The qualitative and quantitative differences in the type of pulsatile release provide evidence that the frequency and magnitude of this release are modulated by ovarian steroids (for review see 545). Although the regulatory mechanism has not been elucidated, there is evidence that the periodic release of gonadotropins from the anterior lobe of the pituitary is controlled by intermittent signals from the CNS via periodic release of LH-RH. This was shown by the parallel follow up of LH-RH in the hypothalamus, and LH in the pituitary and the jugular and peripheral blood of rats and sheep. In monkeys LH-RH has only the permissive action (271a).

The participation of the hypothalamus is also suggested by the fact that catecholamines and $\alpha$-adrenergic blocking drugs modify the pulsatile release of gonadotropins in sheep and monkeys. It cannot be ruled out that steroids act directly on the anterior lobe of the pituitary where they increase the sensitivity to LH-RH.

# CIRCADIAN RHYTHMS IN THE ENDOCRINE SYSTEM

Circadian rhythms are one of the typical properties of all organisms. They depend on automatic periodic processes programmed in the organism. Under normal conditions they are synchronized with external factors of light and darkness in animals, with sleep and wakefulness and social signals in humans.

As to biogenic amines and regulatory peptides, clear evidence was provided of the circadian rhythm of *norepinephrine* with a nocturnal minimum and daily maximum concentration in the cerebrospinal fluid of monkeys, and in the urinary excretion of humans, while evidence in human plasma remains controversial. *Dopamine* and its main metabolite, homovanillic acid, has a similar rhythm in the cerebrospinal fluid of monkeys. *Serotonin* (5-HT) has the reverse rhythm with a maximum concentration in the evening. Because biogenic amines stimulate the formation of adenyl cyclase, the same rhythm is also found in the concentration of *cAMP* with a nocturnal minimum, similar to that in human urine, as well as in cerebrospinal fluid of monkeys. A rhythm of *LH-RH* excretion with a maximum serum concentration and maximum content in the median basal hypothalamus in the morning was found only in rats. There also exists a circadian responsiveness of the hypothalamus-pituitary axis.

As to gonadotropic hormones, in *LH* and *FSH* in serum, during tonic secretion, a circadian rhythm probably does not exist, either in human adults or in lower animals, although in more recent work a sleep-conditioned rhythm of LH was described or a rhythm linked with other conditions. However, raised LH and FSH values in urine are found in children before puberty and during puberty during nocturnal sleep. It is not known why in adult life these differences disappear. There is, however, a circadian rhythm of the cyclic release of LH in the serum of animals as well as in urine of females (for review see 216), the peak being in the evening or during the night. Plasma *prolactin* displays a clear maximum concentration during the night with a minimum near noon, depending on sleep (for review see 12). According to the majority of publications steroids produced by the ovary lack a circadian rhythm, in contradistinction to steroids produced by the adrenals. *Oestrone* and *17β-oestradiol* does not display a circadian rhythm either during the cycle or in castrated women, although it has been demonstrated in monkeys. In pregnant women, however, the *oestriol* and total oestrogen level varied rhythmically with a nocturnal maximum and diurnal minimum. A circadian rhythm of *progesterone* secretion was not found. Plasma *cortisol* displays a marked diurnal rhythm with a maximum in the morning and minimum in the evening. A similar but less marked rhythm is found in the plasma *testosterone* level of females and monkeys, as well as in *androstenedione* and *dehydroepiandrosterone* levels.

A detailed evaluation of the relations between circadian rhythms, sleep and activity are beyond the framework of the present monograph (for review see 12).

# PHYSIOLOGICAL AND MATHEMATICAL MODEL
# OF THE MENSTRUAL CYCLE

Assembling of physiological data, recognition of mutual hormonal relations in particular, which were discussed in previous chapters, and morphological changes were given much attention in the past. Some relationships were elucidated only recently when it was possible to use two different generalizing procedures.

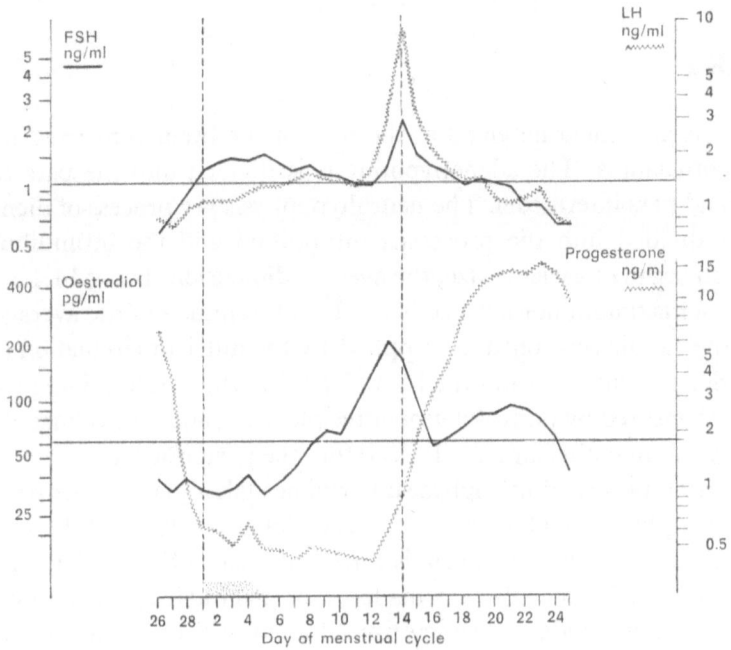

*Fig. 7.* Mutual relationship of gonadotropins and steroids in menstrual cycle (geometric mean values from 11 normal cycles are synchronized both on the first day of the menstrual cycle and around the day of the LH peak) (535a).

The first was the parallel investigation of a large number of parameters in the same woman which made it possible to create a composite picture of processes during the menstrual cycle (Fig. 7). Various authors concurrently investigated plasma levels of FSH, LH, progesterone, 17α-hydroxyprogesterone, 17β-oestradiol by radio-immunological methods or in addition to plasma hormone levels urinary steroids and systemic changes in the organism (339). In other investigations the levels of all detectable steroids in plasma were investigated during the normal female cycle (187). Finally in parallel investigations certain relations in the control of the cycle were studied such as the relations of ovarian and adrenal steroids (109) or the chronological relations of different levels at the time of ovulation (267, 389).

The second generalizing procedure was mathematical modelling of the menstrual cycle using systemic analysis of mechanisms controlling the cycle. Using computers and transformed known experimental data the entire ovarian cycle or parts of it are simulated (139) or other stochastic models of processes of human reproduction are created.

# PITUITARY

The pituitary is an endocrine gland at the base of the brain connected by a stalk with the hypothalamus. The adenohypophysis is divided into the pars tuberalis, pars distalis and pars intermedia. The neurohypophysis is a process of diencephalic tissue and is divided into the processus infundibuli and the infundibulum. In humans it is an organ of variable size, the average dimensions being $14.4 \times 11.5 \times 5.5$ mm, the maximum normal size being 16, 11, 6 mm, and the average weight 0.6 g. As to the vascularization it is supplied by the nutrient circulation (a. hypophysea superior and inferior) and the hypophyseal portal system. The innervation of both lobes is ensured by perivasal vegetative plexuses, and unmyelinated bundles of fibres from the hypothalamic nuclei lead into the posterior lobe.

The production proper of hypophyseal hormones takes place in the pars distalis of the adenohypophysis which is formed by a spatial network of cellular trabeculae, between which are large blood sinusoids lined with cells of the reticulohistiocytic system. The epithelial trabeculae are made up of glandular epithelia. For several decades attempts were made to characterize different cells of the adenohypophysis and to separate the production of seven proteohormones: STH, LTH (PRL), ACTH, TSH, FSH, LH and MSH into different types. The oldest terminology was morphological, based on the shape and functional properties of cells (for review see 294), more recently the international committee for the nomenclature of the pituitary recommended a functional nomenclature. Attempts were also made to characterize the production of pituitary hormones by the size of intracellular secretory granules, as assessed under the electron microscope. Recently immunohistochemical procedures are used for the identification of different cells. The greatest accuracy will probably be achieved by synthesis of morphological, functional and immunohistochemical data. Evidence is being assembled that acidophils contain STH and LTH (PRH), whereby orangeophil acidophil cells of the $\alpha$-type contain LTH and erythrosinophil acidophil cells of type $\varepsilon$ contain prolactin. ACTH and MSH are located into basophil cells type $\beta$, TSH is also produced by basophil cells of the $\beta$-type, LH and FSH are localized in basophil cells type $\delta$.

48

These basophil cells are described as gonadotrophs; after castration their number increases along with the rising concentration of gonadotropins.

Functional changes of gonadotrophs during the menstrual cycle are manifested by changes in the sensitivity and reserve of the adenohypophysis in the response of LH and FSH to LH-RH (see chapter LH-RH, p. 31). For a long time it remained undecided whether the two gonadotropins are produced by one cell (one cell – two hormones) or by different cells (one cell – one hormone). Recently it was revealed, using the immunohistochemical technique, that there are two types of gonadotrophs in human as well as in rat pituitaries (415).

## GONADOTROPINS

Gonadotropic hormones participating in various stages of the physiology of human reproduction are four in number: human follicle stimulating hormone (hFSH), human luteinizing hormone (hLH), human prolactin (hPRL) and human chorion-gonadotropin (hCG). Among them only the first three participate in the physiological regulation of the menstrual cycle, while the two latter are more important during pregnancy. For treatment of disorders of the cycle in addition to hCG human menopausal gonadotropin (HMG), a mixture of hFSH and hLH from the urine of menopausal women, and gonadotropin from the serum of pregnant mares (PMSG) are important. With the exception of hPRL they are glycoproteins with a molecular weight of 20,000 to 35,000; they have similar biochemical and immunological properties, but they differ to such an extent that they can be characterized as separate units.

## HUMAN FOLLICLE STIMULATING HORMONE
## (hFSH, FOLLITROPIN) AND HUMAN LUTEINIZING HORMONE
## (hLH, LUTROPIN)

**Structure.** hFSH and hLH are glycoproteins with a molecular weight of 28,000 and $32,000 \pm 2,000$. Nowadays we know the sequence of amino acids in both hormones and this is gradually being determined for other animal species (sheep, swine, horse). The carbohydrate component accounts for 13–21% of the weight of the molecule and contains mannose, fucose, galactose, glucosamine and galactosamine, which are linked by covalent bonds in the shape of oligosaccharide chains. hFSH contains, as far as hexosamines are concerned, only N-acetyl glucosamine, while hLH contains also N-acetyl galactosamine. At the ends of some carbohydrate chains nonose, sialic acid, is bound (N-acetyl neuraminic acid); hFSH contains 5–6% of this acid, hLH only 1–2%. Sialic acid is important for the biological activity of hFSH but not of hLH. Recently it was revealed that it enhances the metabolic survival of gonadotropins. Both hormones are made up of two different sub-units described as α and β which themselves are inactive. The bond between them is weak, not covalent. The two sub-units can be separated at a strongly acid pH, in practice, however, 8 M urea or propionic acid are used.

The α-sub-unit for hFSH and hLH (hFSHα, hLHα) is identical (479) and is almost identical in other glycoproteins of human origin. It is made up of 89 amino acids arranged in a linear fashion with an amine and carboxylic terminal. It differs from the hCG α-sub-unit only by deletion of three amino acids at the $NH_2$ terminal (Table 2). It has 5 disulphide bridges and a molecular weight of 14,600. The sub-

*Table 2*  Human luteinizing hormone (linear amino acid sequence) (478)

**hLH α-sub-unit**

H₂N-Val-Gln-Asp-Cys-Pro-Glu-Cys-Thr-Leu-Gln-Glu-Asn-Pro-Phe-Phe-Ser-Gln-Pro-Gly-
10
Ala-Pro-Ile-Leu-Gln-Cys-Met-Gly-Cys-Cys-Phe-Ser-Arg-Ala-Tyr-Pro-Thr-Pro-Leu-Arg-
20                                        30
                                          CHO

Ser-Lys-Lys-Thr-Met-Leu-Val-Gln-Lys-Asn-Val-Thr-Ser-Glu-Ser-Thr-Cys-Cys-Val-Ala-
40                              50
                                                        CHO
                                                         |
Lys-Ser-Tyr-Asn-Arg-Val-Thr-Val-Met-Gly-Gly-Phe-Lys-Val-Glu-Asn-His-Thr-Ala-Cys-
60                              70
His-Cys-Ser-Thr-Cys-Tyr-Tyr-His-Lys-Ser-OH
80                              89

**hLH β-sub-unit**

H₂N-Ser-Arg-Glu-Pro-Leu-Arg-Pro-Trp-Cys-His-Pro-Ile-Asn-Ala-Ile-Leu-Ala-Val-Glu-
                                        10
                                        CHO

Lys-Glx-Gly-Cys-Pro-Val-Cys-Ile-Thr-Val-Asn-Thr-Thr-Ile-Cys-Ala-Gly-Tyr-Cys-Pro-
20                              30
Thr-Met-Arg-Val-Leu-Gln-Ala-Val-Leu-Pro-Pro-Leu-Pro-Gln-Val-Cys-Thr-Tyr-Arg-Asp-
40                              50
Val-Arg-Phe-Glu-Ser-Ile-Arg-Leu-Pro-Gly-Cys-Pro-Arg-Gly-Val-Asp-Pro-Val-Val-Ser-Phe-
60                              70                                    80
Pro-Val-Ala-Leu-Ser-Cys-Arg-Cys-Gly-Pro-Cys-Arg-Arg-Ser-Thr-Ser-Asp-Cys-Gly-Gly-Pro-
                                90                                    100
Lys-Asx-His-Pro-Leu-Thr-Cys-Asx-Glx-Pro-His (Ser-Lys-Gly)-OH
                    110                      115

-units of other mammalian species (e.g. pLHα from the swine or oLHα from sheep) are similar but differ by substitution of cca 25–29 amino acids. hFSHα, hLHα, hTSHα, hCGα are completely replaceable although they differ in the carbohydrate portions of the molecule. The α-sub-units are thus a nonspecific or general part of the gonadotropin molecule.

The β-sub-unit for hFSH (hFSHβ) is a specific part of the molecule; it differs in the structure of its amino acids and has different glycoproteins, it determines the resulting hormonal effect when the two sub-units are combined into a dimer and is irreplaceable. The hFSH β-sub-unit was also isolated and the sequence of amino acids assessed (471) (Table 3). It is made up of 115 amino acids and its molecular weight is about 16,000. It displays heterogeneity at the $NH_2$ terminal, i.e. the sequence of amino acids is not constant.

*Table 3*  Human follicle stimulating hormone (linear amino acid sequence) (479)

---

**hFSH α-sub-unit** (identical with hLH α-sub-unit)
**hFSH β-sub-unit**

                                   CHO

$H_2N$-(Asx-Ser)-Cys-Glu-Leu-Thr-Asn-Ile-Thr-Ile-Ala-Ile-Glu-Lys-Glu-Glu-Cys-Arg-Phe-
                                   10
        CHO

Cys-Ile-Ser-Ile-Asn-Thr-Thr (Thr,Asx,Trp) Glu-Thr-Cys-Ala-Gly-Tyr-Cys-Tyr-Thr-Arg-
20                               30
Asp-Leu-Val-Tyr-Lys-Asp-Pro-Ala-Lys-Pro-Arg-Ile-Gln-Lys-Thr-Cys-Thr-Phe-Lys-Glu-
40                               50
Leu-Val-Tyr-Glu-Thr-Val-Arg-Val-Pro-Gly-Cys-Ala-His-His-Ala-Asp-Ser-Leu-Tyr-Thr-
60                               70
Tyr-Pro-Val-Ala-Thr-Gln-Cys-His-Cys-Gly-Lys-Cys-Asp-Ser-Asp-Ser-Thr-Asp-Cys-Thr-
80                               90
Val-Arg-Gly-Leu-Gly-Pro-Ser-Tyr-Cys-Ser-Phe-Gly-Glu-Met-(Glx,Lys)-OH
100                                   110              115

---

The β-sub-unit for LH (hLHβ) contains 115 amino acids (Table 2) (478) where in contrast to the others, tryptophan is in position 8. It is highly homologous with hCGβ which has, however, a longer amino acid chain, of 145. In the carbohydrate component are one or two groups with a N-glycoside bond with aspartine; 3–4 further groups with an O-glycoside bond with serine are lacking. Both are in hCG. The molecule has 6 disulphide bridges and a molecular weight of 15,300. Animal β-sub-units (sheep, ox, swine) have a larger number of amino acids.

Natural hFSH and hLH are thus αβ-dimers the qualitative biological activity of which depends on the nature of the β-sub-unit. In human pituitaries, serum and urine free sub-units were also detected, their role is, however, not known so far.

High-molecular forms were also revealed, for LH so-called "big" LH (100,000), compared with the normal active form "little" LH (30,000) and finally low molecular fragments (1,000), so-called mini LH, in serum (179). A high-molecular form of FSH was also detected. Electrofocusing studies when coupled with RIA thus provide information on different types of heterogeneity of glycoprotein hormones (for review see 36).

**Secretion and metabolism.** Under the control of hypothalamic hormones hFSH and hLH are formed in the gonadotrophs of the anterior lobe of the pituitary where they are deposited in the secretory granules. By migration the granules reach the cell membrane and by exocytosis the pericapillary spaces and finally the blood stream.

The mechanism of LH secretion by the adenohypophysis is as follows: the common $\alpha$-sub-unit circulates independently of the intact hormones and is present in a proportion of developing Graafian follicles. During the late follicular phase, however, when both the hLH$\alpha$- and hLH$\beta$-sub-units are present in follicular fluid, they may recombine in the active form of LH and enhance the steroid production of granulosa cells (189). In the blood they are not bound to plasma proteins. The biological activity of hFSH disappears from blood according to a multiexponential curve — the first phase being rapid, $t_{1/2} = 3.9$ hours, the second phase slow, where $t_{1/2}$ takes 70.4 hours. The first rapid phase corresponds to the disappearance from the circulation and the slow second one to the return of the hormone from the extravascular space. hLH disappears much more rapidly, according to a similar curve, the first $t_{1/2} = 21$ minutes and the second one $t_{1/2} = 234$ minutes. The half-life of the LH$\beta$-sub-unit is cca 15 minutes. The daily production is about 200 IU for hFSH and 1,100 IU for hLH, while according to other data hLH is produced in normal women in amounts of 39.9 IU 24 h and in postmenopausal women $294 \pm 62$ IU/24 h (392). Striking differences are caused by the application of different methods. The values of metabolic clearance (MRC) are greater for hLH (about 35 l/24 h) than for hFSH (about 20 l/24 h) and do not change under different physiological and pathological conditions. Other reports give the figure for hLH of $29.7 \pm 3.7$ ml/24 h for women and $43.5 \pm 8.2$ ml/min for men. Therefore the plasma concentration of hFSH and hLH accurately reflects the secretion of the anterior lobe of the pituitary. From a comparison of data on secretion and excretion it is apparent that only a part ($2-4\%$ or $41-53\%$) of the gonadotropins produced per day is excreted in the urine. From data on the hFSH and hLH content in the adenohypophysis it is estimated that the pituitary contains $50-100\%$ of their daily production. The site of degradation of gonadotropins is not known. There is evidence that the rate of disappearance influencing the biological activity of hFSH and hLH depends on the sialic acid content. After removal of sialic acid the half-life ($t_{1/2}$) declines to less than 1 minute.

**Physiological action.** Both hormones, FSH and LH, circulate in the whole body but nevertheless they have a marked capacity to stimulate only some tissues and cells. They are linked by chemical interaction with receptors of target tissues of the ovary and the testis resp. The physiological action is twofold: gametogenic and steroidogenic.

In women FSH acts on the growth of the primordial follicle up to the formation of the antrum by stimulating the proliferation of granulosa cells. FSH is essential only from the stage when the follicle forms about five layers, as up to that time growth occurs even without gonadotropins (23). LH together with FSH acts on the preovulation follicle, on interstitial and thecal cells and induces oestrogen production, ovulation, the formation of the corpus luteum and progesterone production. More recently, however, evidence was provided that immunologically pure hFSH alone can stimulate oestrogen synthesis in hypophysectomized rats where it causes an increase in the weight of the ovary, stimulates growth and maturation of the Graafian follicle without affecting interstitial cells and luteinization, increases the weight of the uterus and causes cornification of the vaginal mucosa. Granulosa cells from preovulatory follicles of some lower mammals, monkeys and humans luteinize and produce progesterone "spontaneously" in experiments *in vitro* without the further action of gonadotropins. This fact, however, does not rule out the main role of LH after the previous action of FSH on the oocyte, ovulation and the function of the corpus luteum. It rather indicates other intrafollicular factors which *in vivo* inhibit the function of follicular cells. The interpretation of the isolated effect of FSH and LH is difficult, as usually no simple direct action of different gonadotropins is involved. The synergism of the action of FSH and LH is important as well as the interaction of different tissues containing different enzyme systems for steroidogenesis, the interaction between oocytes and follicular cells where the oocyte perhaps produces an inhibitory anti-luteinizing factor, and finally the fact that steroids themselves can act on tissues in which they are formed either directly or by a feedback. Recent experiments in women provided clear evidence that hFSH alone is not able to produce complete maturation of the follicle even when there is a high peripheral level of FSH. hLH is of fundamental importance for the maturation of the follicle and ovulation after previous action of FSH. This conclusion is important for treatment with gonadotropic hormones.

## METHODS FOR THE ASSESSMENT OF GONADOTROPINS

Biological, immunological, radioimmunological and, recently, radioreceptor methods are used. For the evaluation of all methods four general parameters are used which characterize the suitability of the method. These are: precision, accuracy, sensitivity and specificity.

**Biological methods.** These use as criteria the weight of the ovaries, testes, prostate or uterus of the test animal, which is usually an immature mouse or rat.

The total gonadotropic activity (TGA) is so far the most widespread method for the assessment of gonadotropins for clinical purposes. The end-point is an increase in the weight of the infantile uterus of the female mouse.

As to methods specifically assessing FSH, weight increment of the ovary augmented by hCG, as described by Steelman and Pohley, is most widely used. The method is based on the finding that added hCG enhances the action of FSH on the ovary of immature female rats or mice.

There are two specific methods for LH. Greep's method using the weight of the ventral prostate is based on the stimulatory action of LH on testosterone formation which is manifested in the weight of the anterior lobe of the prostate in hypophysectomized, immature male rats. The second method of ovarian ascorbic acid depletion (OAAD) according to Parlow is based on the ability of LH to reduce the ascorbic acid content of the ovaries in immature rats where pseudopregnancy previously has been induced by pretreatment with PMSG and hCG.

*In vitro* biological methods for the assessment of LH are specific and sensitive. Their end-point is the response in the target tissue, e.g. progesterone or cAMP production in the luteinized granulosa of the ovary or testosterone in Leydig cells of the testes (for review see 308).

**Immunological methods.** The general principle of these methods is the quantitative interaction of the antigen with its specific antibody. The antigen is a glycoprotein hormone FSH, LH, hCG. The antibody is a specific antiserum prepared by immunization of rabbits. For the evaluation of the reaction a detectable analogue of the hormone is essential. The reaction involves a competition between unknown amounts of hormone (unlabelled antigen) and a detectable analogue of the hormone (labelled antigen) on the surface of the antibody. The amount of the labelled antigen bound to the antibody depends on the amount of the unlabelled antigen. By addition of the known amount of the unlabelled antigen to the mixture a standard curve is obtained from which readings of the assessed hormone are taken. If we use as detectable hormone analogue an erythrocyte coated with hormone, we speak of methods of haemagglutination inhibition, if we use hormone labelled with radioactive iodine we speak of radioimmunological assay.

**Methods of haemagglutination inhibition.** This method was first suggested for the assessment of hCG in urine and later for LH (536) when it was found that there is an immunological cross-reaction between LH and hCG. The method was improved and simplified by using small hCG-coated latex particles instead of hCG-coated blood cells. The immunological assessment of LH is a very rapid method and renders it possible to assess a large number of samples at a time and thus entire cycles can be tested. Commercial sets with the required constituents are also available (Luteonosticon, Organon). A similar system of haemagglutination inhibition was also elaborated for the assessment of FSH. It contained rabbit antiserum against purified hypophyseal hFSH and ram erythrocytes coated with purified hFSH. Purified urinary FSH was used also for binding with latex particles and for the formation of antibodies. These methods are, however, rarely used for FSH determination.

**Radioimmunological methods (RIA).** These methods were originally introduced for the assessment of insulin. Later they were extended for use not only for high-molecular proteohormones but also for low-molecular steroids (for review see 427). The classical radioimmunological system is based on the ability of the antibody (AB) to bind antigen labelled with a radioactive isotope ($H^x$) and on the competitive inhibition of this reaction with unlabelled antigen (H). The complex of the labelled antigen bound to an antibody ($H^xAB$) is separated from the unbound labelled antigen ($H^x$) and the radioactivity of the complex is assessed. This radioactivity is inversely related to the required concentration of the unbound unlabelled antigen (H). H = hormone assessed in the sample, $H^x$ = highly purified hormone from the pituitary or urine labelled with $^{131}I$ or $^{125}I$. AB = specific antiserum. Schematically the process can be expressed by an equation

$$
\begin{aligned}
H && H \cdot AB + H \\
&+ AB \rightleftharpoons \\
H^x && H^x \cdot AB + H^x
\end{aligned}
$$

The degree of inhibition of the bond which was induced by the tested substance is compared with the appropriate standard. For RIA we need thus: a pure preparation of hormone, a method of iodination, specific antiserum prepared by immunization of laboratory animals (rabbits) with purified hormone, a suitable standard and a method for separation of the complex of hormone linked to antibody ($H^x \cdot AB$) from free hormone ($H^x$) at the end of the reaction. All components needed for the reaction can be prepared in the laboratory or commercial kits can be obtained. The majority of RIA methods differ mainly in the separation of the bound and free fraction. We can use: a) isolation of the bound fraction: either precipitation of double antibodies which is the commonest method, or the method of antibodies in the solid phase, i.e. polymers such as e.g. discs and polyethylene test tubes, Sephadex and cellulose, so-called immunosorbents etc., b) isolation of the free fraction by means of ion exchange resins, active charcoal, cellulose, c) differential migration of the free and bound fraction: chromatoelectrophoresis, gel filtration, etc.

The sensitivity of RIA is many times greater than that of haemagglutination inhibition or biological methods. For LH $2 \times 10^{-9}$ IU/ml plasma are reported, for FSH $4 \times 10^{-9}$ IU ml and for hCG $2.7 \times 10^{-9}$ IU/ml. The accuracy is expressed by index $\lambda = 0.02 - 0.05$ and a variation coefficient for intraassay 2–10% and 2–25% resp. for interassay. As regards the reproducibility of different recommended RIA methods, there is so far a certain lack of uniformity: the use of different standards, different antisera and procedures make the comparison of results difficult.

Furthermore there is the factor of heterogeneity of FSH and LH with the formation of large and small molecules and the presence of sub-units. The immunological activity is not identical with the biological. Clinical data on the absolute magnitude of FSH and LH values differ so far due to the use of different methods. Nevertheless the course of curves is identical and the values are useful in practice (Fig. 8).

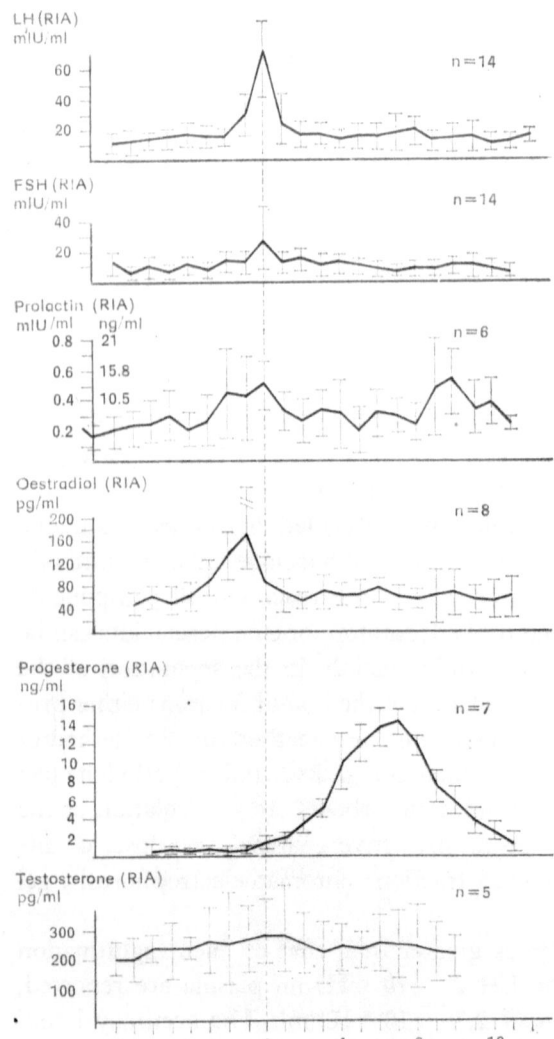

*Fig. 8.* Gonadotropin and sexual steroid plasma levels in normal menstrual cycles (mean values ± ± SD, O day = LH peak) (185a, 219).

**Complement fixation methods.** The third type of immunological methods is complement fixation, based on the direct reaction between the hormone and the specific antibody in the presence of complement. For detection another immunological system is used consisting of red cells and haemolysin which in the presence of the remaining complement leads to haemolysis. The spectrophotometrically assessed extent of haemolysis is quantitatively and inversely proportional to the amount of antigen, i.e. the assessed hormone. This method was elaborated for the estimation of hCG and FSH in urine and serum and was not introduced into practice on a major scale.

**Radioreceptor methods.** Plasmatic membrane receptors are used as specific high-affinity binding agents for the assessment of polypeptide and glycoprotein hormones. The advantage of radioreceptor methods is that they express the hormonal activity more efficiently than RIA and correlate very closely with bio-assays *in vitro* (for review see 458). Isolated membrane receptors from bovine corpus luteum or from luteinized tissue of pseudopregnant rats pretreated with hCG or homogenates from decapsulated rat testes competitively bind either unknown hCG of LH or iodine labelled highly purified hCG or LH after incubation. The bound complex is separated from the free hormone by centrifuging.

The basis of radioreceptor methods for FSH are homogenates from rat testes or partly isolated membrane receptors from bovine testes.

**Reference preparations and standards for FSH, LH and other gonado-tropins.** The WHO Expert Committee on Biological Standardization defined in 1964 the Second international reference preparation of human menopausal gonadotropin (urinary) for bioassay (HMG-IRP-2). The activity of 1 IU equalled 0.25295 mg standard powder and 1 vial contained 40 IU FSH and 40 IU LH. The development of gonadotropin estimations in serum, in the pituitary and the development of immunological methods revealed inadequate parallelism in comparison with this preparation.

Therefore since 1976 when the First international standard for human urinary FSH and for human urinary LH (ICSH) for bioassay came into use 1 IU for FSH and LH are defined as the activities contained in 0.11388 mg and 0.13369 mg of the international standard resp. For practical reasons each vial contains 54 IU FSH and 46 IU LH.

In 1974 moreover the International reference preparation of human pituitary gonadotropins (FSH and LH) (ICSH) for bioassay (coded 69/104 or LER-907) were defined. 1 IU of FSH and 1 IU of LH is the activity of 0.1670 mg and 0.0668 mg of this IRP. One vial contains 10 IU FSH and 25 IU LH.

Furthermore in 1978 the International reference preparation of human pituitary luteinizing hormone for immunoassay (code 68/40) was defined. One vial contains 77 IU. For IRP hCG and sub-units of pituitary FSH, for immunoassay, preparation 68/39 Kabi Stockholm is being prepared.

Since 1963 the Second international standard for human chorionic gonadotropin, for bioassay, is in use, where 1 IU corresponds to 0.001279 mg of the standard powder. One vial contains 5,300 IU. In 1974 the IRP for human chorionic gonadotropin, for immunoassay, was assessed from highly purified urinary hCG and 1 IU is to be defined. For sub-units suitable material and IRP must be obtained (for hLHα MRC 72/20, for hLHβ 71 342) and 1 IU is to equal 1 μg of the sub-unit (535).

Since 1962 the Second international standard for prolactin, ovine, is in use for bioassay. One IU corresponds to an activity of 0.04545 mg standard and 1 vial contains 220 IU. In 1979 the First international reference preparation of human prolactin, for immunoassay has been defined. It has been agreed that the potency allocated to the IRP is by definition 0.650 IU (immunoassay) human prolactin/vial. Up to now local standards were frequently used. 1 µU of the standard MRC 71/222 is equivalent to 0.04 ng of VLS 2 standard NIH.

## HUMAN CHORIONIC GONADOTROPIN (hCG)

**Structure.** hCG is a glycoprotein with a molecular weight of 38,000. The carbohydrate component accounts for cca 31% of the molecular weight and is formed by oligosacharide chains which are linked by covalent bonds to the protein portion of the molecule. They are made up of mannose, fucose, galactose, glucosamine, galactosamine and sialic acid. The content of the latter is approximately 8%, i.e. substantially more than in other glycoproteins. hCG is a heterodimer formed by two sub-units linked by non-covalent bonds, the two individual sub-units being inactive.

hCG α-sub-unit differs only very slightly from α-sub-units of other glycoproteins. It is the common portion of the molecule; it is interchangeable, contains 89–92 amino acids, due to the $NH_2$-terminal heterogeneity and has a molecular weight of about 14,900. It has 5 disulphide bridges and two saccharide units (asparagine-linked N-acetyl glucosamine). The hCG β-sub-unit is a specific part of the molecule. It is made up of 145 and 147 amino acids resp.; it resembles the hLH β-sub-unit but it has additional 30 amino acids on the carboxyl terminal. This group is probably the site where antibodies are linked which differentiate hCG from hLH. At this terminal there are also four of the six saccharide moieties with an O-glycoside bond with serine which is rare in glycoproteins. The biological importance of this part is probably associated with the prolonged half-life of hCG. The hCG β-sub-unit with a molecular weight of 23,000 has six disulphide bridges. The primary structure of sub-units was suggested by two groups of authors (73, 340); they differ in details (Table 4).

There probably also exists a large molecule "big" hCG which as a prohormone is initially synthesized in the placenta.

**Secretion and metabolism.** From histochemical, immunofluorescent and electronmicroscopic investigations (for review see 61) it ensues that hCG is probably synthesized mainly in the cells of the syncytiotrophoblast but also in the cytotrophoblast. Most of it goes into the maternal circulation. The amount of secreted hCG is estimated to be 500,000 to 1,000,000 IU/24 hours in the third month of pregnancy, at the end of pregnancy about 80,000–120,000 IU/24 hours. The factors responsible for the control of hCG secretion are not known. The amount of secretion depends on the size of the trophoblast: there is an enhanced

*Table 4* Human chorionic gonadotropin (linear amino acid sequence) (340)

**hCG α-sub-unit**

H₂N-Ala-Pro-Asp-Val-Gln-Asp-Cys-Pro-Glu-Cys-Thr-Leu-Gln-Glu-Asp-Pro-Phe-Phe-Ser-
                                                     10
Gln-Pro-Gly-Ala-Pro-Ile-Leu-Glx-Cys-Met-Gly-Cys-Cys-Phe-Ser-Arg-Ala-Tyr-Pro-Thr-
20                                    30

                                                     CHO
                                                      |
Pro-Leu-Arg-Ser-Lys-Lys-Thr-Met-Leu-Val-Gln-Lys-Asn-Val-Thr-Ser-Glu-Ser-Thr-Cys-
40                                    50

                                                                      CHO
                                                                       |
Cys-Val-Ala-Lys-Ser-Tyr-Asn-Arg-Val-Thr-Val-Met-Gly-Gly-Phe-Lys-Val-Glu-Asn-His-
60                                    70
Thr-Ala-Cys-His-Cys-Ser-Thr-Cys-Tyr-Tyr-His-Lys-Ser-OH
80                                    90       92

**hCG β-sub-unit**

                                                     CHO
                                                      |
H₂N-Ser-Lys-Glu-Pro-Leu-Arg-Pro-Arg-Cys-Arg-Pro-Ile-Asn-Ala-Thr-Leu-Ala-Val-Glu-
                                             10
                                                     CHO
                                                      |
Lys-Glu-Gly-Cys-Pro-Val-Cys-Ile-Thr-Val-Asn-Thr-Thr-Ile-Cys-Ala-Gly-Tyr-Cys-Pro-
20                                    30
Thr-Met-Thr-Arg-Val-Leu-Gln-Gly-Val-Leu-Pro-Ala-Leu-Pro-Gln-Val-Val-Cys-Asn-Tyr-
40                                    50
Arg-Asp-Val-Arg-Phe-Glu-Ser-Ile-Arg-Leu-Pro-Gly-Cys-Pro-Arg-Gly-Val-Asn-Pro-Val-
60                                    70
Val-Ser-Tyr-Ala-Val-Ala-Leu-Ser-Cys-Gln-Cys-Ala-Leu-Cys-Arg-Arg-Ser-Thr-Thr-Asp-
80                                    90
Cys-Gly-Gly-Pro-Lys-Asp-His-Pro-Leu-Thr-Cys-Asp-Asp-Pro-Arg-Phe-Gln-Asp-Ser-Ser-
100                                   110
    CHO                   CHO                   CHO                   CHO
                                                |                     |
Ser-Ser-Lys-Ala-Pro-Pro-Pro-Ser-Leu-Pro-Ser-Pro-Ser-Arg-Leu-Pro-Gly-Pro-Ser-Asp-Thr-
120                         130                                       140
Pro-Ile-Leu-Pro-Gln-OH
     145

---

secretion in multiple pregnancies, diabetes, erythroblastosis and in trophoblastic tumours; the secretion is low when the trophoblast is damaged. About 10% of the hCG circulating in the blood stream are excreted in the urine in the biologically active form, about 90% are metabolized in the body. hCG has the longest half-life of all gonadotropins — 11 hours in the first stage and 23 hours in the second stage. The low renal hCG clearance is constant during pregnancy (0.95 ml/min). The urinary level of hCG is therefore a reliable indicator of secretion. The hCG concentration in blood and urine takes a parallel course during pregnancy — it is a typical curve with the peak between the 10th and 12th week and a constant low level from the 14th to 40th week which accounts only for cca 1/10th of the peak value.

**Physiological action.** The main action of hCG in humans is its luteinizing and luteotropic effect. During pregnancy the luteotropic action prevents regression of the corpus luteum, while when administered in the course of the cycle it delays menstruation by protracting the function of the corpus luteum. These views already established in the fifties were subjected to criticism. Nevertheless recent findings confirm the luteotropic effect at least *in vitro*: hCG can stimulate progesterone synthesis in corpus luteum sections *in vitro*. After administration of hCG in tissue cultures granulosa cells luteinize after only 2–4 days with a maximum after 6–8 days and luteinization is maintained up to 20 days (80). It remains to be proved yet whether hCG is also the stimulus for steroidogenesis in the corpus luteum during pregnancy *in vivo*.

The second effect exerted by hCG even in highly purified preparations is follicle stimulating. It has been known for a long time, later denied and ascribed to impurities, but today there is evidence that it is the property of the intact molecule. The third effect — thyroid stimulating — is also an intrinsic property of the hCG molecule. All three effects are also properties of the β-sub-unit after recombination.

**Methods of estimation and clinical importance.** hCG can be estimated by biological and immunological methods. Biological methods are based on the observation that in animals hCG causes a so-called complete gonadotropic response: growth and maturation of the follicle and formation of the corpus luteum, and weight increase of the ovary and uterus, while in males a gametokinetic response or a weight increase of the prostate or seminal vesicles are obtained. The criterion for evaluation was thus the formation of corpora lutea in infantile mice (Aschheim-Zondek), ovulation in the infantile rabbit (Friedman) and in amphibians (Hogben), ovarian hyperaemia in infantile rats (Albert), weight of the prostate in rats (Loraine), weight of seminal vesicles (Diczfalusy, Loraine), gametokinesis in male frogs (Galli-Mainini). Diluted urine was used and comparison with a standard solution, or when criteria of constantly variable values were used (weight of organs) a four-point comparison of two volumes of unknown urine with two volumes of standard. Biological methods are laborious, they are not absolutely specific, and have a sensitivity from 0.25 IU to 1 IU (ovarian hyperaemia, weight of organs). A not very sensitive criterion is spermiogenesis in frogs (20 IU). Immunological methods are either based on inhibition of haemagglutination or on complement fixation or on the radioimmunological principle. Because of the similarity of hCG and hLH, these methods have already been discussed (see p. 54).

More recent methods for the assessment of hCG are radioreceptor methods. Some make it possible to assess hCG as early as on the 6th day after conception and could prove useful in the diagnosis of early abortions or in postcoital contraception (interception). They were already discussed (see p. 57). A comparative study using three methods revealed, however, the first rise of hCG only between the 9th–12th day after ovulation, i.e. after the onset of implantation (76).

Today the selective RIA method which assesses the β-sub-unit of hCG and has several advantages is of major importance. It estimates specifically hCG without crossed reactivity, thus hLH does not interfere; in the solid-phase modification (277) it is very rapid, it takes only two hours and can be used for menstrual aspiration as it makes the diagnosis of pregnancy at the time of a missed menstruation in 100%. Commercial kits also exist.

**Clinical importance.** hCG has served for a long time as a qualitative pregnancy test. Quantitative estimation renders it possible to evaluate the prognosis of imminent abortion, diagnosis of extrauterine pregnancy, of choriocarcinoma or to follow up the consequences after evacuation of a hydatidiform mole. For other pathological conditions in pregnancy (diabetes, gestosis, Rh-isoimmunization) hCG estimation is of no value.

New indications are possible due to the introduction of specific methods for assessment of the β-sub-unit of hCG: the diagnosis of early recurrence of choriocarcinoma during follow-up, and as a specific marker for malignancy in ovarian and other carcinomas.

Therapeutic administration of hCG became important for inducing ovulation in females: after administration of follicle stimulating preparations (FSH, HMG) a large dose of hCG is administered (see p. 321). More detailed data will be found in reviews on hCG (for review see 61, 440).

# PROLACTIN (PRL)

**Structure.** Up to 1971 LTH and prolactin were frequently considered equal, at least based on knowledge from animal experiments. At present it appears that a solely luteotropic hormone probably does not exist. The luteotropic effect is comprehensive, incl. the participation of LH and possibly other hormones. Advances in chemistry revealed several species-specific prolactins which differ from other proteohormones with lactogenic action (STH, hPL), although some years ago the opposite view prevailed, i.e. that in humans prolactin alone does not exist.

Human prolactin (hPRL) is a proteohormone with a molecular weight of 21,500 which is formed in one of two types of acidophils in the adenohypophysis, described as lactotrophs. Using physico-chemical procedures two research teams (Lewis, Friesen) obtained highly purified preparations which no matter whether prepared from the adenohypophysis, plasma or amniotic fluid have the same physical and chemical properties. The structure of hPL is a simple polypeptide chain made up of 198 amino acids and three disulphide bridges (480) (Table 5). The difficulty of isolation is due to the heterogenic character of hPRL.

From plasma two types of hPRL were isolated which cannot be differentiated by immunological methods, so-called "little" and "big" hPRL. The big one has

*Table 5*  Human pituitary prolactin (linear amino acid sequence) (480)

H₂N-Leu-Pro-Ile-Cys-Pro-Gly-Ala-Ala-Arg-Cys-Gln-Val-Thr-Leu-Arg-Asp-Leu-Phe-Asp-
                  10                        20

Arg-Ala-Val-Val-Leu-Ser-His-Tyr-Ile-His-Asn-Leu-Ser-Ser-Glu-Met-Phe-Ser-Glu-Phe-Asp-
                  30                        40

Lys-Arg-Tyr-Thr-His-Gly-Arg-Gly-Phe-Ile-Thr-Lys-Ala-Ile-Asn-Ser-Cys-His-Thr-Ser-Ser-
                  50                        60

Leu-Ala-Thr-Pro-Glu-Asp-Lys-Glu-Gln-Ala-Gln-Gln-Met-Asn-Gln-Lys-Asp-Phe-Leu-Val-
                  70                        80

Ser-Ile-Leu-Ile-Leu-Arg-Ser-Trp-Asn-Glu-Pro-Leu-Tyr-His-Leu-Val-Thr-Glu-Val-Arg-Gly-
                  90                      100

Asx-Gln-Glu-Ala-Pro-Glu-Ala-Ile-Leu-Ser-Lys-Ala-Val-Glu-Ile-Glu-Glu-Gln-Thr-Lys-Arg-
                 110                      120

Leu-Leu-Glu-Gly-Met-Glu-Leu-Ile-Val-Ser-Gln-Val-His-Pro-Glu-Thr-Lys-Glu-Asp-Glu-
                 130                      140

Ile-Tyr-Pro-Val-Trp-Ser-Gly-Leu-Pro-Ser-Leu-Gln-Met-Ala-Asp-Glu-Ser-Glu-Arg-Leu-
                 150                      160

Ser-Ala-Tyr-Tyr-Asn-Leu-Leu-His-Cys-Leu-Arg-Arg-Asp-Ser-His-Lys-Ile-Asp-Asn-Tyr-Leu-
                 170                      180

Lys-Leu-Leu-Lys-Cys-Arg-Ile-Ile-His-Asn-Asn-Asn-Cys-OH
                 190                      198

a molecular weight of 56,000. From amniotic fluid four isohormones of hPRL were isolated with a molecular weight from 27,000 to 36,000. It is suggested that chorion decidua may be the source of the large quantities of prolactin in amniotic fluid. So far the biological importance of these facts is not known. The half-life for clearance of endogenous hPRL is 5–15 minutes.

Ovine prolaction (oPRL) is very close to hPRL, its precise structure being known. It is made up of 198 amino acids, it has three disulphide bridges, at one end a —NH₂ group and at the other end a —COOH group, the molecular weight is 22,500. The similarity with hPRL is high, 73% of the amino acid residues being identical. A similar chemical composition with a minor grade of homology is found in human growth hormone (hSTH) and human placental lactogen (hPL) (16 and 13% resp.), both having a known structure with 190 amino acids with two disulphide bridges and a molecular weight of 21,500. Human, ovine and monkey PRL have a complete crossed immunological reactivity which is lacking or only slightly present between hPRL, hSTH and hPL. The chemical similarity led to the hypothesis of an originally common molecule during phylogenesis which explains the overlapping physiological lactogenic and somatotropic action. The different immunological character renders it possible to follow up separately frequently similar physiological effects.

**Control of secretion.** The hypothalamus inhibits prolactin secretion from the anterior lobe of the pituitary. This inhibition is mediated by PIH, a substance, the chemical nature of which has not yet been completely characterized. Its release is controlled from dopaminergic neurons in the hypothalamus. Dopamine can directly reduce prolactin secretion *in vitro* and *in vivo*. It seems that most of the PIH effect is exerted by dopamine or it is dopamine itself. There is also a second route of control via the prolactin stimulating hormone (PRH). In addition to the route via the hypothalamus PRL secretion is affected also by factors at the level of the adeno-hypophysis. In target tissue PRL acts on specific receptors which were found in the mammary gland, liver, adrenal, kidneys, ovaries and testes.

**Physiological action and secretion.** The effects of PRL are numerous and can be divided into several groups: reproduction (luteotropic, lactogenic, mammotropic), osmoregulation, growth, effect on ectodermal structures and synergism with steroid hormones. PRL is thus a pituitary hormone which modifies the response of various target organs to the effect of other endocrine factors. Its secretion and effect in humans will be discussed in more detail. Serum levels of PRL in newborns are on average 200 ng/ml, but soon decline and during childhood they are on average 5 ng/ml, and in adult life they vary in women between 5–25 ng/ml (average 10 ng/ml), while in men they are significantly lower. According to the majority of data the PRL levels do not change in the course of the menstrual cycle. Although some workers drew attention to a significant rise of PRL during the secretory phase, this obviously is only within its relatively wide range of variation. PRL in plasma has a nyctohemeral rhythm with a minimum at noon and maximum after midnight. There is also a relationship with the onset of sleep as the PRL level rises 30–90 minutes after falling asleep and the rise disappears after waking. In contrast to women, rodents have a cyclic course of PRL secretion with the maximum at the time of the LH peak.

Other factors which stimulate and thus raise the PRL level are: stress, hypoglycaemia and tactile stimuli. Surgical operations are also a stress in which anaesthesia probably also participates. Exercise also causes a rise of PRL. Tactile stimuli such as stimulation of the nipples, cause a rise of PRL but not as much as during lactation; a similar effect is produced by sexual intercourse, stimulation of the vagina and uterine cervix and insertion of intrauterine contraceptive devices.

The relationship of PRL and osmolarity is of interest. Its reduction leads to a decline of PRL to $7^0/_0$ of the original value, infusion of a hypertonic solution causes a rise of PRL. This is due to an antidiuretic effect of PRL and an effect on retention of sodium and water was also observed. This effect must be conceived within the wider context of phylogenesis as PRL, being one of the oldest hormones, still plays a role in some fish when changing from sea water to fresh water and vice versa. It may also exert some effect in the regulation of amniotic fluid osmolarity and volume.

The main and in humans best known effect is the lactogenic action. During lactogenesis in the course of pregnancy PRL rises from the 8th week to delivery when it reaches a level of 200 ng/ml. At the onset of lactation soon after delivery the level is high, but during subsequent weeks only double compared with the normal level which is reached after four months. The suckling reflex is the main stimulus for further release of PRL and thus it always rises 15–30 minutes after initiation of suckling to values which are 10–20 times higher than the basal level. It seems that the presence of the infant is not essential. A similar effect is produced by a breast pump, i.e. direct sensory stimulation of the nipple. Episodic secretion of PRL as a result of suckling in lactating women is the main factor which maintains the mammary gland in an active state of lactation. The highest concentration of PRL in pregnant women is recorded at the onset of pregnancy in amniotic fluid (as much as 10,000 ng/ml), with approaching term it declines while the plasma concentration rises. The impact of high PRL levels in amniotic fluid and the foetus resp. is not known.

Prolactin also affects the ovarian activity of women. The low PRL concentration is necessary for the progesterone production by human granulosa cells *in vitro* (328). A high PRL level induces hypogonadism by inhibiting the positive feedback of oestrogens on LH secretion, it inhibits progesterone secretion and leads thus to a short luteal phase or amenorrhoea. The effect on the hypothalamus is probably primary as PRL controls the pulsatile release of gonadotropins and in experiments suppresses LH secretion but a direct effect of a high PRL level on the reduction of progesterone production from the granulosa *in vitro* was also established. In animals PRL has a clear luteotropic effect.

Whether prolactin is as essential for mammotropic action in humans as in animals, is not as yet clear.

**PRL secretion in pathological conditons.** Raised PRL values are found in the following conditions: (1) disorders of the cycle (short luteal phase, anovulatory cycle, amenorrhoea) with hyperprolactinaemia, (2) secreting pituitary tumours, some of which are associated with galactorrhoea, (3) severing of the stalk of the pituitary, (4) hypothyroidism, (5) renal failure and (6) ectopic production in malignant tumours.

Recently much attention was paid to the participation of PRL in the development of carcinoma of the mammary gland. Experimental investigations revealed that PRL is a substantial growth factor of some carcinomas of the mammary gland, either spontaneous or induced by dimethylbenzanthracene. In women with this disease so far raised PRL levels have not been assessed, however, certain data suggest its participation. One third of carcinomas of the breast in tissue tests proved to be sensitive to PRL. PRL receptors were detected in carcinomatous cells. In rare instances therapeutic advances were reported after administration of PRL inhibitors. It seems that there is a relationship with PRL but it is more complicated. Only the participation of other additional factors obviously sensitizes the epithelium of the mammary gland to the action of PRL and thus creates conditions for the development of a neoplasm. Detailed investigations are focused also on the part played by PRL (its synergism with testosterone) in the development of hyperplasia and carcinoma of the prostate.

**Pharmacological action on secretion of PRL.** Secretion of PRL is enhanced by (1) TRH, (2) psychopharmacological preparations, (3) oestrogens, (4) methyl-dopamine and (5) other substances ($PGE_{2\alpha}$, pimozide, sulpiride, metoclopramide, morphine, β-endorphine, enkephalins). Some substances (TRH, chlorpromazine) are used as tests of hypophyseal function. After some centrally acting so-called major tranquillizers (phenothiazines, reserpines, butyrophenones) or thymoleptics and also during central stimulation the rise of PRL is a side-effect, often associated with galactorrhoea. As regards the mechanism of action — competition for a dopamine receptor is involved. The pharmaceutical industry tries to produce substances where this stimulating action will be devoid of other influences; this would be of great value for stimulating lactation. Oestrogens also cause a rise of PRL, the effect depending on the dose, and at the same time they potentiate the stimulating action of phenothiazine substances.

PRL secretion is inhibited as a result of stimulation of dopamine receptors by the following: (1) L-DOPA, (2) derivatives of ergot alkaloids, (3) other substances (barbiturates, clonidine, furosemide, nickel).

L-DOPA and in particular ergot preparations are potent inhibitors of PRL which will be used in practice to an ever increasing extent for the treatment of hyper-prolactinaemia and galactorrhoea. The results attained with bromocryptine, a derivative of the natural ergot alkaloid, are particularly satisfactory. Also equally effective are synthetic derivatives of ergoline (lergotrile, methergoline, lisuride). By treatment with these inhibitors it is possible to modify ovarian function in galactorrhoea with menstrual disorders. Although this is only temporary treatment, the pregnancies achieved are a great success.

## METHODS OF ASSESSMENT OF PRL

Until recently biological criteria were used for the assessment such as changes of the cropsac glands of the pigeon (Riddle's test in many modifications). Much more sensitive and specific were other biological methods based on histological evidence of milk in the mammary gland of mice and rabbits *in vitro* or tests based on the chemical assessment of milk components. However, by none of these methods can normal hPRL levels be assessed in humans but only pathologically raised values. Therefore nowadays radioimmunological methods, in which the sensitivity is steadily improving, predominate. Heterologous or mixed systems assess the human hormone by means of antiserum and labelled PRL of different provenance (sheep, swine, monkey). Most near to perfect are homologous methods where hPRL reacts with antiserum against hPRL and labelled hPRL, or radioreceptor methods. The sensitivity of methods is 40 pg and even 1 ng/ml in human plasma can be assessed. PRL thus opens new ways in the diagnosis as well as treatment in gynaecology and obstetrics (for review see 94, 153, 533).

# MECHANISM OF GONADOTROPIN ACTION

## GONADOTROPINS AND cAMP

A common feature of hormonal molecules which are derived from amino acid precursors is their ability to combine with specific receptor sites in the plasma membrane of their target cells. Binding of gonadotropins to external receptors in the membrane (for review see 81) is followed by rapid activation of individual cellular responses, incl. steroidogenesis and cellular growth. The majority of such

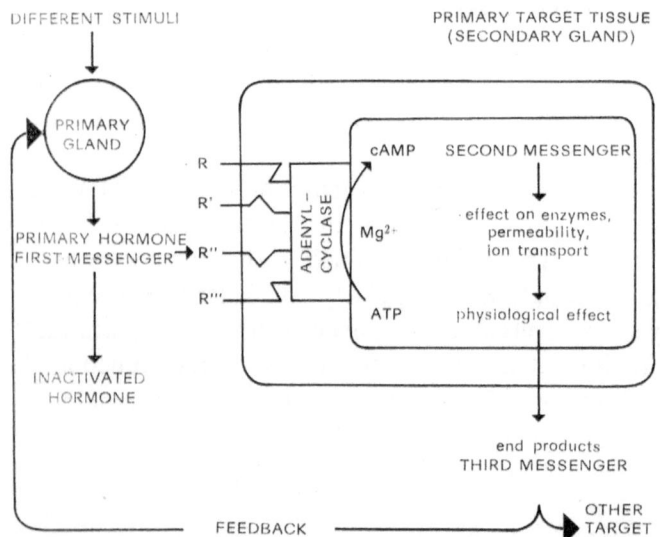

*Fig. 9.* Classical concept of the participation of cAMP (second messenger) in mechanism of gonadotropin action in the cell of the ovarian target tissue. In the two-sub-unit-receptor model on this diagram several regulatory sub-units (discriminators) are projected into one catalytic sub-unit (amplifier) (358).

responses appear to be mediated by the action of cyclic adenosine monophosphate (cAMP) — *the second messenger* being formed by adenylate cyclase on the inner surface of the cell membrane (Fig. 9) (for review see 75).

**Recognition and binding of gonadotropins in the ovary.** *Static models* of the cellular receptor of gonadotropins assume the existence of two or three of its sub-units in the sense that these sub-units are physically proximate and stationary. The two sub-unit model assumes that the receptor is made up of a regulatory substance (discriminator) on the extracellular surface of the membrane, physically related to the catalytic sub-unit (amplifier) on the intracellular surface. Hormone recognition and binding induces a conformative change in the regulatory sub-unit which then activates the catalytic sub-unit to convert ATP to cAMP. The three sub-unit model interposes a transducer sub-unit between the regulatory and catalytic sub-units. The postulated transducer sub-unit could be the site of action which effects hormone binding to the regulatory sub-unit and activation of the catalytic sub-unit. The *fluidity model* is not based upon static relationships but on the fluidity of the lipid matrix of the membrane. In this model the receptor and catalytic units are physically separated. Hormone binding to the receptor induces either transitional movement of the receptor to a juxtaposition favouring complex formation with the catalytic unit, or a field effect in which the structure of the lipid matrix is altered which in turn leads to activation of the catalytic unit. This model would be an alternative to the possibility that each different cyclase has its own receptor (for review see 443).

Data have been presented which indicate that the isolated sub-units of gonadotropins do not bind the receptors nor do they compete with the native molecule for binding or stimulate gonadal steroidogenesis. The relationship of sub-units of the native gonadotropin molecule to the receptor is not yet clearly defined. It is assumed that for recognition and binding of the molecule the β-sub-unit is decisive. It is not known whether it activates also adenylate cyclase. According to an alternative idea it is the α-sub-unit which is common to gonadotropins.

**Properties and number of binding sites for gonadotropins in the ovary.** The isolated ovarian cell receptor at least for LH/hCG is a lipoprotein by nature and has a molecular weight of about 200,000 to 300,000. Its properties are summarized in Table 6. Each receptor site seems to bind a single molecule of the regulatory peptide ligand.

*Table 6* Comparison of cellular receptors for steroids and peptide hormones with plasmatic binding proteins of steroids (483)

| | Plasma binding proteins | Steroid hormone receptors | Catecholamine and peptide hormone receptors |
|---|---|---|---|
| Affinity | low ($K_D^* \simeq 10^{-6}$) | high ($K_D \simeq 10^{-10}$–$10^{-9}$) | high ($K_D \simeq 10^{-10}$–$10^{-9}$) |
| Capacity | high | low | low |
| Location | extracellular (plasma) | intracellular (cytoplasm) | cell membrane |
| Function | unclear | concentrates hormone which alters cell function directly | concentrates hormone which alters cell function indirectly through adenylate cyclase — cAMP |

\* $K_D$ = the dissociation constant, numerically equal to the rate of dissociation of the hormone from its binding protein divided by its rate of association.
A slow rate of dissociation of the hormone coupled with a fast rate of association is indicative of high affinity binding (thus, the lower the $K_D$, the higher the affinity).

Assessment of the number of functional receptor sites in the cell and target organ resp. is difficult. All sites are not functionally active: some are taken up by endogenous hormones, some may be masked in some other way or inhibited. The number of binding sites for gonadotropins in the ovary is certainly limited (142), it varies, however, in different physiological conditions, e.g. the number of hCG binding sites in isolated pig granulosa cells increases during maturation of the follicle from 300 to 10,000 sites cell, respectively (293).

Experimental data suggest that there are more receptor sites than are required for activation of adenylate cyclase and more receptor sites and adenylate cyclase than are necessary for a biological effect such as maximal steroidogenesis. This has led to the hypothesis of "spare receptors" or "receptor excess". If this is not an experimental artefact, these remaining receptor sites which do not have a direct functional relationship with adenylate cylase could serve as "storage sites" to concentrate hormone at the target organ.

Gonadotropins are "utilized" in target cells in a hitherto unknown way: the hLH concentration in blood leaving the human ovary is lower than in venous peripheral blood. Gonadotropins bound to surface receptors of target cells are thought to be internalized and then lysosomally inactivated and degraded. Alternatively, the hormone might undergo only partial breakdown in a hypothetical functionally modified lysosome (regulatory lysosome). Subsequently the hormone or a biologically important fragment is released from the lysosome and will thus be free to interact with various cytoplasmic components or with the nucleus (398). The binding of a radioactive label or the immunoreactive site of gonadotropin to different subcellular components inside the target cell has been repeatedly demonstrated similarly as the presence of hormone fragments in the cytoplasmic cytosol (143).

**Problem of the specificity of gonadotropin action.** The insufficiency of the second messenger hypothesis to account for all the observed effects of many hormones, the variety of responses elicited by a single hormone under physiological conditions, and the simultaneous action of two or more different hormones on the same cell has long been recognized. In this connection observations of intracellular transport of gonadotropins and their sub-units resp. is of interest and so is their interaction with mitochondrial adenylate cyclase and perhaps also guanylate cyclase present in the soluble fraction of cellular cytoplasm. It is assumed that cyclic guanosine monophosphate (cGMP) formed by its action acts on the activity of phosphodiesterase which breaks down cAMP and thus co-determines the cellular cAMP concentration (358).

At present attempts are being made to resolve the open problem of specificity of peptide hormone action by the *unified theory of hormone action (peptide and steroid) at the genomic level*. cAMP as such lacks the chemical and biological specificity to act as a hormone-specific signal. To accomplish this the theory (416) postulates the binding of cAMP to hormone-specific cAMP-binding proteins. These putative, cytoplasmic regulatory proteins are assumed to be constitutive. Upon specific interaction with the receptor – hormone complex the regulatory protein would acquire the ability to bind the effector (cAMP), and as the regulator-effector complex migrate to the nucleus and interact with the chromatin. According to this concept, the only difference between hormones that enter the cell (steroids) and those which do not is that in the former both the receptor and the effector are hormone-specific the effector, in the case of steroids at least, being the hormone itself — whereas in the latter only the receptor is hormone-specific, the effector being a key metabolite (cAMP).

# DEVELOPMENT OF THE SENSITIVITY OF THE OVARY
# TO GONADOTROPINS

The refractory period in the development of the ovary when the gonad does not respond to gonadotropic stimulation and develops autonomously is conditioned by the lack of binding sites for FSH in cells of the granulosa and the absence of target cells for LH, i.e. thecal and interstitial cells. FSH begins to bind in cells of the granulosa at the onset of proliferation of the granulosa sheath of the follicle, LH during the period of differentiation of the theca and primary interstitium. With the further growth of the follicle the number of binding sites increases (410, 411).

Along with the development of binding sites for gonadotropins in the ovary develops also the ability of adenylate cyclase to respond to gonadotropic stimulation by cAMP formation. However, the ovary which does not yet respond to gonadotropins by cAMP production, responds thus to the action of prostanglandin $E_2$. This provides evidence against the idea of prostaglandins as mediators of gonadotropin action on adenylate cyclase and confirms the existence of different receptors for gonadotropins and prostaglandins in the ovary. (Stimulation of ovarian cGMP formation by prostaglandin $F_{2\alpha}$ indicates that prostaglandins $E_2$ and $F_{2\alpha}$ have not only different cellular receptors but also different intracellular mediators.) The reaction of adenylate cyclase to $PGE_2$, while response to gonadotropins is lacking, is explained by the structural or functional immaturity of the gonadotropin receptor.

# Genital Cycle

## OVARIAN CYCLE

The ovary is a paired endocrine gland of flattened ovoid shape 3–5 × 2–3 × × 1.0–1.5 cm in size situated in the fossa ovarica in the lesser pelvis. It consists of surface epithelium, cortex thickened at the surface to form the tunica albuginea, and a vascularized medulla. It serves two reproductive functions: the development and release of the ovum and the production of steroid hormones. Both functions are coordinated and mutually dependent in the regular cycle of adult women, described as the ovarian cycle. The basis of the ovarian cycle is formed by ovarian follicles with oocytes — primordial follicles, growing and atretic follicles which are embedded in the fibrous stroma of the cortex. Their number changes with age, and depends on two basic processes: atresia and follicular growth.

**Atresia** is a continuous degenerative process by which oocytes and follicles disappear from the ovary in a manner other than ovulation. Atresia takes place not only in the foetal ovary but also during postnatal life and ends after the menopause. Loss of follicles during life is considerable, whereby during the postnatal period primordial follicles predominate over growing follicles (9:1).

In the nucleus of oocytes chromatin is condensed, the nuclear membrane wrinkles, and the nucleus undergoes karyolysis. During the reproductive life of women only some 400–500 follicles ovulate.

The first signs of atresia appear in the oocyte. Atresia of the follicular walls begins by activation of hydrolytic enzymes in the lysosomes of follicular cells sooner than histological changes can be detected. Follicular cells in the vicinity of the oocyte and antrum are released, in the cells numerous vacuoles and fat droplets appear, the nuclei undergo karyorrhexis and karyolysis. The basal membrane becomes thickened and hyalinized, and the follicular wall collapses. The degenerating oocyte and follicular cells disintegrate into debris (cytolysis) and are taken up by phagocytes which penetrate into the follicles.

The final fate of these follicles varies. Primordial follicles disappear completely without any remnant. In growing follicles further atresia is more complicated. In addition to the degenerative changes of the oocyte and granulosa described, there is hypertrophy and hyperplasia of the cells of the theca interna. Thus luteinization may develop or a formation resembling the corpus luteum but without granulosa and luteal cells (corpora lutea atretica in animals). Blood vessels and connective tissue septa penetrate into the layer of proliferated thecal cells. In the cytoplasm of thecal cells lipid droplets are deposited. The thickened and hyalinized basal membrane which originally separated the theca and granulosa persists for a long time but is impaired. In a similar manner

71

as during the destruction of the corpus luteum, the cavity of the follicle is filled with fibrous tissue, diminishes in size, and the whole atretic follicle undergoes hyalinization and eventually disappears.

The fate of cystic atresia is different. A cyst develops during this atresia, which is sometimes of considerable size and lined with simple epithelium and filled with watery fluid.

Lobules of interstitial tissue in the stroma are sometimes formed from hypertrophic and surviving cells of the theca interna. Atresia is influenced by many factors such as age, pregnancy, hormone deficiency or excess. From experiments it is known that excessive action of FSH leads to cystic atresia, and excessive action of LH to persisting luteinization of the theca. Many basic problems, however, still remain unresolved. We do not know for instance why one follicle starts to grow and the other remains in a quiescent stage, why one growing follicle ovulates and another ceases to grow and undergoes atresia.

The second basic process which governs primordial follicles is **follicular growth.**

*Primordial follicles* (30–40 μm) are made up of oocytes in the diplotenic stage (oocyte of the first order), from a single layer of spindle-shaped granulosa cells and the basal membrane. These so-called quiescent follicles are found in large numbers in the cortex of ovaries near the surface. Follicular growth starts by mitotic activity of follicular cells. The follicles are divided with regard to size, shape and growth rate into three stages: primary, secondary and tertiary (150). The nomenclature is not uniform. The following terms are also used: at rest, growing, maturing and mature or preovulatory follicle. Occasionally the term secondary is used up to the time of ovulation, conversely the primordial follicle is sometimes described as primary. Sometimes size is used as criterion and small (up to 20 granulosa cells), medium (up to 200) and large follicles ( >200) are differentiated.

*Primary follicles* (0.2 mm) differ from primordial ones: (1) by an increased oocyte, (2) by proliferation of granulosa cells and the development of one and later as many as five layers of cuboidal cells near the oocyte — so-called membrana granulosa, (3) by formation of a layer, the zona pellucida between the oocyte and the granulosa, which at first is discontinuous, later continuous, made up of mucopolysaccharides. The growth of the primary follicle is continuous and autonomous and requires no gonadotropic impulse.

*Secondary follicles* develop only as a result of FSH impulses. In the late foetal period these impulses are placental gonadotropins, during the period before puberty hypophyseal FSH plays a part. Only after puberty during every proliferative stage of the cycle the growth of up to 50 follicles to a size of 1 mm is stimulated. Of these not more than 2–3 reach the size of 8 mm and only one achieves ovulation, while the remainder undergo atresia. Contrary to former views, in every cycle a new group of follicles grows and matures resp.

The secondary follicle is characterized by overall growth, growth of the granulosa layers (preantral follicles) and the formation of cavities which fuse to form the antrum folliculi which contains follicular fluid (antral follicle). The liquor is at first a secretion of the granulosa, later mainly a serous exudate of the thecal capillaries. The oocyte with the compact portion of granulosa cells in the follicle is pushed sidewards by the enlarging antrum and forms near the follicular wall the cumu lus oophorus, which is as a rule at the base of the follicle turned away from the ovarian surface. The follicular theca which already began to develop in the second half of the primary stage is separated from the granulosa by the basal membrane. Simultaneously with the formation of the antrum it differentiates into the theca interna with glandular cells and vascularization and the theca externa with cells of a fibroblastic type which do not differ much from cells of the surrounding stroma. The antral follicle is usually described as the maturing or Graafian follicle.

Under the influence of regularly controlled hormonal conditions at the end of the proliferative stage of the cycle the *tertiary follicle* develops, i.e. the preovulatory or mature follicle which is characterized in addition to further growth (1.5–2 cm) mainly by continued meiosis; shortly before ovulation the first meiotic division is completed and an oocyte of the second order is formed with a first polar body.

In the meantime the antrum takes up most of the follicle and compresses the granulosa which forms only a narrow layer at the border. The oocyte with the cumulus oophorus gradually separates from the association with the granulosa. The follicular cells in its vicinity form a protective layer, the corona radiata, round the oocyte which before ovulation floats freely in the antrum. The entire follicle penetrates to the surface of the ovary and a portion of it bulges above the surface as a flat protuberance. In women and some mammals only one follicle per cycle attains the stage of ovulation.

The morphological changes of the ovarian follicle during the cycle correlate with gonadotropin and steroid levels in peripheral plasma (see p. 56), however, less is known about the correlation with levels in ovarian venous blood or inside the follicle during different stages of its development (for review see 441). In venous effluent from both ovaries in the early follicular stage there is 1000 times more oestrone and oestradiol than in the peripheral blood stream and during the late follicular phase the ovary with the follicle which will ovulate has much higher levels of oestradiol as well as of 17$\alpha$-hydroxyprogesterone, which provides evidence of its secretory activity. In the luteal phase the ovary with the corpus luteum contains in addition to the substances mentioned more androgens and progesterone. Further results were obtained from assessment of gonadotropins and steroids in the follicular fluid from the antrum. LH had maximum values before ovulation, FSH had higher values in the large follicles, the oestrogen levels in the late follicular phase being high, while androgen levels were lower than in the early follicular phase.

Direct quantitative estimation of the production of 17$\beta$-oestradiol from the isolated follicle in cultures *in vitro* revealed the highest values in preovulation follicles of women and these values increased further after HPG or hCG. The site of 17$\beta$-oestradiol in the follicle has not been conclusively determined. Some work on animals provided evidence that cells of the theca and granulosa act synergically as regards oestrogen synthesis, recently it has been, however, reported that the theca interna itself can synthesize oestrogens and the granulosa only when androgen and FSH are present (198).

Androgens are produced in the theca interna and are important for the normal development of the follicle because first of all testosterone and dihydrotestosterone stimulate progesterone secretion in granulosa cells of both antral and pre-antral

73

follicles, and secondly in the presence of FSH granulosa cells convert testosterone to a considerable amount of oestrogens (454).

It seems thus that FSH influences the biosynthesis of oestrogens by specific stimulation of aromatizing enzymes and becomes bound to cellular receptors of the granulosa. LH participates in steroidogenesis by conversion of cholesterol to pregnenolone, mainly in the granulosa (342) and becomes bound to cellular receptors in the theca and granulosa. FSH stimulates accumulation of cGMP and LH stimulates cAMP in preovulatory follicles (318). During the period of follicular maturation and ovulation thus significant changes occur in the cell structure and steroidogenic function.

## OVULATION

The first external sign of incipient ovulation is thinning of the follicular wall at the site where this wall bulges above the ovarian surface. At this defined site the vascularization becomes reduced and a translucent stigma develops made up of the basal membrane between the granulosa and theca interna. In the centre of the stigma develops, pointing outwards, a conic process which persists for some time as a thin avascular membrane. The conus is torn, a circular opening develops through which the follicular fluid escapes along with the oocyte surrounded by cells of the corona radiata. Although the intrafollicular pressure in the tertiary follicle increased, the pressure is no higher than that in the capillaries. Shortly before ovulation this rise ceases. The process of ovulation was followed up and recorded on films by many authors in different animal species and humans. A gradual release of the oocyte always occurred and the rupture never had an explosive character. Between the formation of the stigma and the penetration of the oocyte in women about $1^1/_2$–2 minutes elapse. The blood loss at the site of rupture is minimal because the stigma is avascular. After penetration of the oocyte gradual collapse of the follicular wall occurs.

**Alternating monoovulation.** Clinical and morphological evidence that the ovaries alternate in their ovulating function and only one follicle from the maturing series ovulates, has been long known (for review see 214). Both was explained by Halban's thesis that "incretions and lipoids of the corpus luteum during the cycle and during pregnancy inhibit maturation of the follicle". More recent experimental work rendered the idea on the direct local action of oestradiol and progesterone on inhibition of the ovary which at the time does not contain a corpus luteum, more accurate (214). The inhibiting action of oestradiol administered by the intraovarian route, and under certain conditions also of progesterone, has been demonstrated. It seems that the control of alternating monoovulation takes place in two consecutive stages. During the early luteal phase of the previous cycle in both ovaries a series of new follicles begin to grow. Steroids of the corpus luteum, however, locally inhibit the growth of follicles in an ovary which contains a corpus luteum; thus the growth of follicles in the contralateral ovary is more advanced. During the follicular stage of the subsequent cycle the growing follicles produce in increasing amounts oestrogens which locally induce the process of follicular atresia, except for one follicle which by some unknown selective mechanism reaches the most advanced stage and proceeds as far as ovulation (367).

After unilateral ovariectomy in the remaining ovary the same number of ova ovulate as in intact subjects. The mechanism responsible for the compensatory ovarian hypertrophy is not fully understood. Consistent with data in the literature a raised FSH serum level is found for a short time after operation and prolongation of the preovulatory surge of FSH in subsequent cycles. The reason is, however, not a reduction of oestrogens but it could be inhibin deficiency (69).

*Many theories attempted to explain the mechanism of ovulation proper.* As causal factors the following were emphasized: osmotic pressure, contractility, vascular changes, proteolytic enzymes, chemical changes and the effect of hormones (for review see 302). Many views were speculative and were ruled out later by facts. Recently many objective data and relationships have been revealed on which new hypotheses are based, so far, however, the mechanism of follicle rupture has not been completely explained. It only seems that the main factors are increased distensibility and local enzymatic destruction of the follicular wall.

**A raised intrafollicular pressure** was for long considered to be the main cause of rupture. This mechanistic theory dates back to the last century. The increase of pressure was explained either by the action of smooth muscles in the ovarian stroma or by hypertrophy of the theca interna. Later it was assumed that the colloid osmotic pressure rise occurs as a result of depolymerization of acid mucopolysaccharides due to an increased amount of hyaluronidase in the follicle. Only when accurate measurement proved that the intrafollicular pressure did not rise, this theory was abandoned.

**Smooth muscles and their increased contractility** were also for long considered causal factors. Although no muscle fibres were found in the theca interna, they were found in the theca externa along with adrenergic and cholinergic nerves in the neighbourhood of follicles. In intact ovarian follicles, as in strips of ovarian stroma from women before and after the menopause, the spontaneous motility under the influence of various pharmaceutical preparations was studied. Norepinephrine, acetylcholine, 5-hydroxytryptamine and $PGF_{2a}$ caused sustained tonic contractile tension in the strips. Whole follicles responded by an increased follicular resting tension to norepinephrine, acetylcholine, $PGF_{2a}$ and move mildly to $PGE_2$. On the other hand, $PGE_1$ had an inhibitory effect on contraction and the basal tonus. It seems, however, that ovarian contractility plays only an adjuvant or modifying role during ovulation.

**Vascular changes** which were observed more frequently before rupture of the follicle in various mammals were overestimated and considered by some authors as evidence of active tissue decomposition during ovulation.

**Changes of the tension of the follicular wall** are found before ovulation. By several different methods a reduced modulus of elasticity and thus enhanced distensibility of collagenous tissue in the follicular wall was observed closely before rupture. On this basis and on the assumption of semipermeability of the follicular wall also mathematical models of follicular rupture were elaborated (for review see 302), based on the idea of an increasing tension of the follicular wall.

**Enzyme theories** assumed first the participation of diastase, later of hyaluronidase, more recently proteases and collagenases are studied which could be the cause of breakdown of the follicular wall (for review see 136). Attention is paid also to precursors of collagenase such as zymogen. Recently a rise in the number of bodies resembling lysosomes at the site of rupture of the follicular wall was observed, however, subsequent investigations did not confirm a causal relationship with ovulation.

Several concepts of the mechanism of ovulation using the above mentioned and other assessed data were elaborated. All remain to be conclusively confirmed. However at present it may be said that rupture of the follicle is the final result of histo-morphological changes (enzymatic destruction) and of biophysical changes (increased distensibility) which affect a defined site in the follicular wall.

## PHYSIOLOGICAL ANOVULATION

Ovulation occurs every month during the fertile period of women. There are three periods where it is regularly or irregularly absent under physiological conditions. During the initial period after menarche when regular function is not yet established. We speak of so-called physiological (adolescent) infertility. At that time the first cycles are frequently anovulatory (see p. 13). At the end of the fertile period before the menopause anovulatory cycles also occur. Finally ovulation is absent during pregnancy and after childbirth during lactation.

The majority of authors maintain that ovulation does not occur sooner than six weeks after delivery. During the period between 7–12 weeks 56% women ovulate, and between 13–24 weeks 86% of women. During lactational amenorrhoea ovulation occurs only rarely (0–1.5%). In women who do not breastfeed ovulation occurs on average after 10.2 weeks, while in mothers who breastfeed it depends on the period of breastfeeding: in those who breastfed for 4 weeks ovulation occurs on average after 10.6 weeks, after three months breastfeeding on average after 17 weeks. The relationship with the first menstruation after delivery is manifested by frequent anovulatory cycles. Shortly before the first menstruation ovulation occurs in 28.1% women, before the second menstruation in 66.6%. Figures reported by others are 16%, 50% and before the third menstruation 83%. The problem why physiological anovulation occurs after delivery has not been fully explained, although many facts are known. The early period after delivery is characterized by a low LH level which only later reaches that of the follicular stage. After delivery refractoriness of the ovaries to stimulation by exogenous gonadotropins has also been proved. However, the main feature is a reduced or even lacking receptivity of the anterior lobe of the pituitary to stimuli from the hypothalamus which was assessed after exogenous administration of LH-RH. Six weeks after delivery the response to LH-RH as regards LH output returns to normal. It seems that the main cause of anovulation is prolactin which inhibits progesterone production.

# CORPUS LUTEUM

After ovulation changes take place in the follicle by which it develops into a temporary endocrine gland: the corpus luteum. The changes are due to a high LH level. The function of the corpus luteum is progesterone production which is needed for pregnancy and the control of the length of the ovarian cycle, as progesterone inhibits further gonadotropin release. The inhibitory properties of progesterone are known: it blocks maturation of the follicle and ovulation during the cycle and during pregnancy and this is made use of in contraception. For the development of the corpus luteum during the cycle LH is needed, however, not at as high a level as for ovulation. During pregnancy this luteotropic function is taken over by hCG. During the cycle the corpus luteum persists for only 8–10 days and then gradually degenerates. Its function develops fully only after fertilization and during pregnancy.

**Histological changes during the development of the corpus luteum** have been known since the beginning of the century (Meyer, 1911). As to the structure there are no substantial differences between the corpus luteum menstruationis and the corpus luteum graviditatis. After rupture of the follicle during ovulation its wall collapses, it becomes folded and the follicular cavity acquires a star-like shape. In the cavity a fibrin nucleus is formed by the action of fibrinogen from remnants of follicular fluid and clotted blood which penetrates from capillaries of the theca interna. The cells from the membrana granulosa hypertrophy, they acquire a polyedric shape and change into granulosa-lutein cells. They contain lipid droplets, the lipochromic pigment lutein, numerous vesicles of smooth endoplasmic reticulum and mitochondria in a form typical for steroid-producing cells. The capillaries of the theca penetrate through this tissue and create a network which extends up to the fibrin nucleus. Along with the capillaries processes of sparse connective tissue penetrate and later replace the fibrin nucleus by a thin tissue of fibroblasts and fibrils. The cells from the theca interna also hypertrophy but to a less extent and penetrate along with the capillaries into the granulosa. They form, however, only septa which fill the folds and surface of the granulosa-lutein wall in an interrupted layer. The theca-lutein cells differ from the granulosa-lutein cells in particular by being about half their size. Both lutein cells give positive histochemical reactions with enzymes and precursors of steroid synthesis. However, most of the steroid production in humans originates from granulosa-lutein cells. If impregnation does not occur, the corpus luteum undergoes rapid lytic degeneration. The secreting cells atrophy, stromal fibroblasts grow rapidly and gradually replace the corpus luteum by fibrous tissue. The fibrous tissue undergoes hyaline degeneration and a small fibrous scar is formed, the corpus albicans, which persists for a long time in the deep layer of the ovarian cortex.

# ACTIVITY OF THE CORPUS LUTEUM AND ITS DEGENERATION (LUTEOLYSIS)

**Control of hormonal activity in the corpus luteum.** The hormonal activity of the mammalian corpus luteum differs greatly from one species to another, from complete autonomy and independence of the adenohypophysis (in sows) to

77

dependence on the third pituitary gonadotropin, luteotropic hormone (LTH), identical with PRL (in rats). In humans it also depends on the pituitary. Clinical trials on hypophysectomized females provided evidence that for the maintenance of normal function of the corpus luteum after ovulation for its steroidogenesis and persistence of its activity pituitary LH is essential. The apparent autonomy of the corpus luteum after ovulation caused by a single administration of a sufficient amount of hCG following administration of HMG explains the substantially longer biological half-life of circulating hCG in women than that of pituitary LH.

The above mentioned experiments on hypophysectomized women revealed moreover that for the function of the corpus luteum in females hypophyseal PRL is not needed. It did not prove possible to stimulate the activity of the corpus luteum in a woman with hypophyseal PRL and inhibition of PRL release did not shorten its life span. Even *in vitro* hypophyseal PRL did not stimulate steroidogenesis in the human corpus luteum. Human PRL in the non-pregnant female apparently is not the genuine luteotropic hormone; probably in humans this phylogenetically very old hypophyseal proteohormone also plays a rather specific extragonadal role (for review see 49). Nevertheless, some recent reports suggest a specific role, perhaps a modulatory one, of PRL even in the human corpus luteum function. The human ovary contains specific binding sites for PRL (for review see 153, 533).

**Regression of hormonal activity of the corpus luteum in primates.** The mechanism of regression of the ovarian corpus luteum and factors which regulate the duration of its functional activity in subhuman primates and in man remain so far obscure.

hCG or human hypophyseal LH raise the level of circulating progesterone in the non-pregnant female. At the same time they prolong the life span of the corpus luteum. However, even during continuous administration of large amounts of hCG or LH it did not prove possible to prolong the functional activity of the corpus luteum by more than nine days. The position is similar in monkeys.

In the hypophysectomized female after ovulation induced by exogenous gonadotropins hPL alone does not replace the luteotropic effect of hypophyseal LH.

If the continuous administration of hypophyseal LH in the non-pregnant female is unable to prevent regression of the corpus luteum, this implies that its involution is caused by another factor or factors.

The existence of a uterine luteolytic factor in man is ruled out by the fact that hysterectomy does not alter substantially the duration of the luteal phase of the ovarian cycle nor the level of circulating progesterone. The same was observed in monkeys.

After implantation of a small amount of oestradiol into the human ovary which contains a corpus luteum marked shortening of the menstrual cycle results. In monkeys the postovulation increase of circulating oestradiol above the normal level (by implantation or a single injection) caused premature functional regression of the corpus luteum; at the same time the concentration of prostaglandin $F_{2\alpha}$ in the peripheral blood stream increased. The same effect is produced in women e.g. by a single sufficiently large dose of oestrogen after spontaneous ovulation, recommended in exceptional cases as postcoital contraception ("morning-after-pill") (for review see 471). If conception has occurred, only administration started within 7 days after ovulation is effective. Administration at the time of implantation is without effect, the action of oestrogen probably being blocked by the action of hCG. It seems that in the menstrual cycle of primates physiological luteolysis is started by oestrogens produced by the corpus luteum. The site of their action is probably the corpus luteum itself. An early breakdown of the level of circulating progesterone caused by oestrogen is not always associated with a decline of plasma LH. Therefore the term "autodestructive mechanism" of the corpus luteum is used (for review see 270). In the venous blood leaving the ovary containing a corpus luteum the $PGF_{2\alpha}$ concentration is significantly higher than in venous blood of the "inactive" ovary; the latter does not differ from the peripheral venous blood (9). No doubt, the human corpus luteum produces $PGF_{2\alpha}$. Reversal of oestrogen-induced luteolysis in the rhesus monkey by administration of indomethacin implicates PG as a possible intermediary between increased oestrogen concentration and resulting luteolysis in primates (14).


## OVARIAN STEROIDOGENESIS

Steroids are heterocyclic lipid substances derived from cyclopentanoperhydro-phenanthrene and are very widely distributed in the plant and animal kingdom. Steroids are classified either according to the number of carbon atoms or according to function: into oestrogens ($C_{18}$ steroids), androgens ($C_{19}$ steroids), corticosteroids and gestagens ($C_{21}$ steroids). Systematic nomenclature of steroids is based on the maternal hydrocarbons: gonan, estran, androstan, pregnan, cholan, cholestan, etc. (Fig. 10) supplemented by prefixes and suffixes. The spatial localization of carbon atoms is expressed by the Greek letters alpha, beta. Sex steroids are those which are primarily excreted by the gonads of higher vertebrates (in particular mammals) and which are responsible for the phenotype, physiology and behaviour which differentiates males and females. They comprise three groups: **oestrogens, gestagens** and **androgens.**

## STEROID BIOSYNTHESIS

The main sites of steroid biosynthesis in normal individuals are: the ovary, the testicle and the adrenal cortex. The onset of synthesis is the same in all tissues. The final hormones differ to a considerable extent, depending on the type of tissue: the ovary produces mainly oestrogens and progesterone, the testis mainly testo-

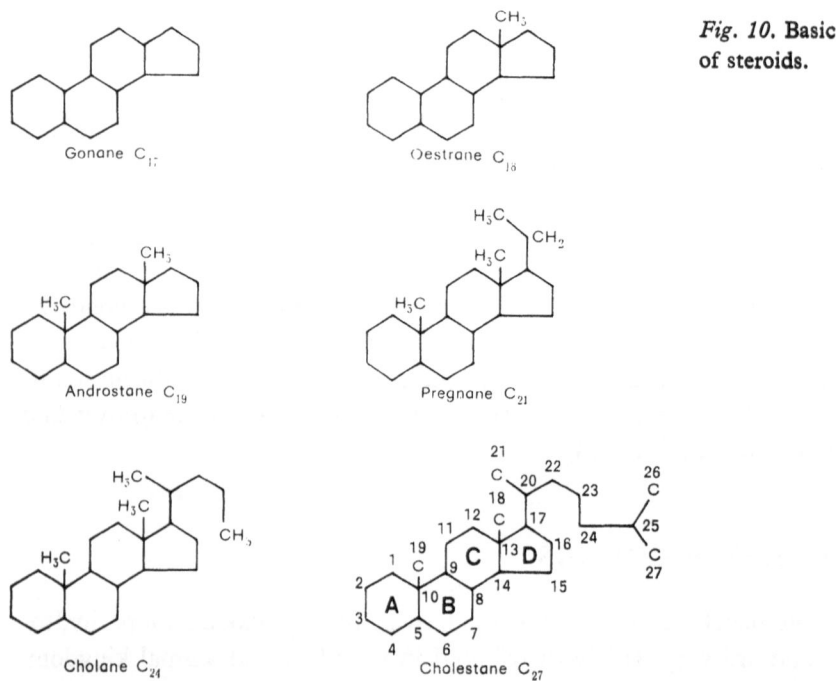

*Fig. 10.* Basic hydrocarbons of steroids.

Gonane $C_{17}$

Oestrane $C_{18}$

Androstane $C_{19}$

Pregnane $C_{21}$

Cholane $C_{24}$

Cholestane $C_{27}$

sterone, and the adrenal cortex mainly corticosteroids. During pregnancy there is a further site of steroid synthesis, the placenta. The basic unit of steroid synthesis is acetate. Molecules of acetyl CoA form by condensation and reduction mevalonic acid, and by other condensations a 30-carbon substance squalene. By a further series of reactions lanosterol and finally cholesterol is formed. It is a 27-carbon alcohol where all four circles (A, B, C, D) in space are in one plane. It is synthesized in the majority of tissues as a building constituent of membranes or is deposited in lipid droplets. Cholesterol is the main material for steroidogenesis in cells where it is either newly formed or conveyed by the plasma (mainly from the liver). It seems that its esterified form is this primary source and LH by one of its actions promotes the mobilization of esterified cholesterol. Subsequently carbon atoms are gradually lost and changes occur mainly in circle A. The first step is the splitting off of the side chain of cholesterol. This occurs as a result of the introduction of hydroxyl groups on the 20th and 22nd carbon atoms by means of hydroxylases and

80

*Table 7* Major metabolic pathways involved in biosynthesis of sex steroids (334)

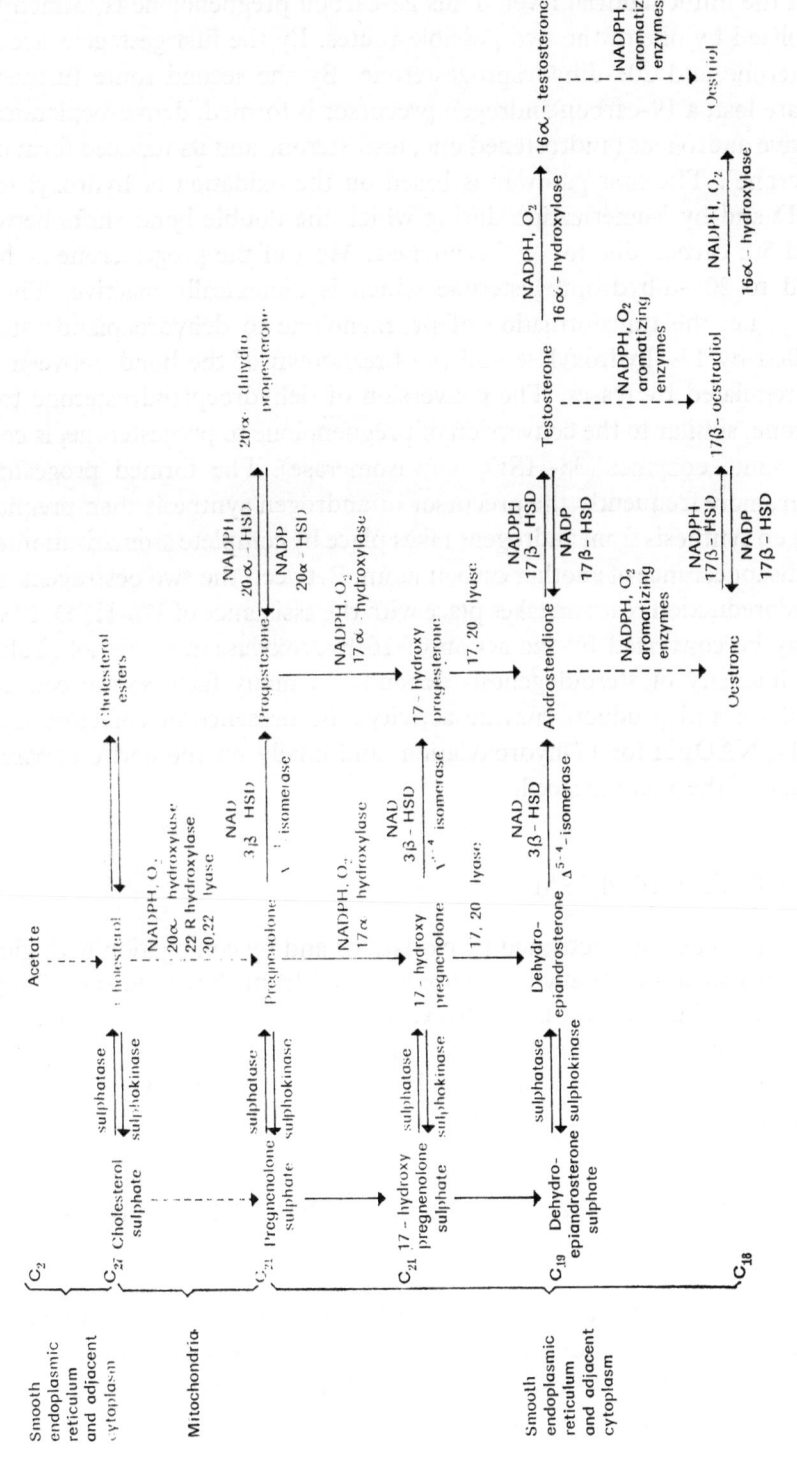

lyase at the mitochondrial level. Thus 22-carbon pregnenolone is formed which is metabolized by one of the two possible routes. By the first gestagens are formed: progesterone and 20α-dihydroprogesterone. By the second route further carbon atoms are lost, a 19-carbon androgen precursor is formed, dehydroepiandrosterone and active androgens (androstenedione, testosterone and its reduced form dihydrotestosterone). The first pathway is based on the oxidation of hydroxyl to $C_3$ via 3β-HSD and by isomerization during which the double bond shifts between the 4th and 5th carbon due to $\triangle^{5-4}$ isomerase. Most of the progesterone is, however, reduced to 20α-dihydroprogesterone which is biologically inactive. The second pathway, i.e. the transformation of pregnenolone to dehydroepiandrosterone, is controlled by 17α-hydroxylase and the breakdown of the bond between $C_{17}$ and $C_{20}$ is regulated by lyases. The conversion of dehydroepiandrosterone to androstenedione, similar to the conversion of pregnenolone to progesterone, is controlled by the same enzymes (3β-HSD, $\triangle^{5-4}$ isomerase). The formed progesterone is, however, more frequently the precursor of androgen synthesis than pregnenolone. Oestrogen synthesis from androgens takes place by complete aromatization of circle A and disappearance of another carbon atom. Between the two oestrogens a reversible oxidoreduction reaction takes place with the assistance of 17β-HSD. 17β-oestradiol may be converted by the action of 16-hydroxylase into oestriol (Table 7).

The intensity of steroidogenesis depends on many factors: the concentration of substrate and product, enzyme activity, the presence of cofactors (NAD for 3β-HSD, NADPH for 17-hydroxylation) and finally on the entire apparatus and processes of the secreting cell.


## STEROID CATABOLISM

Effective steroids are inactivated by oxidations and by conjugation with glucuronic or sulphuric acid and as such they are excreted from the organism. The primary site of steroid inactivation is the liver. The main form of inactivation to which almost all steroids are subjected is saturation of double bonds in the grouping of $\triangle^{4-3}$ ketone where both double bonds are eliminated by liver hydrogenases as a result of oxidation.


## SECRETION, TRANSPORT AND METABOLIC DYNAMICS OF STEROIDS

The steroid levels circulating in plasma are the result of many factors: the secretion of gonadal and adrenal steroids, peripheral conversion of one steroid into another, relative bonds with plasma proteins, metabolism and conjugation in liver, kidney and other tissues, excretion and reabsorption by bile and urine, and distribution in the body.

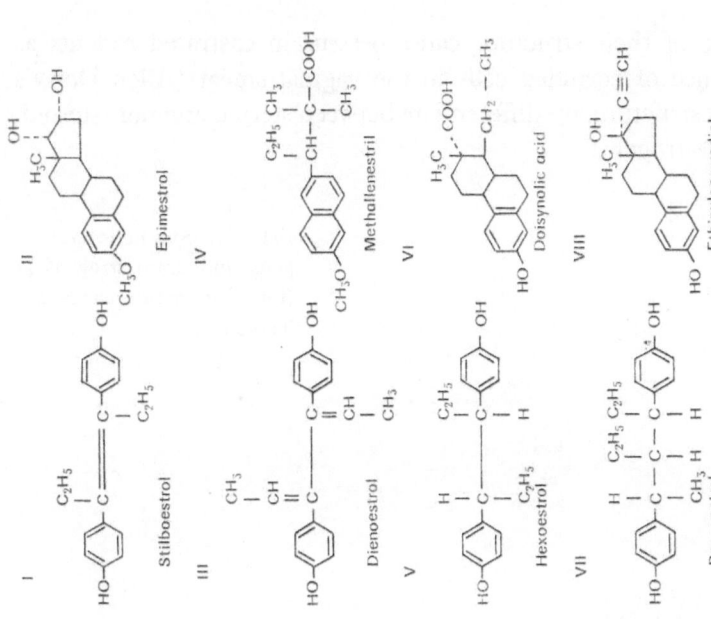

Fig. 12. Synthetic oestrogens and anti-oestrogens I (systematic names): I. 3,4-di-p-hydroxyphenylhex-3-ene; II. 3-methyl-1,3,5(10)-estratrien-3,16α,17α-triol; III. 3,4-di-p-hydroxyphenylhexa-2,4-diene; IV. β-(6-methoxynaphth-2-yl)α,α-dimethylvaleric acid; V. 3,4-di-p-hydroxyphenylhexane; VI. 1-ethyl-1,2,3,4,4a,9,10,10a-octahydro-7-hydroxy-2-methyl-2-phenanthrene carboxylic acid; VII. 3-ethyl-2,4-di-(p-hydroxyphenyl) hexane; VIII. 17α-ethinyl-1,3,5(10)-estratrien--3,17β-diol.

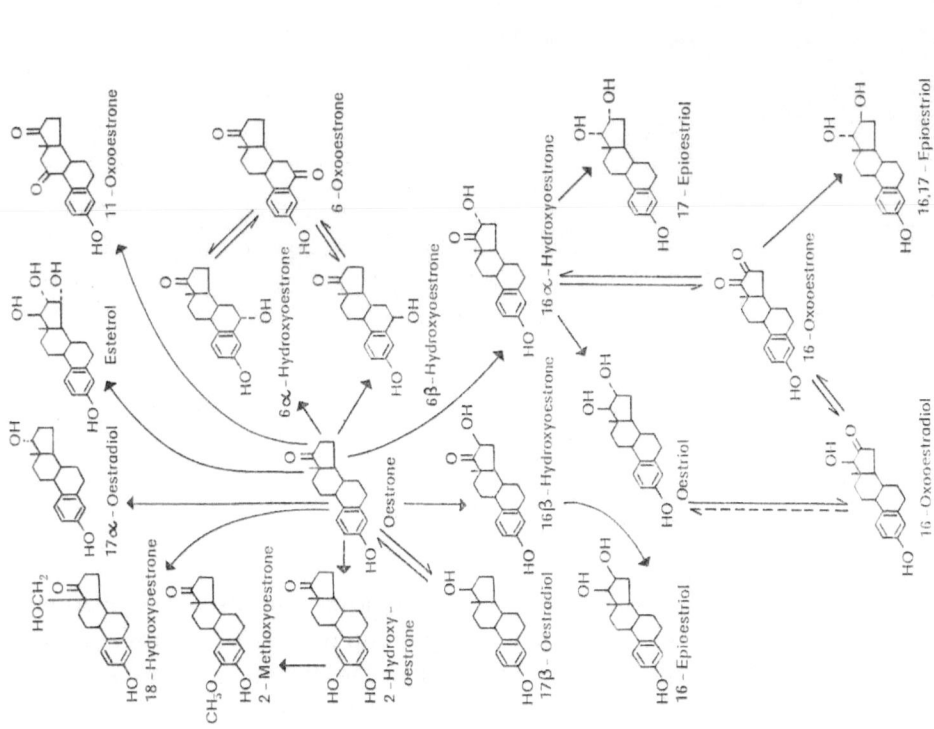

Fig. 11. Natural oestrogens and their metabolism.

83

# OESTROGENS

Oestrogens, irrespective of their structure, cause oestrus in castrated rodents as indicated by the presence of cornified cells in the vaginal smear (Allen-Doisy's test). As to the chemical structure, we differentiate between steroid and non-steroid, natural and synthetic oestrogens.

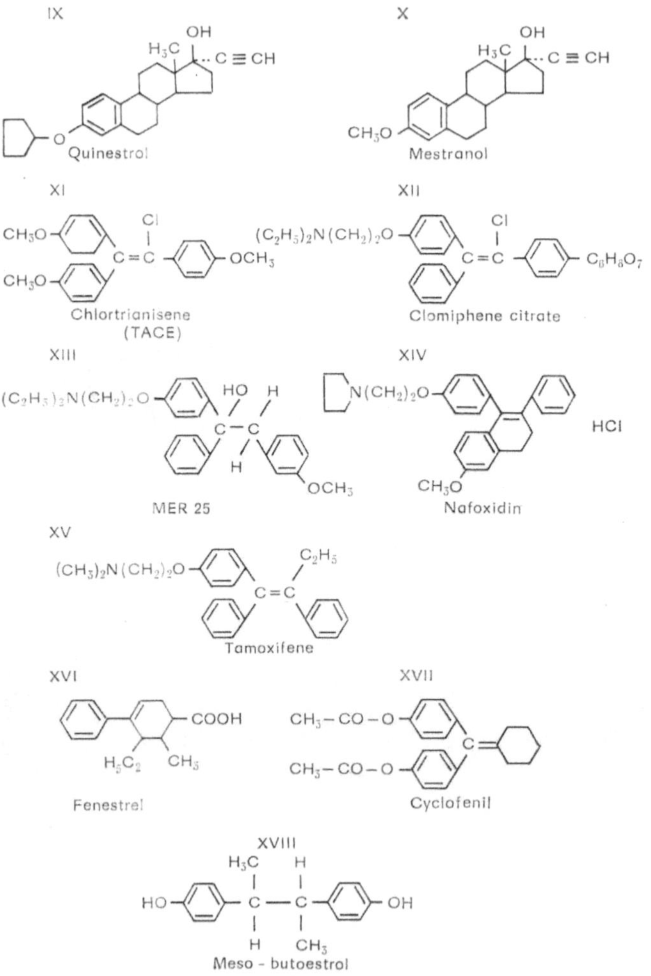

Fig. 13. Synthetic oestrogens and antioestrogens II (for systematic names see Table 8).

IX Quinestrol

X Mestranol

XI Chlortrianisene (TACE)

XII Clomiphene citrate

XIII MER 25

XIV Nafoxidin

XV Tamoxifene

XVI Fenestrel

XVII Cyclofenil

XVIII Meso - butoestrol

**Natural oestrogens** mostly contain a steroid oestran nucleus with a methyl group on $C_{13}$, an aromatic ring A and a hydroxyl group on $C_3$. A large number of oestrogens were isolated and defined chemically (Diczfalusy mention 75). In humans alone 25 different oestrogens were found. The so-called classical oestrogens are three in number: 17β-oestradiol [1,3,5(10)-oestratrien-3,17β-diol], oestrone [1,3,5(10)-oestratrien-3-ol-17-one] and oestriol [1,3,5(10)-oestratrien-3,16α,17β--triol]. Many others are formed by hydroxylations in positions 2, 6, 11, 16 and 18, and are mostly metabolites of the three main oestrogens with slight or almost absent biological activity (Fig. 11).

**Synthetic oestrogens** form the second group of oestrogens which is, however, heterogeneous. Part is derived from stilbens (stilboestrol, dienoestrol, hexoestrol), part from allenolic acid, part from triphenylchloroethylene (chlorotrianisene). A steroid nucleus in a synthetic steroid is found in 17β-ethinyloestradiol, its methyl ether mestranol and quinestrol. Ethinyloestradiol is nowadays the most potent oestrogen, while quinestrol due to its deposition in adipose tissue is an important depot oestrogen (Fig. 12, 13).

## SOURCES AND FORMATION OF OESTROGENS

Oestrogens are very widely distributed in nature. In mammals we find them mainly in the ovary and placenta, with smaller amounts in the adrenals and testes. Ovarian oestrogens are formed in the theca interna and in the stratum granulosum of the maturing Graafian follicle and in the corpus luteum after ovulation. The main route of their formation in the ovary leads from pregnenolone to DHEA. The primary product is oestradiol and oestrone. Their concentration in the ovary is 0.10–0.16 μg/g and 0.25–0.41 μg/g resp. The low concentration at the site of formation is explained by the fact that oestrogens are not stored. Their biological "turnover time", i.e. the time necessary for the exchange of the circulating volume of hormone, is very short: 6 min. Natural oestrogens are, however, also found in lower animals and in the plant kingdom, e.g. so-called phytooestrogens: genistein, kumestrol, mirestrol and others. They are also found in carboniferous layers, in lignite, bituminous slate, etc.

## SECRETION, CIRCULATION AND METABOLISM OF OESTROGENS

Oestrogens are substances which are soluble in alcohol, chloroform and acetone, insoluble in water. In an aqueous alkaline medium or in water they dissolve only after conjugation. The daily oestradiol production depends on the cycle and is 50–500 μg/24 hours. In the whole cycle this is as much as 5 mg. According to other data in the proliferative phase of the cycle it is 51 μg/24 hours for oestrone, and 70 μg/24 hours for oestradiol. In the secretory phase the production is treble; oestrone 178 μg/24 hours, and oestradiol 202 μg/24 hours. In women after the menopause 20 μg oestrone are formed and 14.5 μg/24 hours oestradiol. The daily production in males is lower than in females: 40 μg/24 hours oestrone and oestradiol are produced. In addition to production in the ovary a considerable proportion of oestrogens is formed by extraglandular peripheral conversion of androstenedione to oestrone, and to a minor extent also of testosterone to oestradiol. The same holds true for men (for review see 309, 482). Thus androstenedione becomes a prehormone from which in the periphery not only most of the testosterone is formed but also oestrone. Oestrone sulphate is thus the main circulating oestrogen in plasma. Peripheral conversion takes place mainly in the liver (21, 307). It was found also in adipose tissue, although views reported in the literature are still controversial (48); nevertheless the consumption of oestrogens by adipose tissue *in vitro* and *in vivo* in obese women is substantially elevated. In clinical medicine this could explain disorders of the cycle in obese women and the therapeutic effect of weight loss.

Formerly it was assumed that the low oestrogen production in the postmeno-pausal period is of adrenal origin. It seems, however, that the adrenals contribute only a small direct oestrone secretion but mainly produce the precursors, DHEA and androstenedione. It was proved that the oestrone content was three times, and that of oestradiol and oestriol twice as high in the plasma of the adrenal vein as in the peripheral veins (530). Most of the oestrogens, and according to some all oestrogens in postmenopausal women, originate from the extraglandular peripheral conversion of androgens into oestrogens (184).

The main physiologically important oestrogen in the female is 17β-oestradiol. It is released in the free form into venous blood, but bound immediately with plasma proteins, and specifically with high affinity or non-specifically with low affinity. The plasma contains 2%, of free oestradiol fraction, 38% of specifically TeBG-bound and 60% non-specifically protein-bound oestradiol fraction. Biologic events related to cyclic changes of total plasma oestradiol throughout the normal menstrual cycle may be caused by fluctuations in the free oestradiol and in the non-specifically protein-bound oestradiol. High affinity binding to TeBG seems to render oestradiol inactive (542). This TeBG has the greatest affinity for testo-sterone and a smaller affinity for oestradiol and the least affinity for oestrone and oestriol. The clearance (MCR) of oestrogens is the amount of blood cleared from oestrogens per unit of time. For oestrone it is the same for men and women, i.e. 2,000 1/24 hours, for oestradiol 1,360 1/24 hours in women but 1,600 1/24 hours in men. Expressed per square meter it is for oestrone 1,230 $\pm$ 30 l/24hours/sq.m and for oestradiol 790 $\pm$ 30 1 24 hours/sq.m (309). The clearance is directly pro-portional to the amount produced and inversely proportional to the blood con-centration.

The main organ where the metabolism of oestrogens takes place is the liver. Oestrogens are metabolized there and also conjugated. From the liver about 50% reach the kidney and are excreted in the urine, while about 50% come with the bile into the gut. Only 7–10$^{\circ}_{0}$ are excreted in the faeces, the remainder returning via the enterohepatic circulation to the liver. In the liver the oestrogens are metabolized mainly by oxidoreduction and hydroxylation and thus are mostly inactivated. The main final product which is formed by 16-hydroxylation is oestriol and a series of other hydroxylated oestrogens (see Fig. 11). Recently it was found that in oestrogen metabolism 2-hydroxylation and formation of catechol oestrogens (2-hydroxyoestrone and 2-hydroxyoestradiol) are from both the quantitative and functional aspect more important than 16-hydroxylation (for review see 145).

The intestinal oestrogen metabolism is characterized by the fact that 16-hydroxy-oestrone is transformed in the portal venous plasma into 15-hydroxyoestrone.

Conjugation is another process for inactivation of oestrogens. They become thus soluble in water and can be excreted by the kidneys. Conjugation is a bond of oestrogens with glucuronic and sulphuric acid. Double conjugates are also formed. Glucuronoside complexes have a rapid clearance and are filtered by the glomerulus, sulphates have a slow clearance and are partly reabsorbed in the tubule.

About 25% of exogenous oestradiol is lost without trace in the organism. A small portion passes into the lungs as $CO_2$, 7–10$^{\circ}_{0}$ are excreted in the faeces, and about 50–65$^{\circ}_{0}$ in the urine. The main products are oestrone, 5%, oestradiol, 2$^{\circ}_{0}$, oestriol, 9$^{\circ}_{0}$, i.e. 15–16$^{\circ}_{0}$ which are detected by routine estimation of oestrogens in urine.

The oestrogen metabolism and steroidogenesis in the placental unit is a special chapter which is beyond the framework of the present monograph. The mechanism of action of oestrogens in the cell is the subject of a separate chapter (see p. 113).


## PHYSIOLOGICAL ACTION OF OESTROGENS

Oestrogens have a wide range of action, and may be described as morphogenetic hormones with a stimulating proliferative action on genital organs, secondary sex signs and secondary organs of reproduction. They have also some systemic metabolic effects in the organism. (1) The external genitalia increase in size after administration of oestrogens, the labia minora and maiora develop and grow, and the secretory activity of the sebaceous glands of the vulva increases as well as the thickness and turgor of the epithelium. In animals the manifestations of oestrogens in the vulva are much more marked (opening of the vagina, changes in the vulvo-perineal region in monkeys — sex skin). (2) The vaginal mucosa proliferates under the influence of oestrogens, the epithelial layers undergoing periodic changes during the cycle, while glycogen formation is potentiated as is its breakdown by lactobacillus to lactic acid which raises the acidity of the vagina (pH 5.7). (3) In the uterus oestrogens cause softening of the mucosa, hyperaemia and cellular growth in the cervix, myometrium and endometrium. In the cervix they promote the secretion of thin mucus in mid-cycle with a high "Spinnbarkeit" and arborization, and stimulate its growth and motility and sensitize it for the action of oxytocin. In the endometrium they cause proliferation of the glands, enhance the mitotic activity in the glandular epithelium, the softening of the stroma and vascularization by blood vessels. (4) In the oviduct they promote the growth of musculature and tubal motility. (5) At the trigone of the urinary bladder oestrogens cause desquamation of the epithelium and thus the cells of the urinary sediment display similar cyclic changes to vaginal cells. (6) On the ovary they act not only indirectly via gonadotropins but also directly as they stimulate the initial growth of follicles *in vitro* and *in vivo*. (7) At the level of the hypothalamus the feedback effect of oestrogens is manifested by changes in the release of LH-RH and by changes in the sensitivity of adenohypophysis; the result are changes of the LH and FSH release during the cycle. (8) They participate in the development of secondary sex characteristics, in the development of the female stature, typical shape of the skeleton and female distribution of adipose tissue. They participate in the development of the breasts, mainly the growth and branching of the gland ducts. They influence the thickening of collagen bundles in the skin, the distribution of hair, the character of the voice, and the psychic make up, behaviour and action. (9) Oestrogens influence a) the water and mineral metabolism: they retain $K^+$ in the cell and $Na^+$ in the extracellular space which leads to retention of water in the tissues and to the development of oedema. This rise of K affects muscular function by participation in the formation of contractile actomyosin; b) the carbohydrate metabolism: they reduce glucose utilization in rats, but they have a hypoglycaemic effect in monkeys, the action being species dependent; c) the lipid metabolism: oestradiol reduces the plasma concentration of β-lipoproteins and cholesterol; d) calcium metabolism and ossification: they cause retention of calcium phosphate by promoting the activity of osteoblasts, enhance the maturation of ossification centres and the closure of epiphyseal cartilage, and prevent the development of osteoporosis; e) the thyroid and adrenals: oestrogens in plasma increase the concentration of globulin which binds thyroxin and cortisol and thus both hormones are inactivated. (10) They act on the vegetative system in the parasympathicotonic sense. (11) Oestrogens have a favourable effect on the capillary resistance and fragility by reinforcing the vascular wall by polymerization of mucopolysaccharides. Other effects could be listed: on phagocytosis, inhibition of haematopoiesis, etc.

Contrary to the action of oestradiol and oestrone, some so-called weak oestrogens, in particular oestriol and its epimers (16-epioestriol and 17-epioestriol) have different effects. By competition at receptor sites they block the action of oestradiol and exert an inhibitory effect on the growth of the uterus, by their antiandrogenic action they inhibit the growth of the testes, and the weight increment of the prostate and seminal vesicles. Oestriol exerts an oestrogenic effect on the uterine cervix and vagina, urethra and trigone of the urinary bladder with the exception of the endometrium. It acts on the tissues of the genitals which develop from the ectoderm and have a different enzymatic equipment. Oestriol treatment therefore hardly ever causes unpleasant uterine bleeding as does therapy with other oestrogens.

Catechol oestrogens are not only excretory oestrogen products but antioestrogens with a physiological action devoid of all oestrogenic action. The site of formation in addition to the liver and placenta is the central nervous system. Catechol oestrogens have a marked affinity for soluble oestrogen receptors in the hypothalamus, pituitary and uterus. They may be naturally occurring antioestrogens regulating the actions of oestrogens *in situ*. This includes the control of pituitary hormone release, the onset of puberty, feeding and sexual behaviour and others (145).

## OESTROGEN LEVELS IN URINE AND PLASMA

In practice either total urinary oestrogen values are used or their individual fractions. The level varies typically during the menstrual cycle (Fig. 14) and thus rises during the proliferative phase from low values to the preovulation maximum which precedes the preovulatory surge of LH (positive feedback). After ovulation the level declines sharply and on approximately the 20th–24th day the second maximum occurs which is lower than the first and coincides with the maximum progesterone level at the peak of function of the corpus luteum. The values vary from 10 to 100 $\mu$g/24 hours. Values lower than 10 $\mu$g/24 hours suggest that production in the ovary has ceased. Oestrogen plasma levels are assessed mainly by new methods. Nowadays in particular the plasma oestradiol level is assessed which has a similar course as the urinary excretion curve but the values are expressed in pg/ml. The values vary in the course of the cycle from 50 to 200 pg/ml with a peak of cca 300 pg/ml. If we omit women in reproductive age, the oestrogen level is raised during the first days of life, because in the foetus oestrogens of placental origin circulate, which are responsible for the so-called neonatal hormonal period. During the quiescent period commonly used methods usually assess zero levels in plasma, although subthreshold amounts are excreted in the urine. Several years before menarche the concentration of plasma and urinary oestrogens rises gradually to normal levels. After the menopause the oestrogen levels are low. Excessive levels are recorded in feminizing tumours of the ovary and some carcinomas of the adrenals. In clinical practice it is moreover important to follow the oestrogen concentration after gonadotropin therapy.

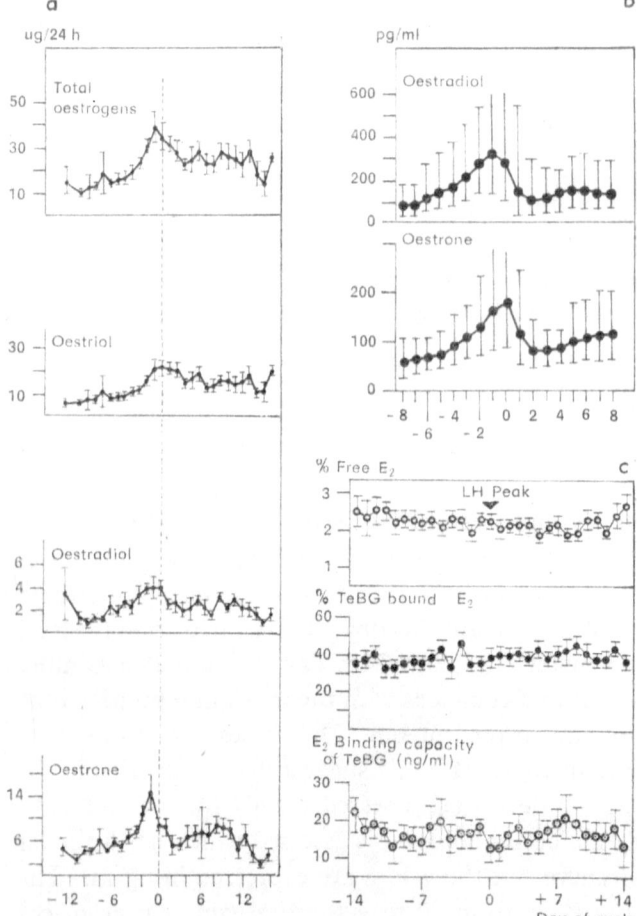

*Fig. 14.* Urinary and plasma oestrogen levels in cycle a) urine — n = 10, mean values ± SE (339); b) plasma — n = 17, mean values ± ± 90 % CL (108a); c) plasma free E₂ (%), TeBG bound E₂ (%), E₂ binding capacity of TeBG (ng/ml), n = 5, mean values ± SE (542).

## METHODS FOR THE ASSESSMENT OF OESTROGENS

Biological methods of oestrogen assessment belong to the past. Nowadays chemical methods are used, gas chromatography, competitive protein-binding, immuno-enzymatic and radioimmunological methods. Chemical methods are based mainly on Kober's colour or fluorescent reaction given by oestrogens with sulphuric acid. The dye is extracted with *p*-nitrophenol in chloroform or acetylene tetrabromide. Urine enters the reaction after acid hydrolysis, ether extraction, purification and chromatography. The most widely used methods are Ittrich's and Brown's method. Conjugated oestrogens are assessed by Beling's method. Gas chromatography is not very much used because it necessitates a tedious procedure to purify the extract. Much more sensitive are the double isotope method and protein binding methods

(125). Protein binding methods use competitive binding of an unknown amount of oestrogen and labelled oestrogen with serum or tissue proteins described as macromolecules or ligands. The yield of these methods is 75–100%, the coefficient of variation less than 10% and the sensitivity 20 pg. It is thus possible to assess plasma oestradiol during the cycle. Radioimmunological methods are most sensitive and are based on a similar principle of competition, however, for the bond anti-bodies against the conjugate of the appropriate hormone are used. Only by the use of highly specific antisera, against 17β-oestradiol-6-carboxymethyloxime BSA or against 11α-hydroxyoestradiol-11-succinyl BSA the specificity of this method was improved. Its sensitivity is high — it can detect even amounts of 5 pg, the accuracy of the method is given by a variation coefficient below 10% (131). Enzyme immuno-assays (EIA, ELISA) of oestradiol and oestriol using peroxidase as marker have also been reported.

## ANTIOESTROGENS

Antioestrogens in the wider sense of the word are substances which suppress some or all effects of oestradiol (165). They include so-called antagonists or inhibitors. For testing of the antioestrogenic action either uterine growth is used (uterotropic action) or vaginal smears (Allen-Doisy's test) in experimental animals. According to the site of action antioestrogens can be divided into a) substances interfering with the synthesis, metabolism and elimination of oestradiol, b) substances which act at the level of the target organ, where they either competitively block oestradiol receptors or other sites in the target cell. The first group includes e.g. antibodies, enzymes, factors which influence the bond with plasma proteins, etc. The second group comprises antioestrogens in a strict sense which interfere at the site of the receptor in the cytosol of the cell. Apart from the receptor in the cell antioestrogenic action is also exerted by the group of steroids such as testosterone, progesterone, cortisol, etc. The majority of antioestrogens proper also have oestrogenic effects and are divided according to these into four groups: (1) obvious oestrogens (cis- and trans- clomiphene ICI 46,474, a derivative of diphenylindene U-11,555 A); (2) so-called impeded oestrogens such as oestriol, dimethylstilboestrol and ent-oestradiol; (3) a partial oestrogenic effect is exerted also by naphoxidin -U- 100 A and nitrostyryl derivatives CN-55, 945-27; (4) ethamoxytriphetol (MER-25) and catechol oestrogens are oestrogenically inactive substances. Impeded oestrogens and cis-clomiphene are weak antioestrogens which is explained by the short period of competition and persistence on the receptor. Substances of the MER-25 type have a much more marked antioestrogenic action because they take up the receptor for a longer period of time. Usually the grade of oestrogenic action proceeds parallel with the grade of antioestrogenic action. Based on both effects, in most of

*Table 8*  Non-steroid antioestrogens (403)

1. Derivatives of triphenyl ethylene:
   a) MER-25, ethamoxitriphetol: 1-[p-(β-diethylaminoethoxy)-phenyl]-1-phenyl-2-(p-methoxyphenyl) ethanol
   b) MRL-37: 1-[p-(β-diethylaminoethoxy)phenyl]-1-phenyl-2-(p-methoxyphenyl) ethane
   c) MRL-41, clomiphene: 1-[p-(β-diethylaminoethoxy)-phenyl]-1,2-diphenyl-2-chloroethylene citrate
   d) ICI-47,699, ICI-46,474, cis- and trans-tamoxifen: 1-(p-β-dimethylaminoethoxyphenyl)-1,2-diphenyl but-1-ene

2. Derivatives of dihydronaphthaline and diphenylindene:
   a) U-11,100A, naphoxidine: 1-(2-[p-(3,4-dihydro-6-methoxy-2-phenyl-1-naphthyl)-phenoxy]ethyl)-pyrrolidine hydrochloride
   b) U-11,555A: 2-(6-methoxy-2-phenyl inden-3-yl)-phenoxytriethylamine hydrochloride

3. Oxazolidinethione:
   U-11,634: 5-(α-α-α-trifluoro-m-tolyloxymethyl)-2-oxazolidinethione

4. Derivatives of diethylstilboestrol:
   a) DMS, dimethylstilboestrol: 2,3-di-p-hydroxyphenylbut-2-ene
   b) Meso-DMA, meso-butoestrol: meso-2,3-bis (p-hydroxyphenyl) n-butane
   c) Threo and erythro MEA: threo and erythro-α-ethyl-α-methyl-4,4' dihydroxybibenzyl

5. Diphenylbenzofuran series:
   DBF: 2-phenyl-3-diethylpyrrolidinoethoxy-6-methoxy-benzofuran hydrochloride

6. Derivatives of 4-phenylcyclohexencarboxylic acid:
   ORF 3858, fenestrel: 2-methyl-3 ethyl-4-phenyl-4-cyclohexencarboxylic acid

7. Nitrostyryl compounds:
   CN-55,945-27: 1-[2-(p-[α-(p-methoxyphenyl)-β-nitrostyryl]phenoxy)ethyl]pyrrolidine monocitrate

8. Aromatic sulphur derivatives:
   66/179: 2-phenyl-3-p-(β-pyrrolidinoethoxy)phenyl-2,1(b)naphthofuran
   67/20: trans-2,2-dimethyl-3-phenyl-4-(p-β-pyrrolidinoethoxy)phenyl-7-methoxychroman hydrochloride

9. Diphenylethylene derivatives:
   F 6066, cyclofenil: bis(p-acetoxyphenyl)cyclohexylidene methane

the substances an antiimplantation and antifertility effect develops. Antioestrogenic substances are nowadays in the foreground of clinical interest in three spheres: non-steroid postcoital contraception, induction of ovulation and treatment of hormone-dependent mammary carcinoma. As to their chemical nature, they come from different spheres and new ones are being discovered (for review see 311a, 403) (Table 8). Many of these substances are only in the stage of clinical tests, while others already exist as commercial preparations. In clinical practice clomiphene citrate and cyclofenil are used for inducing ovulation, naphoxidine and tamoxiphene for the treatment of malignant tumours of the breast, and centchromate is being tested clinically in population control in India.

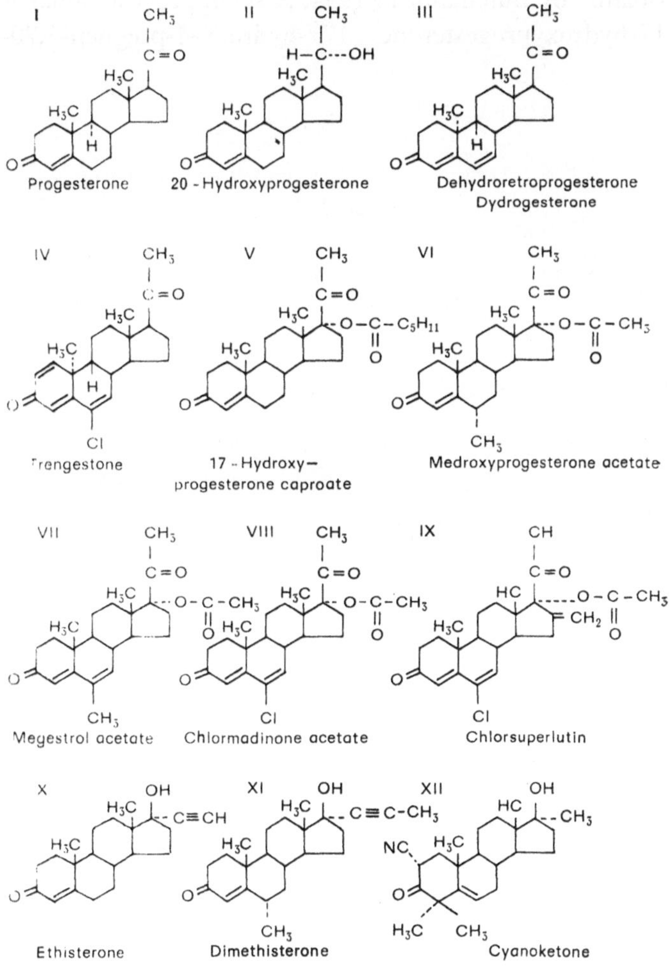

Fig. 15. Natural and synthetic gestagens and their metabolites I (systematic names):
I. 4-pregnen-3,20-dione;
II. 20α-hydroxy-4-pregnen-3-one; III. 9β,10α-4,6-pregnadiene-3,20-dione;
IV. 6-chlor-9β,10α-pregna-1,4,6-triene-3,20-dione;
V. 17α-hydroxy-4-pregnen-3,20-dione caproate; VI. 17α-hydroxy-6α-methyl-4-pregnen-3,20-dione acetate; VII. 17α-hydroxy-6-methyl-4,6-pregnadiene-3, 20-dione acetate; VIII. 6-chloro-17α-hydroxy-4,6-pregnadiene-3,20-dione acetate; IX. 16-methylene-6-chloro-17α-hydroxy-4,6-pregnadiene-3,20-dione acetate; X. 17α-ethinyl-17β-hydroxy-4-androsten-3-one; XI. 17α-(1-propinyl)-6α-methyl-17β-hydroxy-4-androsten-3-one; XII. 2α-cyano-4,4-17α, trimethyl-17β-hydroxy-5-androsten-3-one.

93

# GESTAGENS

Gestagens or progestogens can induce the progestation response in the endometrium which is the preparation for the nidation of the fertilized ovum. Biologically this progestation response is tested on the endometrium of castrated rabbits after pretreatment with oestrogens and after local, oral or subcutaneous administration (McGinty's, Clauberg's, Hooker-Forbes'test). In women the test is the secretory transformation of the endometrium or delay of bleeding. Chemically these substances are steroids derived from the pregnane nucleus. There are natural and synthetic gestagens. The term progestogens is sometimes restricted to synthetic contraceptive gestagens.

As opposed to oestrogens, there are few **natural gestagens.** The main and physiologically most important is progesterone (4-pregnen-3,20-dione) first isolated by Butenandt in 1934. A small progestational activity is also possessed by 17-hydroxyprogesterone (17α-hydroxy-4-pregnen-3,20-dione) and 20-hydroxy-

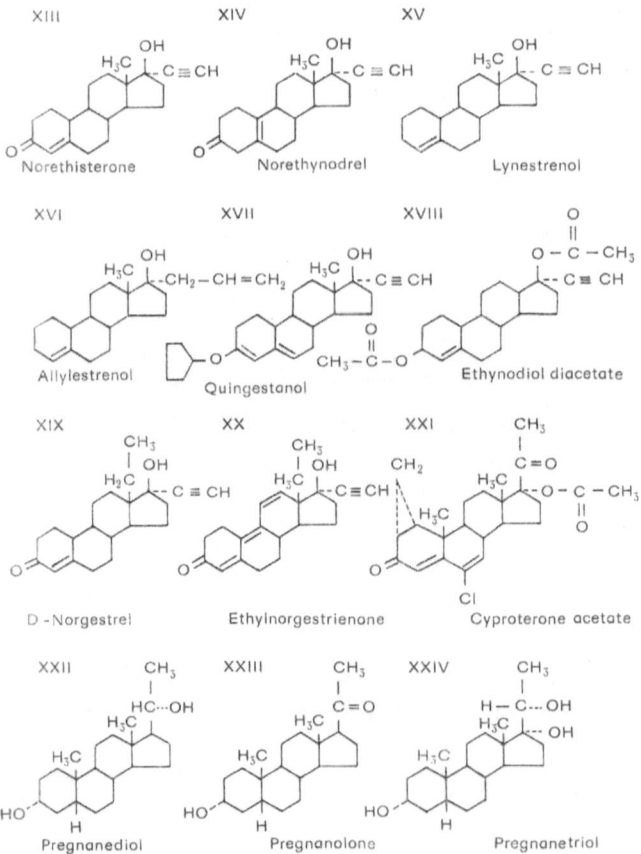

Fig. 16. Natural and synthetic gestagens and their metabolites II (systematic names): XIII. 17α-ethinyl-17β-hydroxy-4-estren-3-one; XIV. 17α-ethinyl-17β-hydroxy-5(10)estren-3-one; XV. 17α-ethinyl-17β-hydroxy-4-estren; XVI. 17α-allyl-17β-hydroxy-4-estren; XVII. 3-cyclopentylenolether-17α-ethinyl-17β-hydroxy-4-estren; XVIII. 17α-ethinyl-3β, 17β-dihydroxy-4-estren-diacetate; XIX. d-13β-ethyl-17α-ethinyl-17β-hydroxy-4-gonen-3-one; XX. 13β-ethyl-17α-ethinyl-17β-hydroxy-4,9,11-gonatrien-3-one; XXI. 1,2α-methylen-6-chloro-17α-hydroxy-4,6-pregnadien-3, 20-dione acetate; XXII. 5β-pregnan-3α,20α-diol; XXIII. 3α-hydroxy-5β-pregnan-20-one; XXIV. 5β-pregnan-3α,17α,20α-triol.

94

progesterone or 20-dihydroproges-
terone (20α-hydroxy-4-pregnen-3-
-one and its isomer 20β-hydroxy-
-4-pregnen-3-one).

There are many **synthetic gestagens** mainly due to the pharmaceutical industry which sought substances with a rising progestational
activity for contraception and therapy (Fig. 15, 16). The principles
of modification which increased the
activity were as follows: a) substitution of the ketone and methyl
group on $C_{20}$ and $C_{21}$ by ethinyl
group; b) suppression of the methyl
group on $C_{19}$, thus forming so-called
norsteroids; c) esterification of the
hydroxyl group on $C_{17}$; d) methy-
lation or halogenation on $C_6$. Today
we recognize four series of synthetic
gestagens: (1) progesterone derivatives (6-dehydroretroprogestero-
ne); (2) derivatives of 17α-hydro-
xyprogesterone (17α-hydroxypro-
gesterone caproate and enanthate
with a depot action, 17α-hydroxy-
progesterone acetate or acetoxyprogesterone, the chlorinated derivatives of which are among the
most effective gestagenic preparations); (3) testosterone derivatives
(17α-ethinyl testosterone or ethisterone, 6,21-dimethylethisterone or
dimethisterone, cyanoketone, danazol); (4) nortestosterone derivatives,
so-called norsteroids (17α-ethinyl
nortestosterone acetate or norethisterone acetate, 17α-ethinyl-5(10)es-
tren-17β-ol-3-one or norethynodrel, allylestrenol, lynestrenol, ethynodiol diacetate, norgestrienon, nor-

*Table 9* Activity spectrum of some progestagens (359)

| Compound | Endometrial transformation | Oestrogenic | Androgenic | Anti-oestrogenic | Anti-androgenic | Anti-gonadotropic | Gluco-corticoid like | ACTH stimulation | Virilization | Feminization |
|---|---|---|---|---|---|---|---|---|---|---|
| Progesterone | + | − | − | + | ± | + | + | − | − | − |
| Norethisterone | + | ++ | ++ | ++ | − | ++ | − | ++ | ++ | − |
| Lynestrenol | + | ++ | ++ | ++ | − | ++ | − | ++ | ++ | − |
| Norgestrel | + | − | ++ | ++ | − | ++ | − | − | ++ | − |
| Norethynodrel | ± | + | ± | − | − | + | + | + | ± | ± |
| Medroxyprogesterone acetate | + | − | − | ++ | ± | ++ | ± | − | − | ± |
| Chlormadinone acetate | + | − | − | ++ | ++ | ++ | + | − | − | + |
| Cyproterone acetate | + | − | − | ++ | +++ | ++ | + | − | − | + |
| Megestrol acetate | + | − | − | ++ | + | ++ | + | − | − | + |
| Hydroxyprogesterone caproate | + | − | − | ++ | − | ± | − | − | − | − |
| Gestonorone caproate | + | − | − | ++ | − | + | − | − | − | − |

gestimat, and at present the most potent gestagen — norgestrel). Synthetic gestagens have in addition some other effects, e.g. norsteroids have an androgenic, oestrogenic and antioestrogenic in addition to the gestagenic effect (Table 9). Cyanoketone is a potent inhibitor of 3β-hydroxysteroid dehydrogenase and thus interferes with progesterone synthesis. Cyproterone acetate is an antiandrogen. Danazol and norgestimat are strong antigonadotropins. Gestonorone caproate is a depot gestagen, five times more potent than 17α-hydroxyprogesterone caproate.

## SOURCES AND FORMATION OF GESTAGENS

The site of progesterone formation is mainly in luteal cells of the corpus luteum. Its amount in venous ovarian blood of women is proportional to the degree of ovarian luteinization. A small amount is also formed by thecal cells of the maturing follicle before ovulation, and the tissue and fluid of the follicle may contain equal or greater amounts than the functional corpus luteum. It is also produced in small amounts by the adrenals as a precursor of adrenal hormones. Large amounts of progesterone are formed in the trophoblast and placenta. Progesterone in the ovary is formed from cholesterol and its precursor is pregnenolone (see p. 81). Some experiments revealed, however, that animal ovaries produce progesterone rather from acetate and thus this route must also be considered.

## SECRETION, CIRCULATION AND METABOLISM OF GESTAGENS

Progesterone is a crystalline substance insoluble in water but readily soluble in organic solvents. The progesterone content of the corpus luteum is 20 μg/g, of the placenta 2–4 μg g. This relatively low content, as compared with the total secretion, indicates that progesterone disappears very rapidly from the site of formation. The daily progesterone production during the proliferative stage is 2.5–5.4 mg/ 24 hours, in the luteal phase 22–43 mg 24 hours, in men 1.1–6.5 mg/24 hours. Recently reported values give the daily progesterone production as 0.75–2.5 mg/day during the proliferative phase, 15.0 to 50.0 mg/day in the luteal phase (301a). Data on the biological half-life of endogenous progesterone vary. The original values were 25–29 minutes, for men and ovariectomized women 15.8 and 10.7 min resp., for pregnant women 3–6 min. Later it was revealed that progesterone disappears in a biphasic manner. The first part of the curve $t_{1/2} = 6$ minutes reflects the metabolism and steady state in plasma, the second slower part reflects the metabolism, excretion and return from tissue, in which $t_{1/2}$ occupies 95 min.

Progesterone in blood is partly free, and partly bound to albumins and α₁-globulins. The bond with globulins is much stronger than that with albumins and specific for progesterone and hydrocortisone. This protein carrier is described as a corticoid-binding globulin (CBG) or transcortin; it is formed in the liver and the bond with progesterone makes it biologically ineffective. There exists a dynamic equilibrium between the free and bound fraction in blood, the bound fraction being a reserve of the hormone. A further reserve is the rapid deposition of progesterone in adipose tissue.

After injection of progesterone about 25% disappears by routes yet unknown, 3% is expired through the lungs as $CO_2$, and 5–10% is excreted through the gut and faeces, while a portion returns from the gut by the enterohepatic circulation into the liver. 35–55% of the administered amount is excreted by the kidneys. The values of metabolic clearance of progesterone (MCR) during the whole menstrual cycle are 2,500 – 135 1/24 hours which is more than in men (2,080 1/24 hours). The time required for the exchange of the entire amount of progesterone, i.e. the turnover time, is 3.3 minutes. Another natural gestagen 20α-hydroxy-4-pregnen--3-one has in biological tests about one quarter to half the effect of progesterone, its MCR is slower, and the daily production is 1.83–15.6 mg/day. About 5% are converted to progesterone and conversely progesterone contributes towards 24–73% of its production (for review see 304).

The metabolism and breakdown of progesterone takes place mainly in the liver. The metabolic product is pregnanediol (5β-pregnane-3α,20α-diol) and pregnanolone (3α-hydroxy-5β-pregnane-20-one). Small amounts of isomers of the following series are also formed: allopregnanedione, allopregnanolone, allopregnanediol as well as hydroxylated metabolites on $C_6$ and $C_{16}$. A small amount of pregnanetriol (5β-pregnane-3α,17α,20α-triol) in plasma is formed from 17α-hydroxyprogesterone of adrenal origin. Not all pregnanediol is of ovarian origin, a small amount is formed during the metabolism of corticosteroids and is described as so-called residual pregnanediol in the proliferative stage of the cycle or after castration. From radioisotope studies following administration of ³H-progesterone it appears that 6–27% of the administered amount is excreted in the urine as pregnanediol, 1.6–5% as pregnanolone and 0.5–2% as pregnanedione, while the other metabolites account for less than 1%. In the liver progesterone metabolites are conjugated with glucuronic acid and are excreted in urine as sodium glucuronosides. Other organs of progesterone metabolism are the brain, kidneys, endometrium, myometrium and mammary gland. While during the metabolism in the liver 5β-derivatives are mainly formed, the endometrium and myometrium have a different progesterone metabolism and form mainly 5α-derivatives (alloderivatives). All progesterone metabolites excreted in the urine are biologically inactive.

# PHYSIOLOGICAL ACTION OF GESTAGENS

The main function of gestagens is the preparation and maintenance of pregnancy, and on this their effects on the organs of reproduction are focused. In addition they have, however, metabolic effects on other organs. In the uterus gestagens act on the endometrium, myometrium and uterine cervix. In the endometrium they cause transformation and secretion of the glands of the endometrium, prepared by the proliferative action of oestrogens. The glands curl into spirals, the lumen enlarges, and glycogen is formed in the glands which then passes into the lumen and subsequently into the uterine secretion. The stromal cells of the mucosa undergo pseudodecidual transformation and are preparing for nidation. In the myometrium gestagens inhibit the motility of smooth muscles and during pregnancy they cause the so-called progesterone block. The reduced ability of myometrial cells to contract while the contractility of actomyosin is preserved, prevents according to Csapo's theory the onset of premature contractions during pregnancy. In the uterine cervix gestagens cause reduction of the amount of mucus and its condensation. In the vagina they act against the effect of oestrogens and influence changes in the vaginal cytology, staining, and morphological characteristics (curled-up cells in clusters from medial and surface epithelia). In the mammary gland they promote the development of alveoli, while oestrogens stimulate the development of ducts. In the feedback via the hypothalamus they inhibit LH secretion after ovulation. They reduce fertilization by impaired transport of the ovum and by inhibiting the capacitation of sperm cells. They reduce libido.

Many metabolic effects of gestagens are mostly secondary, i.e. they develop as a result of the effect on controlling organs, the brain, kidneys and liver. They have a protein catabolic action and promote urinary nitrogen excretion. They increase body weight. They stimulate urinary excretion of $Na^+$ and $Cl^-$ in a significant way. Urinary electrolyte losses occur because gestagens inhibit the action of aldosterone on renal tubules, and at the same time after gestagen administration a compensatory increase in the aldosterone level occurs. Gestagens influence respiration by reducing alveolar $p_{CO_2}$. This probably takes place by a direct increase of the sensitivity to $CO_2$ in the respiratory centre. The thermogenetic effect of gestagens is involved in the development of the biphasic basal body temperature. Finally they exert an inhibitory action on the central nervous system and in large doses they have an anaesthetic action (for review see 359).

Progesterone and progestational substances have thus above all a *progestational action*. The mechanism of this action is implemented in specific organ receptors which were detected in the uterus of some animals and humans, in the oviduct of the chick, and in the ovary, pituitary and hypothalamus of the rat (see p. 114).

Some of the modes of action of progesterone mentioned are *antioestrogenic*. The mechanism of the antioestrogenic action of progesterone may, according to present knowledge, be implemented in two ways. Progesterone reduces the concentration of receptors for oestradiol and on the other hand raises the level of 17β-oestradiol dehydrogenase in tissue. Both ways lead to a reduced sensitivity of tissue for oestradiol, in one instance because of deficiency of receptors, in the other instance because of inactivation of oestradiol which is metabolized to oestrone. So far this has been confirmed for the endometrium, and it may, however, explain the antioestrogenic action of progesterone in general. In clinical practice these antioestrogenic effects of progesterone are widely used in the treatment of endometriosis, benign mastopathies, premenstrual syndrome, menometrorrhagia due to a disorder of the corpus luteum and these antioestrogenic effects probably play a role also in the protection against the carcinogenic action of oestrogens on the endometrium.

Another effect of gestagens is *antiandrogenic*. Only recently experimental evidence was provided (1960) that progesterone inhibits the stimulating action of testosterone on the cock's comb and reduces, when administered subcutaneously, the growth of accessory sex organs in mice. Local administration of progesterone inhibits growth and activity of sebaceous glands which were stimulated by testosterone. The mechanism of action is a disorder of the transformation of testosterone to 5α-dihydrotestosterone (DHT). It is thus antiandrogenic in action, in particular in those target organs which have DHT-dependent receptors (sebaceous glands, prostate, and urogenital sinus). In clinical practice thus new therapeutic indications in dermatology develop (alopecia and acne).

Finally gestagens are known to possess *androgenic* and *oestrogenic* effects. They ensue from their closely related chemical structure and metabolism. A simultaneous androgenic and oestrogenic action is displayed e.g. by norsteroid derivatives.

Some synthetic gestagens have certain effects inhibited while others are more marked, thus some derivatives of acetoxyprogesterone are antiandrogens and are used to suppress precocious puberty. Other gestagens, such as cyproterone acetate, are also antiandrogens, while others such as norsteroids cause haemostasis in dysfunctional haemorrhage, similarly as oestrogens.

Derivatives of synthetic gestagens also include danazol (17α-hydroxy pregn-4--en-20-yno-2,3-d-isoxazol-17-ol). It is a derivative of ethisterone which has a marked *antigonadotropic effect*, it lacks, however, a progestational, oestrogenic, antiandrogenic effect and only in large doses it has also an androgenic effect. It reduces the LH and FSH plasma level and its action is reversible. In women it suppresses menstruation, ovulation and causes regressive changes in the vaginal cytology and atrophic changes of the endometrium. In clinical practice it is used for treatment of endometriosis, fibrocystic mastopathy, gynecomastia and precocious puberty.

# URINARY AND PLASMA LEVELS OF GESTAGENS

*Progesterone* is found mainly in plasma, the urinary level being very low. During the proliferative stage of the cycle its concentration is low, usually not exceeding 1 ng/ml and corresponds to values assessed in men, and women after the menopause. In the middle of the cycle, concurrently with the peak of LH, a rise of the level begins with a maximum 5–8 days after ovulation when it reaches 8–15 ng/ml at the functional peak of the corpus luteum, and then before menstruation it declines to the initial low level (Fig. 17). Assessment of its levels is useful in the diagnosis of impaired function of the corpus luteum. The urinary progesterone level assessed by RIA gives a similarly shaped curve as in plasma, only at a low level (average 0.2 g/24 hours) during the proliferative phase and 1.4 g/24 hours during the secretory phase.

*17α-hydroxyprogesterone* in plasma varies between 0.3 to 2 ng/ml and the shape of the secretory curve imitates to a certain extent the oestradiol and progesterone curve. The preovulatory peak was described by some authors as significant, but according to others it is not constant. The idea that the preovulatory peak of 17α-hydroxyprogesterone is of physiological importance for the gonadotropin output, and its levels are important for the diagnosis of impaired luteal function was not confirmed. It is rather an intermediary metabolite in steroid conversion.

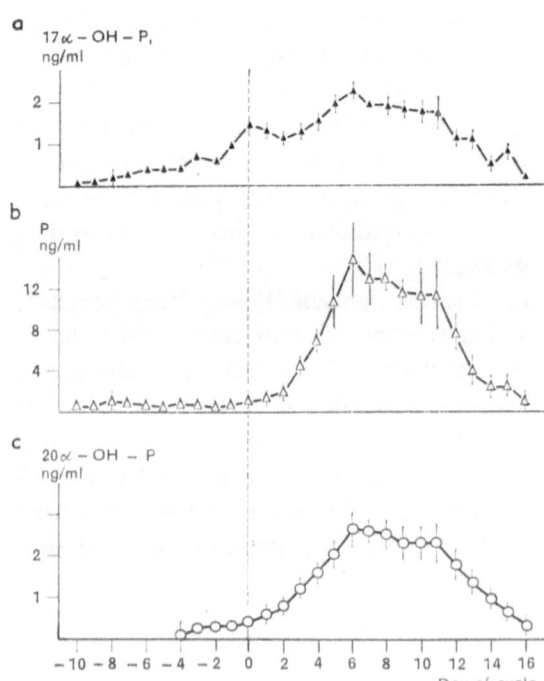

*Fig. 17.* Gestagen plasma levels during the cycle: a) 17α-hydroxyprogesterone, b) progesterone, c) 20α-hydroxyprogesterone, n = 7; mean values ± SE (310a).

100

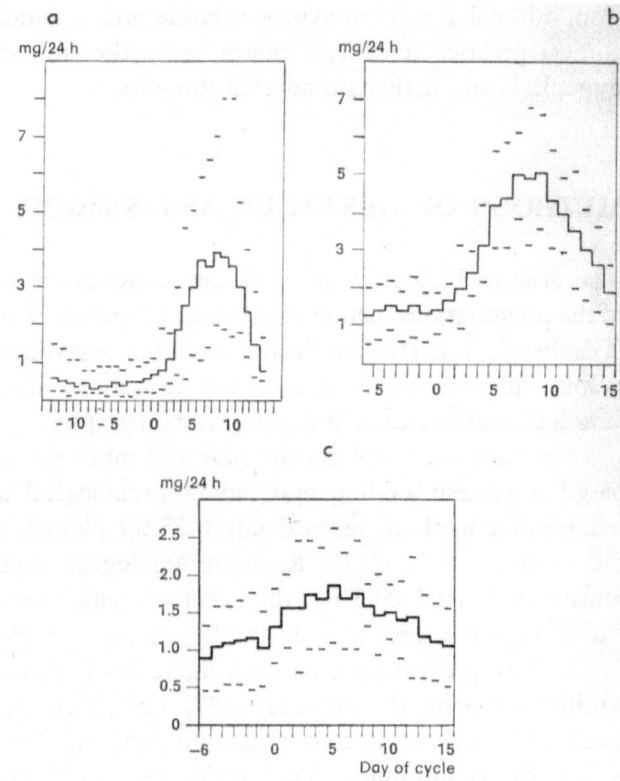

*Fig. 18.* Urinary pregnanediol and pregnanetriol levels during the cycle: a) pregnanediol by the method of gas chromatography, n = 15, mean values ± ± max.min. (27); b) pregnanediol by the method of thin layer chromatography, n = 6, mean values ± SD; c) pregnanetriol by the method of thin layer chromatography, n = 6, mean values ± SD (147a).

The function of another metabolite, *20α-hydroxy-4-pregnen-3-one*, in the female organism is obscure. Its values in the course of the cycle are low. (On the other hand, in the rabbit it is the main gestagen in plasma.) In women its values are not indicative of corpus luteum function.

In urine the main metabolic product of progesterone is *pregnanediol*, till recently the only steroid from which conclusions on progesterone values could be drawn. The curve of urinary pregnanediol excretion has the same shape as the curve of progesterone excretion. In the follicular stage of the cycle its values do not exceed 1 mg/24 hours, and after ovulation it rises to levels between 3–8 mg/24 hours with a maximum on the 5th–8th day after ovulation. Assessment of pregnanediol in urine was used in clinical practice to evaluate corpus luteum function, for the diagnosis whether ovulation has taken place, i.e. as an ovulation test. Although there is a close correlation between progesterone values in plasma and pregnanediol in urine, it must be born in mind that on average only 15% of the administered progesterone appears in the urine as pregnanediol (Fig. 18).

*Pregnanetriol* in urine has low levels with a slight maximum in the middle of the luteal phase of the cycle (it rises from 1.0 to 1.5 mg/24 hours). It originates mainly from adrenal 17α-hydroxyprogesterone and a minor portion from the ovary. In clinical practice its raised values serve the differential diagnosis of congenital hypoplasia and malignant adrenal tumours.

## METHODS OF GESTAGEN ASSESSMENT

The original biological methods for progesterone assessment serve only as tests of the progestational action of different preparations in the pharmaceutical industry (Glauberg's test, Hooker-Forbes'test). For assessment in plasma paper chromatography, fluorometry and double isotope methods are used. These methods are very laborious and intricate, as is gas chromatography.

They have been replaced by new and much more accurate and rapid methods based on protein binding, and radioimmunological techniques. Competitive protein binding methods require only 0.25 ml plasma, the sensitivity is 0.1 ng, and the accuracy 8% (243). Radioimmunological methods further increased the sensitivity to 0.02–0.05 ng, the accuracy remaining equal. So far in all methods chromatography meant a delay. By the use of more specific antisera (against 11α-hydroxyprogesterone hemisuccinate BSA) chromatography could be omitted without reducing the accuracy (488, 525). New enzyme-linked immunosorbent assays (ELISA), using a conjugate progesterone 11α-hemimaleate-β-galactosidase to identify the immunological reaction are specific and simple.

Pregnanediol in urine was long assessed by means of chemical methods, mainly by Klopper's where after hydrolysis and extraction chromatography and acetylation with final colorimetry were necessary. Recently, however, gas chromatography has predominated. It is more rapid and more accurate (27).

## ANTIPROGESTATIONAL SUBSTANCES

This term implies substances which inhibit the action of progesterone and are recently in the foreground of interest as substances with an antifertile effect. The antiprogestational effect may have a different mechanism. In a strict sense this term covers some gestagens such as danazol (see p. 99) or R 2323 (13β-ethyl--17α-hydroxy-18,19-dinor-17α-pregna-4,9,11-trien-20-yn-3-one). These substances bind with a progesterone receptor and the steroid-receptor complex enters into the nucleus but does not activate the chromatin template, and thus the resulting effect is antiprogestational (504). Other antiprogestational steroids are ORF 9326 [17β-acetoxy-2α-chloro-3(p-nitrophenoxy)imino-5-androstan] and RMI 12,936 (17β-hydroxy-7a-methyl-androst-5-en-3-one) which have so far been investigated in animal experiments. They block progesterone synthesis and have an antifertile effect in pregnant animals. They also block ovulation by causing reduction in hypophyseal sensitivity to LH-RH (261).

## ANDROGENS

Androgens stimulate the development of the male genital apparatus and secondary male sex characteristics. They are derived from androstan and therefore are sometimes described as $C_{19}$ steroids. There are natural and synthetic androgens.

**Natural androgens** comprise: testosterone and dihydrotestosterone, androstenedione, dehydroepiandrosterone and androsterone (for systematic names of androgens see Fig. 19 and 20).

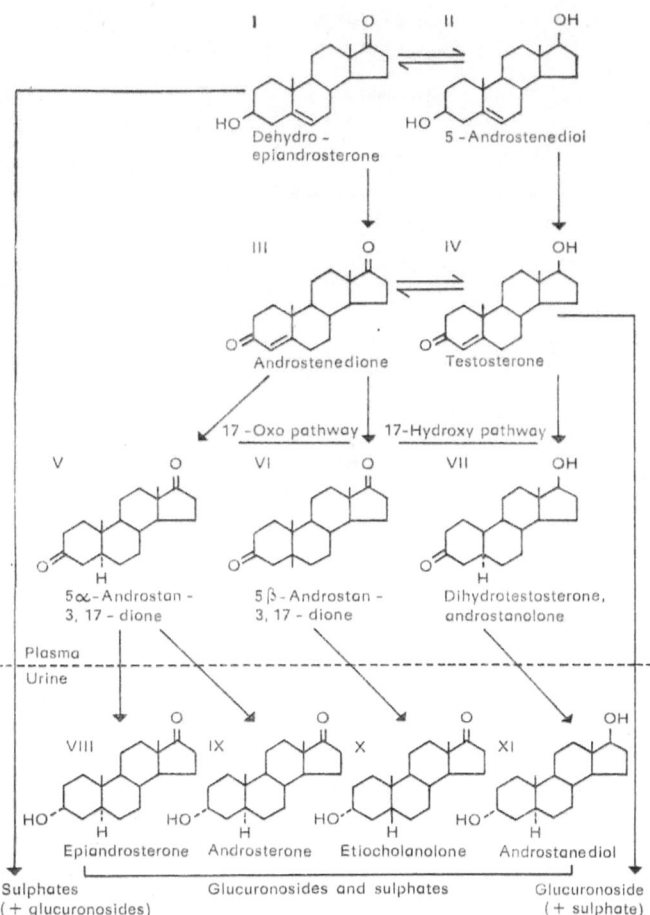

*Fig. 19.* Natural androgens and their metabolites (systematic names): I. 3β-hydroxy-5-androsten-17-one; II. 5-androsten-3β,17β-diol; III. 4-androsten-3,17-dione; IV. 17β-hydroxy-4-androsten-3-one; V. 5α-androstan-3,17-dione; VI. 5β-androstan-3,17-dione; VII. 17β-hydroxy-5α-androstan-3-one; VIII. 3β-hydroxy-5α-androstan-17-one; IX. 3α-hydroxy-5α-androstan-17-one; X. 3α-hydroxy-5β-androstan-17-one; XI. 5α-androstan-3α,17β-diol.

103

**Synthetic androgens** are: (1) testosterone esters (propionate, phenylacetate, enanthate, undecylate); esterification potentiates or protracts their effect, (2) oral or perlingual forms of testosterone derivatives (methyltestosterone, mesterolone), (3) testosterone derivatives which are formed by 14-dehydrogenation; by re-

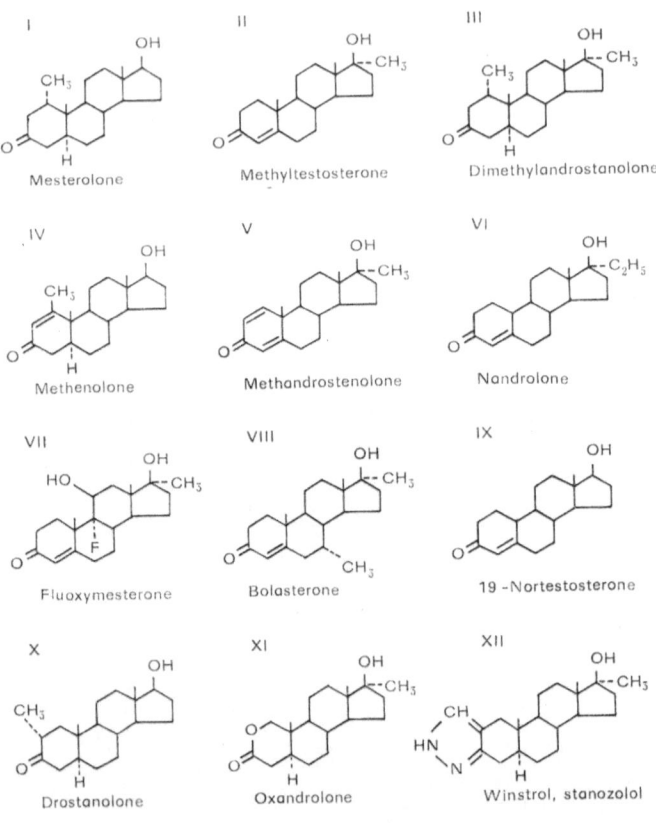

I. Mesterolone
II. Methyltestosterone
III. Dimethylandrostanolone
IV. Methenolone
V. Methandrostenolone
VI. Nandrolone
VII. Fluoxymesterone
VIII. Bolasterone
IX. 19-Nortestosterone
X. Drostanolone
XI. Oxandrolone
XII. Winstrol, stanozolol

*Fig. 20.* Synthetic oral androgens and anabolic preparations (systematic names): I. 17β-hydroxy-1α--methyl-5α-androstan-3--one; II. 17α-methyl-17β--hydroxy-4-androsten-3--one; III. 1α,17α-dimethyl--17β-hydroxy-5α-androstan-3-one; IV. 17β-hydroxy-1α-methyl-5α-androst--1-en-3-one; V. 17α--methyl-17β-hydroxy-1,4-androstadien-3-one; VI. 17α-ethyl-17β-hydroxy-19--nor-4-androsten-3-one; VII. 17α-methyl-9α-fluoro--11β,17β-hydroxy-4--androsten-3-one; VIII. 7α,17α-dimethyl-17β-hydroxy--4-androsten-3-one; IX. 17β-hydroxy-19-nor-4--androsten-3-one; X. 2α--methyl-17β-hydroxy-5α--androstan-3-one; XI. 17α--methyl-17β-hydroxy-2--oxo-5α-androstan-3-one; XII. 17α-methyl-17β--hydroxy-(3,2-c)-pyrazole--5α-androstane.

moval of the 10β-methyl group (nor-) and by 7α-methylation their androgenic activity is enhanced; thus the most potent androgen known at present was formed, i.e. 7α-methyl-14-dehydro-19-nortestosterone, which is 100 times more effective in biological tests than testosterone, (4) anabolics (methenolone, methandrostenolone, nortestosterone etc.) with a high anabolic effect where the androgenic action is suppressed to a minimum.

# SOURCES AND FORMATION OF ANDROGENS

Androgens are formed in three different endocrine glands: the testes, the adrenal cortex and the ovary. In males 60% of all androgens are produced in the testes, and the remaining 40% in the adrenals. In women at least 40% of the androgens originate in the ovary, and the remaining 60% in the adrenals. As to androgens, the testes produce mainly testosterone, the adrenal cortex mainly dehydroepiandrosterone, and the ovary androstenedione. In the testis the main site of androgen production are Leydig's interstitial cells. Here testosterone accounts for 90% of the production, a small amount of dehydroepiandrosterone and even less androstenedione is produced in the testis. The concentration of these three androgens in the blood of the spermatic vein is 47.9, 4.4 and 2.9 µg/100 ml. Thus the contribution of other androgens to the clinical androgenic action as well as to conversion into testosterone in man is negligible. Recently it was demonstrated that also Sertoli cells in humans produce testosterone. The formation of testosterone in the testis proceeds from pregnenolone by two pathways: either via progesterone and 17-hydroxyprogesterone ($\triangle^4$ pathway) or via 17-hydroxypregnenolone and dehydroepiandrosterone ($\triangle^5$ pathway) and also via 4-androstenedione or via 5-androstenediol. Other pathways of testosterone formation directly from progesterone were detected or the so-called sulphate line which is a sort of safeguard mechanism. It is very difficult to assess the main routes of actual formation on the basis of interpretation of assessed factors *in vitro* and *in vivo*. The assumption that $\triangle^4$ and $\triangle^5$ pathways are organ or species-specific was not confirmed.

The normal ovary secretes androstenedione, testosterone and dehydroepiandrosterone. According to the concentration in the ovarian vein they are produced at a ratio of 23:1:13 (307). Androstenedione is thus the main ovarian androgen. In the formation of the total circulating androstenedione the ovary participates by 40–70%, depending on the phase of the cycle, and the adrenal cortex by 30–55%. In the total circulating testosterone the ovary participates by 33–66%, 40–66% is of adrenal origin. In the total circulating dehydroepiandrosterone the ovary participates by 20% and the adrenal cortex by 80%. The ovarian ratio of peripheral testosterone, androstenedione and dehydroepiandrosterone sulphate varies with the stage of the cycle and is highest in the middle of the cycle (1). The site of androgen formation in the ovary are the hilar stromal cells, the theca of the growing follicles and the corpora lutea (22). The androgen formation in the human ovary takes place by two pathways as in males, either via progesterone (so-called $\triangle^4$ pathway) or via dehydroepiandrosterone (so-called $\triangle^5$ pathway). Based on experiments *in vitro* it is estimated that by the second pathway three times as much androstenedione is formed than via 17α-hydroxyprogesterone.

# SECRETION, CIRCULATION AND METABOLISM OF ANDROGENS

The evaluation of the daily secretion of different androgens is complicated by the extraglandular conversion of precursors to the final product. This means that not all circulating final androgen in plasma is secreted. This extraglandular conversion is of greatest importance for the formation of plasma testosterone or oestrogen from androstenedione in females. Extraglandular conversion to testosterone takes place mostly in the liver $(15^{o}{}_{o})$ but also in the skin. While in the ovarian plasma the ratio $A/T \approx 23 \cdot 1$, in peripheral plasma it is only 3–4/1 (307). The original values of daily secretion obtained by methods of isotope dilution in urine proved erroneous. For the characterization of secretion at present values of blood production are used $(P_B)$, assessed on the basis of plasma concentration and metabolic clearance (MCR). Furthermore we must know the ratio of conversion of the precursor to the final product. Then the actual secretion in blood $(S_B)$, e.g. of testosterone, is obtained according to the formula

$$S_B^T = P_B^T - P_B^{A-\!\!-T} - P_B^{DHA-\!\!\to T}$$

If extraglandular conversion does not take place, $S_B^T = P_B^T$. Values of the daily plasma production of testosterone in men are on average 7 mg (5–10 mg/day), and in women 20 times less, 0.23–0.34 mg day. The daily production of androstenedione in men is 1.4 mg/day, in women 3.4 mg/day. The daily production of dehydroepiandrosterone in men is 0.15 mg day, in women about 8 mg/day incl. 0.3–3 mg from ovarian secretion, the remainder being of adrenal origin. The metabolic clearance (MCR) of testosterone in men is approximately 1100 l plasma/day, in women 650–700 litres per day. MCR for androstenedione in men is 2,300 l/day and in women 2,000 l day. More recently the MCR is given in litres per sq.m day; then $MCR^T$ in men is 516, and in women 304 l/sq.m/day. The half-life of testosterone disappearance from plasma $(t_{1/2})$ in the initial component is cca 7 minutes, in the late component about 35 minutes. When assessing the actual secretion $(S_B)$, it was revealed that in men $95^{o}{}_{o}$ testosterone in blood are actually secreted as testosterone, in androstenedione $60^{o}{}_{o}$ are secreted as such and $40^{o}{}_{o}$ originate from the peripheral conversion of testosterone and dehydroepiandrosterone. In women only $40^{o}{}_{o}$ testosterone are secreted, $50^{o}{}_{o}$ come from the peripheral conversion from androstenedione and $10^{o}{}_{o}$ from dehydroepiandrosterone (for review see 21).

Circulating androgens in plasma are mostly bound to four plasma proteins. Under normal conditions $98–99^{o}{}_{o}$ of testosterone are bound to β-globulin described as TEBG, testosterone binding globulin (synonyms: TeBG, SBP, SHBG, SBβG). This globulin has a high affinity but low capacity for testosterone, it also binds oestradiol, but with a three times smaller affinity. Part of the testosterone is also bound to an $\alpha_1$-globulin called orosomucoid, another portion to CBG, in the same way as cortisol. Also part of androstenedione is bound to CBG. Finally a small portion of both androgens is also bound to albumins (for review see 30). From various publications ensues that testosterone in men is distributed as follows: $2\%$ free, $40\%$ bound to albumin and $58\%$ to TEBG, and in women: $1\%$ free, $18\%$ bound to albumin and $81\%$ to TEBG. The bond with plasma proteins is very important. It is accepted nowadays that only unbound androgen in plasma is biologically active. Recently therefore the TEBG concentration is expressed quantitatively in mIU/ml, the percentage of binding capacity of TEBG and the index of free androgen is assessed or free androgen is estimated directly. Either free testosterone is assessed or total androgens (17$\beta$-hydroxysteroids). Both are a better characteristic of the androgenic activity than assessment of the total hormone in plasma. The bound hormone in blood represents the inactive reserve which protects the hormone against metabolic and chemical changes and is by reversible dissociation a protection against sudden changes in the concentration of the active hormone. It serves for the elaboration of methods for assessment of testosterone by means of competitive inhibition.

In addition to testosterone ($100\%$ effect) and androstenedione potent androgens also include dihydrotestosterone ($125\%$), androstanediol ($50\%$) and androstenediol ($33\%$). Dihydrotestosterone is an important intracellular androgen. In some tissues (ventral prostate, seminal vesicles, epididymis) it is formed mainly by $5\alpha$-reduction of testosterone and is bound to the cytoplasmic receptor much more firmly than testosterone. In other tissues (kidneys, uterus, ovary, hypothalamus and pituitary) it is formed only to a very small extent from testosterone and binds as readily as testosterone and thus both are effective. Finally in other tissues (testis, levator ani) it is formed in minimal amounts or not at all; at these sites only testosterone is linked with the receptor (299). The diurnal production of dihydrotestosterone in plasma ($P_B^{DHT}$) in men is 0.39 mg/day, whereby $50\%$ originate from testosterone. In women 0.05 mg/day are produced, however, only $10\%$ originate from testosterone and most of it is formed from androstenedione as the prehormone.

The metabolism proper of androgens takes place mainly in the liver. It may take place also in the prostate, kidneys, skin, mammary gland. Testosterone as well as androstenedione are reduced step by step. Androsterone, etiocholanolone, epiandrosterone, epietiocholanolone and $5\alpha$-androstanediol and $5\beta$-androstanediol are formed. The former two are most important. The final metabolites conjugate in the liver with glucuronic and sulphuric acid and are excreted as sodium salts by the kidneys into the urine. Part is excreted with bile into the intestine, where most is reabsorbed and only a small portion excreted with the faeces. Most of these metabolites have a 17-oxo group and are described as 17-ketosteroids, and more recently as 17-oxosteroids. 17-oxosteroids in urine were formerly considered, often erroneously, as a test of the androgenic function of the gonads. However, only one third

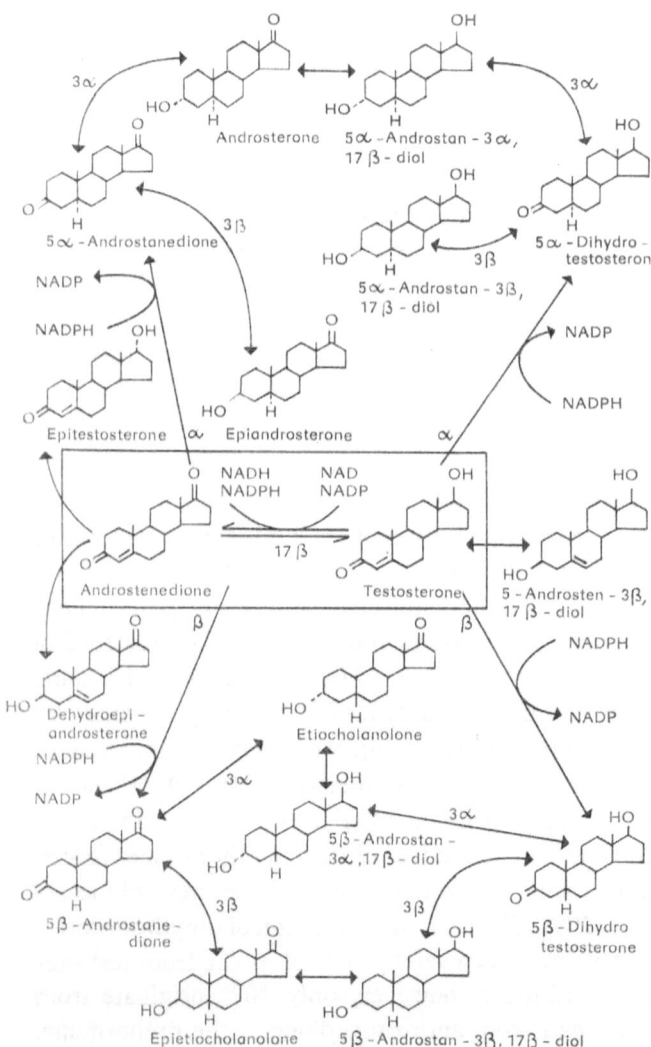

*Fig. 21.* Testosterone metabolism ($\alpha = 5\alpha$ reductase, $3\alpha = 3\alpha$-hydroxysteroid dehydrogenase, $\beta = 5\beta$ reductase, $3\beta = 3\beta$-hydroxysteroid dehydrogenase, $17\beta = 17\beta$-hydroxysteroid dehydrogenase).

originates from the production of the testes or ovaries as most is of adrenal origin, mainly dehydroepiandrosterone, 11β-hydroxyandrosterone, 11β-hydroxyetiocholanolone, 11-oxoandrosterone, 11-oxoetiocholanolone (see Fig. 19 and 21).

## PHYSIOLOGICAL ACTION OF ANDROGENS

Testosterone and dihydrotestosterone are the most effective androgens. The androgenic action of androstenedione is substantially smaller and, dehydroepiandrosterone is a very weak androgen of minor clinical importance (Table 10). The effects of testosterone are a) androgenic, b) protein anabolic.

*Table 10*  Relative androgenic and anabolic activities of some naturally occurring androgens (300)

| | Rat, i.m. | | | |
| | Ventral prostate | Seminal vesicle | Levator ani muscle | Chick comb by inunction |
| --- | --- | --- | --- | --- |
| Testosterone | 100 | 100 | 100 | 100 |
| Dihydrotestosterone | 268 | 158 | 152 | 228 |
| Androstenedione | 39 | 17 | 22 | 121 |
| 4-Androstene-3β,17β-diol | 124 | 133 | 95 | |
| 5α-Androstan-3,17-dione | 33 | 13 | 11 | 115 |
| 5α-Androstan-3α,17β-diol | 34 | 24 | 30 | 75 |
| 5α-Androstan-3β,17β-diol | | 10 | | 2 |
| 5α-Androstan-13α-ol-17-one | 53 | 8 | 10 | 115 |
| Testosterone propionate | 161 | 146 | 187 | |
| Methyltestosterone | 103 | 100 | 108 | 300 |
| 17α-Methyldihydrotestosterone | 254 | 78 | 107 | 480 |

a) *Androgenic action* of testosterone is already manifested in the foetus as the foetal testis has a decisive effect on the normal development of the male foetus (see p. 6 and 8). During puberty testosterone is essential for the growth and function of male sex organs, secondary sex organs, the development of secondary sex characteristics and the growth of axillary and pubic hair. Testosterone in adult life influences spermatogenesis, perhaps indirectly, perhaps by local production in the Sertoli cells. The psychological effect of testosterone is its influence on libido, the male type of behaviour and action. Another target area of testosterone is the CNS. By a negative feedback it regulates the tonic secretion of gonadotropins.

b) General *protein anabolic action* of testosterone involves enhanced protein synthesis and reduced catabolism of amino acids. It increases muscular mass, causes retention of $K^+$, $Na^+$, $Cl^-$ and water. By increasing calcium retention it prevents osteoporosis. After puberty in inhibits general growth by influencing the closure of epiphyseal cartilages.

The effects of androgens in females were till recently considered pathological (virilization, masculinization of the sex organs etc.). Today we know the actual physiological importance of androgens in women: (1) they control the growth of axillary and pubic hair, (2) they maintain libido, and (3) they are precursors of oestrogens in normal biosynthesis as well as during extraglandular production of oestrone from androstenedione.

## URINARY AND PLASMA ANDROGEN LEVELS

Formerly mainly *17-oxosteroids* in urine or plasma were assessed. In men between 20–40 years the values of total 17-oxosteroids vary between 12 and 17 mg/24 hours. In childhood the values are low, in puberty they rise and reach the peak at the age of 25 years and in old age they decline again. In women the values are lower than in men and vary between 7 and 12 mg/24 hours. The lower borderline of normal values is about 5 mg, and the upper 15 mg/24 hours. In women there are similar variations with age as in men. Raised values are found in adrenal tumours, in adrenogenital syndrome, in some cases of Stein-Leventhal syndrome, and reduced values in panhypopituitarism and hypogonadism. The diagnostic value of total 17-oxosteroids is not great and only liminal values — high and low — can be used. Assessment of fractionated 17-oxosteroids, some of which are of adrenal origin, and others mainly of gonadal origin, did not improve their diagnostic importance because some predominating fractions originate from both sites. The stimulatory action of ACTH, hCG and the inhibitory action of dexamethasone on the 17-oxo-steroid level is employed in functional tests, but even these are not very helpful in diagnosis, although they are recommended in different modifications by some authors.

The urinary *testosterone* level gives a better but also inaccurate picture of androgenic activity, as much of the urinary testosterone glucuronoside does not originate directly from the testosterone produced but by peripheral conversion from androstenedione, dehydroepiandrosterone and 17α-hydroxyprogesterone. The mean values in men are from 40 to 90 μg/24 hours, in women from 6 to 11 μg/24 hours (for review see 309a). The plasma testosterone level is also influenced by peripheral conversion. In men we find values of 5,000–7,000 pg/ml, in women 300–600 pg/ml. The androstenedione plasma levels in women are 1,300 to 2,000 pg/ml, 5α-dihydrotestosterone 150–220 pg/ml, androstenediol 680 pg/ml, dehydroepiandrostenedione 2,800–7,800 pg/ml, free testosterone 2–7.5 pg/ml, TeGB capacity 11–37 μg l (438). Because it is nowadays accepted that only free testosterone exerts a biological action, i.e. testosterone not bound to plasma proteins, the level or the index of free testosterone is assessed. It seems that they latter allow a better interpretation of results than total testosterone in plasma. In hirsute women they often give higher values than total testosterone.

Physiological variations include cyclic variations of androgen levels during the menstrual cycle and their diurnal variations. Usually raised testosterone values are found in urine, but less frequently in plasma, during the preovulation or luteal stage. The cyclic changes are even more obvious in the *androstenedione* levels where there are significant correlations between the androstenedione and 17β-oestradiol levels in peripheral as well as ovarian blood (22). From initial values the andro-stenedione values in the ovarian vein rise before ovulation to a double, and at the time of corpus luteum function to a 20fold level.

The plasma *dihydrotestosterone* level does not change in the course of the cycle. The daily rhythm of androgen secretion discussed in the chapter on the mutual relations of gonadotropins and steroids records a morning maximum and minimum in the evening. Episodic fluctuations of androgens do not depend on the feedback of gonadotropins. Their level does not depend on phases of sleep or on body position. Surgical stress raises the concentration of circulating androgens. During pregnancy testosterone values double or treble, with wide variations but without a definable trend.

Testosterone levels can be influenced by a number of pharmacological substances. According to some authors hCG causes a mild rise. Clomiphene citrate (100 mg/day for a period of 10 days) causes a significant increase of testosterone in men and women. ACTH stimulates, and dexamethasone reduces the plasma testosterone level. Gestagens (medroxyprogesterone and norethindrone) cause a decline of the level and at the same time reduce the amount of TEBG. Testosterone propionate and other esters cause a rise of testosterone values after 24 hours but reduce the concentration in the testes and thus inhibit spermatogenesis, which requires a considerable local concentration. 17α-methyltestosterone does not raise the testosterone level. Androgens reduce the TEBG and CBG level, on the other hand, oestrogens cause its rise and thus should also cause a rise of the testosterone level. Doses of oestrogen and progesterone which in contraception block ovulation reduce testosterone levels by restricting ovarian production.

Changes in the total plasma level, and in particular in that of free testosterone, are also found in some pathological conditions. They are raised in congenital adrenal hyperplasia, arrhenoblastoma, hyperthyroidism, in some cases of hirsutism and in the majority of polycystic ovary syndromes. In Addison's disease they are reduced. In testicular feminization the values correspond to normal levels in men.

## METHODS OF ANDROGEN ASSESSMENT

Biological methods: test on the cock's comb, test of the weight of seminal vesicles and weight of prostate in rats are used nowadays only for testing preparations and not for the assessment of androgens. Methods which determine *17-oxosteroids* in urine involve hydrolysis, extraction, washing of the extract and colorimetric estimation of Zimmerman's reaction with *m*-dinitrobenzene. 17-oxosteroid fractions are obtained moreover by separation on a thin layer. Colorimetry can be nowadays replaced by gas chromatography. *Testosterone* in urine was originally estimated by a colorimetric method, but nowadays gas chromatography or a protein binding method are used. For assessment of testosterone in plasma, methods of double isotope dilution were previously used and till recently gas chromatography (specific, sensitive to 1 ng, time consuming), while at present competitive protein binding methods and radioimmunological estimations predominate. Competitive protein binding methods use for binding of the hormone plasma from pregnant women or plasma with a raised TEBG after administration of oestrogens, and to a smaller extent cytosol from target organs. The separation of the free and bound fraction was

111

effected by means of florisil, or charcoal, but nowadays mainly by centrifuging. For the purification of steroids paper chromatography was used. The coefficient of variation is $10\%$, and the sensitivity 0.5–20 mg. A disadvantage was the rather large amount of plasma needed for estimation (10 ml) and the variable value of the macromolecule or cytosol. Radioimmunological methods after extraction and after chromatographic isolation use antisera of rabbits immunized with testosterone-3--carboxymethyloxime BSA, and for the separation of the free and bound fraction dextran-coated charcoal are used. The sensitivity is 10 pg, the coefficient of variation $8\%$, and sample size 0.1–0.5 ml plasma. The preparation of new antigens for immunization, where the steroid is bound by some carbon atom in the B or C ring to protein and the functional groups in rings A and D are left free, will lead to such an improvement of the specificity that the chromatographic purification of steroids will be eliminated which will shorten the method of estimation. In other methods chromatography is avoided by binding with TEBG. Radioimmunological methods are nowadays the most accurate, most sensitive, specific and rapid way of testosterone assessment. Alternative RIA methods are enzyme-linked immunoassays (ELISA) for testosterone which use peroxidase-testosterone or glucoamylase-testosterone complexes for the antigen-antibody reaction. The resulting complex is assessed spectrophotometrically. Enzyme methods are less sensitive but rapid and simple.

## ANTIANDROGENS

Antiandrogens are substances which block the biological action of androgens in target tissues. The mechanism and site of their action may differ: a) by interfering with the process of accumulation, this is the mechanism of action of gestanorone caproate (17-hexanoyl-oxy-19-norpregn-4-ene-3,20-dione); b) by inhibition of DHT formation, i.e. by substrate competition for $5\alpha$-reductase, this is the mechanism of action of progesterone and some of its derivatives such as megestrol acetate, medrogestone (6,17-dimethyl-pregna-4,6-diene-3,20-dion) and SC 14207 (17$\beta$-hydroxy-16,16-dimethyl-estr-4-ene-3-one); c) by inhibition of receptor binding and nuclear retention of DHT, which is the mechanism of action of the majority of new antiandrogens: cyproterone acetate (6-chloro-17-acetoxy-1,2$\alpha$--methylene-4,6-pregnadien-3,20-dione), BOMT (6$\alpha$-bromo-17$\beta$-hydroxy- 7$\alpha$--methyl-4-oxa-5$\alpha$-androstane-3-one), SKF 7690 (17$\alpha$-methyl-B-nortestosterone), R-2956 (17$\beta$-hydroxy-2$\alpha$,2$\beta$,17$\alpha$-trimethyl-8$\alpha$-estra-4,9,11-triene-3-one) and finally the nonsteroid androgen flutamide ($\alpha$-$\alpha$-$\alpha$-trifluoro-2-methyl-4'-nitro-$m$--propiono-toluidine). (For review see 360.)

Cyproterone acetate in animal experiments causes atrophy of the accessory sex glands and in humans inhibits in some cases the growth of prostate carcinoma; it delays the closure of the epiphyseal cartilages and inhibits the function of sebaceous glands and thus can be used for the treatment of acne and hirsutism; it inhibits libido and this is used in clinical practice for the treatment of hypersexuality and sexual deviations; further its action on inhibition of spermiogenesis is beginning to be used in male oral contraception. Because cyproterone acetate has also a strong progestational effect, it is also used in combination with oestrogens for female contraception, as it inhibits gonadotropin release after ovulation by a negative feedback mechanism. On the other hand, pure cyproterone has merely an anti-androgenic effect and does not inhibit ovulation or fertility. The effect of cypro-terone acetate on embryonic differentiation is intersexuality of male foetuses and the development of testicular feminization.

Flutamide is one of the pure antiandrogens which have no effect other than antiandrogenic, i.e. are not even antigonadotropic and are suitable for treatment of carcinoma of the prostate. The clinical importance of antiandrogens is only recently increasing and thus the clinical indications are not yet firmly established and research into further pure and possibly non-steroid antiandrogens is pro-ceeding.

# MECHANISM OF ACTION OF OVARIAN STEROIDS ON TARGET TISSUE

The common property of steroid hormones is their ability to combine with specific receptor sites in the cytoplasm of their target cells. Binding to intracellular recep-tors (see Table 6) is followed by rapid activation of individual cellular responses, among which undoubtedly the regulation of protein synthesis in the target tissue is the principal. Generally, the hormone–receptor complex is transferred to the nucleus, in an "activated" form, where it interacts with the chromatin at the genomic level — the selected segment of DNA is activated so that RNA encoding the information in those genes is synthesized. In addition to this primary mechanism of the action of ovarian steroids (for review see 78) other effects of hormones can be initiated by entirely different, extragenomic mechanisms (e.g. steroid hormones have been reported to effect changes in the cAMP concentration of cells in the target tissue).

## MECHANISM OF OESTROGEN ACTION

The cytoplasmic oestrogen receptor is a protein of the cytosol fraction probably made up from several sub-units one of which is oestrophil. Each macromolecule of the receptor protein binds one molecule of the hormone. By the bond of the oestrogen the cytoplasmic receptor is "activated", i.e. after transformation the hormone–receptor complex is translocated into the nucleus and is able to bind with nuclear acceptor sites. Their prime components are acidic non-histone proteins rather than histones. Interaction with the hormone–receptor complex leads to activation of gene transcription and enhanced RNA synthesis.

## MECHANISM OF PROGESTERONE ACTION

The cytoplasmic progesterone receptor is a dimeric protein molecule made up of two unequal sub-units A and B (molecular weight 110,000 and 117,000 resp.). Each macromolecule of the receptor protein binds two molecules of the hormone. By the bond with progesterone the "activated" cytoplasmic receptor migrates as the hormone–receptor complex to the nucleus; the sub-unit B is bound to chromatin at the site of the non-histone acceptor. It then dissociates and sub-unit A interacts with DNA and renders its transcription and the promotion of mRNA possible.

## MECHANISM OF ANDROGEN ACTION

In the majority of target tissues testosterone as the prohormone is converted by $5\alpha$-reductase into biologically more effective $5\alpha$-dihydrotestosterone (androstanolone). In others, however, testosterone acts directly and in others still it plays a part only after aromatization to oestradiol. So far it is not known whether there exists more than one type of cytoplasmic receptor for both androgens or a single type of receptor which forms functionally different complexes by interactions with both androgens. It is also possible that the cellular response differs as a result of different uptake, metabolism, non-receptor bond and excretion of different androgens (e.g. the rapid formation of DHT and its slow metabolism ensure that the predominant form of active androgen in the target cell is DHT and conversely, slow formation of DHT and its rapid metabolism or the lack of $5\alpha$-reductase are the reason why the main active androgen in the cell is testosterone). According to Ohno's hypothesis (376) the cytoplasmic androgen receptor has a double function. In its free form it acts as a repressor of translation of certain enzymes. The bond with testosterone and DHT respectively releases this translation block and the androgen–receptor complex migrates into the nucleus where, similar to other steroids, due to the acceptor molecule, it plays a specific role in the regulatory functions of gene activity.

# TISSUE LOCALIZATION, PHYSIOLOGICAL CHANGES AND REGULATION OF SEX STEROID RECEPTORS

So far it is not known whether cytoplasmic receptors for the same steroid in different target tissues are identical. It is certain that in one cell at the same time receptors for different steroids may be present. Probably, one cell may contain different receptors for a single steroid, e.g. oestradiol is also bound with the androgen receptor, although the affinity of this receptor for oestradiol is smaller than the affinity of the oestrogen receptor (this leads to the known anti-androgen effect of oestradiol). The oestrogen receptor, on the other hand, does not bind any androgens.

The presence of a high concentration of cytoplasmic steroid receptor proteins is considered a typical property of target tissues, determining their responsiveness to the hormones. Receptors are, however, present also in organs which are generally not classified as steroid target organs but which definitely respond to hormones (e.g. oestrogen receptors were also demonstrated in the liver, kidney and fibroblasts). Target organs of the sex steroids include also the ovary. There is evidence of the role of oestrogens, androgens and progesterone in the *intragonadal control of ovarian function*. Their action is probably direct via the classical receptor mechanism where a one-cell type within the ovary appears to be the target for the action of a steroid hormone produced within the same organ, as well as indirect action mediated by modulation of the ovarian action of gonadotropins.

The concentration of the cytoplasmic receptor protein for steroids in the cell of target tissue is not constant, it was shown to vary according to different physiological conditions and periods (e.g. the number of binding sites for oestrogens varies from 10,000 to 100,000 per cell in the immature rat uterus). Oestrogens, probably by interfering with protein synthesis, control the intracellular concentration of their own receptor protein. In oestrogen deficiency the molecules of the receptor protein degenerate or become inactivated. At the same time the nuclear acceptor activity declines. These findings explain e.g. the reduced reaction of the endometrium to exogenous oestrogens in long-lasting hypoestrogenic amenorrhoea. Moreover, oestrogen administration results in a multiple increase in the cellular content of the progesterone receptor. Conversely, the withdrawal of oestrogen is followed by a decline of the progesterone receptor level. Atrophic human endometrium appears to be completely devoid of specific progesterone-binding capacity. Therefore for the development of progesterone action on the endometrium its adequate oestrogenic stimulation is essential. In turn, progesterone induces a decrease of cytoplasmic oestrogen receptors. This anti-oestrogen effect in the endometrium explains the development of "progesterone withdrawal bleeding". It is also known that human proliferative endometrium contains significantly higher levels of cytoplasmic receptors for oestradiol than does secretory endometrium. It is a remarkable fact that progesterone decreases the concentration of its own cytoplasmic receptor. It may thus be assumed that there is an autolimitation of progesterone action. Moreover, progesterone inhibits dihydrotestosterone formation by competing for the 5α-reductase enzyme in testosterone target cells, particularly the skin.

The hormone–receptor complex has a finite half-life before its dissociation back into the individual components. If the stability of the bound complex is great, since the rate of dissociation is slow, a low circulating level of hormone can maintain a maximum rate of biological stimulation of target cells, as in the case of oestrogens. The progesterone–receptor complex, however, has a very short half-life. Thus the target cells require a high level of circulating hormone to achieve a maximum biological response. Similarly the half-life of binding of the hormone–receptor complex to nuclear chromatin (i.e. the retention of the hormone–receptor complex in the nucleus) determines the intensity of the sex steroid effect in terms of promotion of cellular growth and replication.

# PROSTAGLANDINS

## BIOSYNTHESIS AND METABOLISM OF PROSTAGLANDINS

Prostaglandins (PG) are biologically effective fatty acids with 20 C which contain a cyclopentane ring derived from the hypothetical molecule of prostanoic acid (Fig. 22). Their precursor are unsaturated fatty acids which, as glycerol and cholesterol esters, are building stones of phospholipids in the cellular membrane. After release by phospholipase e.g. arachidonic acid, dihomo-γ-linoleic acid etc. are transformed by microsomal synthetase to primary PG.

There are six so-called primary PG (PGE and PGF) which occur naturally and were thought not to be precursors of other PG.

The biological half-life of $^3$H-PG administered by the i.v. route is very short, 1–3 min. 50%, of radioactivity is excreted in the urine within 2 hours, and 90% within 5 hours.

The initial stage of PG metabolism is oxidation, catalyzed by PG-specific dehydrogenase. There exist considerable interspecific differences in the final products (in humans these are dicarboxylic acids) as well as in the routes of excretion.

PG synthesis is inhibited by indomethacin and acetylsalicylic acid whereby the efficiency of indomethacin is about 20–50 times greater.

Prostaglandins were given their name because of the original erroneous assumption that they are formed mainly in the prostate. In humans they are secreted mainly into the seminal vesicles and from there they penetrate into the ejaculate.

116

A similar synthetase system is present, however, also in various other tissues and organs, incl. the central nervous system. PG release is rather "biosynthesis *in situ*" than release of preformed stores. Obviously their action is as a rule at the site of their formation or in the close vicinity, in the same way as their metabolism.

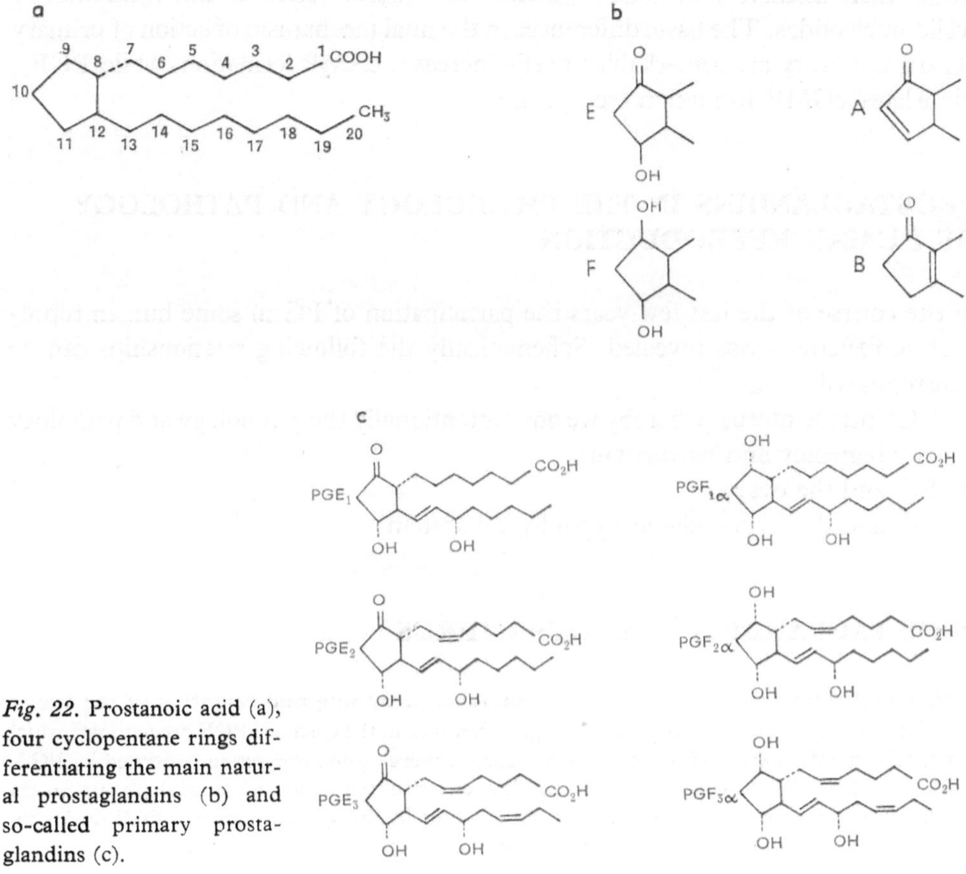

*Fig. 22.* Prostanoic acid (a), four cyclopentane rings differentiating the main natural prostaglandins (b) and so-called primary prostaglandins (c).

The highest PG concentration and the largest number of PG in humans is in the seminal plasma, where it varies within the range of μg/ml. The plasma concentration of PG in peripheral venous blood is lower by two orders. Plasma PGF do not display cyclic variations during the menstrual cycle, and the mean concentration ranges approximately between 40 and 100 pg/ml. The plasma level of PGE is statistically significantly higher in the luteal than in the follicular phase; the mean concentration ranges approximately from 135 to 330 pg/ml. No relationships were detected between the types of PG nor between the PG and plasma LH or FSH. There exists an extremely high interindividual variability of plasma PG (520).

## MECHANISM OF PROSTAGLANDIN ACTION

Ideas on the mechanism of action of PG are so far very incomplete and certainly simplified. It is beyond doubt that PG are closely related to another ubiquitous group, the cyclic nucleotides, cAMP and cGMP. They are assumed to modulate rather than mediate hormonal regulation of cellular function and formation of cyclic nucleotides. The basic differences in the final mechanism of action of primary PG on the ovary are remarkable: $PGE_2$ increases cAMP formation, while $PGF_{2\alpha}$ stimulates cGMP formation (see p. 69).

## PROSTAGLANDINS IN THE PHYSIOLOGY AND PATHOLOGY OF HUMAN REPRODUCTION

In the course of the last few years the participation of PG in some human reproductive functions was revealed. Schematically the following relationships can be differentiated:
A. PG and the uterus (whereby we omit intentionally the physiology and pathology of pregnancy and parturition),
B. PG and the ovary,
C. PG and the hypothalamo-hypophyseal system.

## PROSTAGLANDINS AND THE UTERUS

**Prostaglandins and migration of spermatozoa, trapping and retention of the ovum.**
PG of the ejaculate are absorbed from the vagina. Because in the ejaculate PGE predominate which inhibit the spontaneous motility of the non-pregnant uterus (the same action is exerted by PGA; PGB, and their 19-OH derivatives are only less effective) the action of seminal plasma on the musculature of the human non-pregnant uterus is mainly inhibitory. This effect of PGE during the ovulatory period is more marked; the sensitivity of the myometrium thus varies during the menstrual cycle and is influenced by hormones. It is assumed that PG of the ejaculate play a physiological part during coitus: inhibition of uterine contractions perhaps facilitates the migration of spermatozoa in the uterus.

During orgasm the uterus contracts, the contractions having an expulsive character. The inhibitory action of PG of the seminal plasma can be involved only during the subsequent stage of resolution.

The control of transport of sperm cells through the oviduct, trapping of the ovum from the open Graafian follicle and its migration through the tube, retention in the amply adrenergically innervated ampullo-isthmic portion (in women at the junction of the inner and middle third of the oviduct) and finally the passage through the uterotubal junction into the uterine cavity depends on a very complicated harmony of contractions of the fimbria and the utero-ovarian ligament, the musculature of the oviduct and in particular the movement of epithelial cilia, where PG play only a subsidiary part.

118

The migration of the ovum through the oviduct in humans takes about four days after ovulation (the ovum can be fertilized about 12–24 hours), the morula and initial blastula respectively cannot be implanted, and it develops in contact with the endometrium in the uterine cavity during the following 3–4 days before nidation of the blastocyst occurs. Hastening of the transport of the ovum with premature opening of the uterotubal junction or conversely its "locking" in the ampullo-isthmic part (where impregnation takes place) leads to destruction of the conceptus or to pathological implantation (for review see 193, 194, 273).

**Prostaglandins and the endometrium.** In menstrual blood the PG concentration is, as compared with peripheral blood, considerable (on average 56 ng/ml); PGF which stimulate the contraction of the smooth muscles of the non-pregnant uterus predominate (the pregnant uterus is about ten times more sensitive). The concentration of $PGF_{2a}$ is about ten times higher than that of $PGE_2$. The concentration of PG in menstrual blood is higher than in the endometrium. In the late secretory phase the concentration of endometrial PG is more than double, as compared with the early follicular phase; the $PGF_{2a}/PGE_2$ ratio increases also. The concentration of the two PG is even higher in the endometrium during menstruation; the formation of endometrial PG is obviously controlled by hormones. The higher concentration in menstrual blood is explained either by the formation of larger amounts of PG shortly before the onset of menstruation or during menstruation or by a reduction of their metabolism in the blood. The total PG "loss" during one menstruation is estimated to amount to 5 μg.

During menstruation PG are absorbed into the blood stream and this leads to an enhanced motility of the gastrointestinal musculature (with nausea, vomiting and diarrhoea), to a greater liability to develop asthmatic attacks, syncopes, diarrhoea in infants fed milk from menstruating mothers, etc. As to clinical aspects the direct action of endometrial PG on uterine muscle is more marked. Its sensitivity is influenced by ovarian hormones, thus e.g. during the premenstrual period the stimulating response to $PGF_{2a}$ is greater.

Excessive formation of endometrial PG (probably as a result of excessive stimulation of the uterine mucosa by progesterone) is considered one of the pathogenetic factors in primary dysmenorrhoea (see p. 162). Although the PG concentration in menstrual blood of these women does not differ significantly from that in eumenorrhoeic women, a change of the PG ratio in favour of PGF is described. The PGF concentration in fluid obtained by lavage of the uterine cavity during menstruation is in these women significantly higher than in normal women. The therapeutic use of inhibitors of PG synthesis which is a logical step is actually successful in some cases. The favourable effect of dilatation of the uterine cervix is explained by facilitated expulsion of the menstrual decidua which prevents increased absorption of PG.

## PROSTAGLANDINS AND THE OVARY

The participation of PG in the control of ovarian function was discussed in conjunction with the mechanism of gonadotropin action (see p. 66) and luteolysis (see p. 77) and the innervation of the ovary (see p. 25).


## PROSTAGLANDINS AND THE HYPOTHALAMO-HYPOPHYSEAL SYSTEM

The problem of PG participation in the control of gonadotropic hypophyseal activity is at present the subject of intensive studies. Results available so far were as a rule not obtained in primates but only in laboratory rodents and sheep.

Typical stimulatory (positive) feedback release of LH after a single injection of oestradiol in sheep can be blocked by inhibition of PG synthesis by indomethacin. It is possible that PG modulate the action of neurotransmitters in the CNS as regards the control of synthesis and secretion of GnRH; they participate thus in the nervous control of release of hypophyseal gonadotropins.

Conclusive evidence of the decisive participation of PG in the physical process of ovulation, i.e. in the rupture of the follicle, was also provided in monkeys. Indomethacin, when administered suitably, blocks ovulation in monkeys after HMG and hCG without inhibiting maturation of the follicle and the typical increase of progesterone and oestradiol secretion.


# UTERINE CYCLE

In its different tissues the uterus contains specific receptors of oestrogen and progesterone action. In the uterus therefore striking changes occur in conjunction with the menstrual cycle. We speak of target organs of steroid action and differentiate between an endometrial, myometrial and cervical cycle.


## ENDOMETRIAL CYCLE

The endometrium and its secretion plays an important part in the reproductive process. On the endometrial secretion depend: spermatozoa on their path to fertilization, the fertilized ovum before implantation, and finally the embryo depends on the vascular supply of the endometrium after implantation. The endometrium is characterized by cyclic growth and secretory changes in conjunction with oestrogen and progesterone levels. It is made up of a basal and functional

120

layer which undergoes changes. Vascularization is ensured by two types of arterioles which originate from short straight arteries in the myometrium. The aa. basales, which anastomose, supply the basal layer of the endometrium and do not undergo cyclic changes, the aa. spirales, which supply the functional layer, grow and disappear cyclically. The height of the endometrium changes from 0.5 mm at the onset to 3.5 mm at the peak of secretion. The chronological relationship of endometrial changes was confirmed in many ways: by observation of implants in the anterior chamber of the eye, by histology of timed biopsies, by correlation with other indicators of ovarian function. The endometrial cycle is divided into a proliferative (under the influence of oestrogens) and secretory phase (under the influence of progesterone and oestrogens); the menstrual phase precedes the proliferative phase and its onset is taken as the first day of the cycle.

**Proliferative phase.** It begins approximately on the fifth day of menstruation and is manifested by proliferation of glands, stroma, arteries and surface epithelium. The proliferating epithelium is at first thin, the surface epithelium cuboidal, and the glands sparse, straight and narrow, while the stroma is compact and made up of small fibroblasts. The proceeding proliferation is manifested by numerous mitoses of glandular and stromal cells, by pseudostratification of the nuclei of the glandular epithelium, release of the stroma and oedema. At the end of proliferation the glands are very elongated and begin to assume a spiral form.

**Secretory phase.** It begins on the 15th day of the cycle if we take the 14th day as that of ovulation. The first day of the secretory phase is morphologically inert and only on the 16th day, i.e. 36 hours after ovulation, in the majority of glandular cells basal vacuoles appear which press the nuclei towards the lumen. On the subsequent day the nuclei form a continuous rim near the lumen and the vacuoles beneath it a continuous light layer, the zona lucida. On the fourth or fifth day after ovulation the subnuclear vacuoles, i.e. the sites left after dissolved glycogen move round the nucleus into the apical end of the glandular cell and the nuclei drop to the base. On the sixth day the lumina of the glands increase due to the increasing glycogen secretion and they become more spiral. The apical ends of the cells are eroded as a result of apocrine secretion. During the first week after ovulation only slight changes occur in the stroma, while during the second week its imbibition and oedema in conjuction with the second peak of oestrogen secretion rises. The maximum oedema is on the 8th day after ovulation. On the 8th and 9th day after ovulation the glands have diverticula, a saw like crossection, the pseudodecidual (predecidual) reaction develops mainly round the spiral arteries in the stroma. The stromal oedema diminishes and the pseudodecidual reaction expands on the 10th–11th day after ovulation beneath the surface epithelium. Among the pseudodecidual cells small endometrial granular cells appear in similar numbers. From the 12th day after ovulation when the entire compact layer of the endometrium is differentiated into pseudodecidual and granular cells wrinkling and degenerative processes begin. First we can observe numerous capillaries with lacunar enlargement parallel with the surface, and after a decline of the hormonal levels the glands collapse. The glands still have a saw-like crossection which Moricard describes as "épines conjonctives". Regression of the Golgi apparatus of cells and complete loss of RNA occurs. On the 13th and 14th day after ovulation dissociated stromal and vacuolized granular cells appear.

The **menstrual phase** starts on the first day by blood imbibition into the surface layers of the stroma. The pseudodecidual character of dissociated cells can still be differentiated, as well as remnants of the collapsed glands, while haemorrhages and a leucolymphocytic infiltration develop. On the second day of menstruation there is advanced desquamation which is completed after 60

121

hours. Regeneration begins as early as 36 hours and is complete 140 hours after the onset of menstruation (368).

The changes described during the normal cycle serve in the diagnosis of phases of the cycle, and deviations from normal in the diagnosis of different disorders of the cycle.

*Histochemistry of the endometrium* reveals more subtle cyclic changes of some substances and enzymes. The latter include: glycogen, ascorbic acid, alkaline glycerol phosphatase, β-glucuronidase, nucleic acids and mucopolysaccharides. Glycogen is found as a typical substance of the secretory phase and thus proves the progesterone effect. Ascorbic acid is lacking in the proliferative phase but is an integral part of secretion. The alkaline phosphatase activity is greatest near ovulation, while acid phosphatase is lowest during this period and rises before menstruation. β-Glucuronidase has its peak of activity during the proliferative phase. DNA has its peak, consistent with proliferation and mitotic activity, during the second week of the cycle before ovulation. The content of acid mucopolysaccharides reaches its maximum during the proliferative phase in the stroma and in the glands during the secretory phase. Conversely the content of neutral mucopolysaccharides is highest in stroma in the secretory phase. Cyclic changes of enzymes and some substances render the functional diagnosis of the endometrium possible (Fig. 23). On the whole it may be said that in some the character of changes is similar to the course of plasma oestrogen levels (with the maximum during ovulation), in some it is similar to the progesterone level (with the maximum in the middle of the secretory phase).

The changes described correspond to an ideal cycle, there exists, however, a range of variations of histological and histochemical changes. The ideal cycle which lasts 28 days, with ovulation on the 14th day, was taken as the basis of methods for dating the endometrium for diagnostic purposes (372). Histological and histochemical changes during the cycle were described by many authors (for review see 95).

In recent years *ultrastructural cyclic changes* in the glandular epithelium and in the villous processes of the surface epithelium were described under physiological, as well as under experimental conditions after administration of different doses of steroid hormones. In investigations of the ultrastructure of glandular cells of the endometrium it is possible to classify subcellular changes during the menstrual cycle with regard to the functions in which it participates. Five main systems serve the following: protein synthesis and transport, secretion, synthesis of glycogen – of carbohydrates and their transport, proliferation, reproduction and genetic control, and finally digestion. Changes in the cycle have a periodic character (77).

Recently, in addition to the above changes, in the endometrium cyclic *quantitative biochemical changes* were also demonstrated. These changes are also associated with the action of oestrogens and progesterone. The water content of the endo-

122

metrium increases before ovulation, declining after ovulation, and rises again during the fourth week. Potassium and chlorides are highest during the proliferative phase. Cholesterol in stroma rises typically during the secretory phase, as does the glycine content. It seems that both substances are a preparation for the nutrition of the embryo. The rise of catecholamines assessed in the rat endometrium during oestrus is probably important for the implantation of the ovum. Different enzyme activities are raised, in particular during the proliferative phase. This is associated with active growth and the preparation of anabolic reactions for the secretory phase.

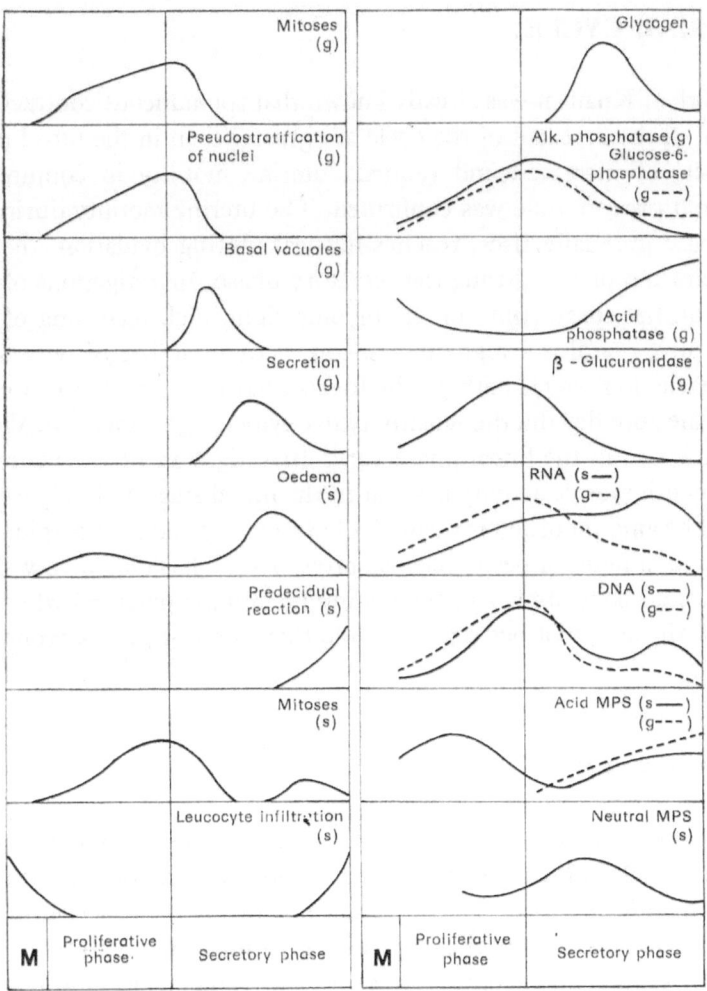

*Fig. 23.* Histological and histochemical changes on the endometrium in the course of the menstrual cycle (s — stroma, g — glands) (371).

123

Oxidative enzymes are involved: DPN-diaphorase and TPN-diaphorase, succinic dehydrogenase, enzymes of the intermediary carbohydrate metabolism (LDH, glucose-6-phosphate dehydrogenase, isocitric dehydrogenase and transdehydrogenase). In the secretory phase the total prostaglandin content (mainly $PGF_{2\alpha}$) is fourfold as compared with proliferation, although their concentration does not change in the two phases.

In the endometrium specific receptors for oestradiol and progesterone were also detected. Their number changes and is dependent on the cycle (see p. 113).

## MYOMETRIAL CYCLE

From the work of Knaus it was already known that spontaneous contractions of the myometrium in the first half of the cycle are greater than in the luteal phase. The dynamic cycle of increased and reduced uterine motility in conjunction with oestrogens and progesterone was confirmed. The uterine motility during the proliferative phase gradually rises, reaches its peak during ovulation, then declines and disappears completely during the secretory phase. Investigations of the action of oxytocin on the contractility of the myometrium, incl. recording of the intra-uterine pressure, revealed a high spontaneous activity and sensitivity to oxytocin during menstruation which both gradually receded from the 6th to the 20th day and only on the 26th day did the sensitivity to oxytocin again increase. Views on the type of contraction in the luteal phase vary. Investigation of the neuroendocrine control of smooth muscle activity is so far in the initial stage and only isolated facts are known. The amount of actomyosin, ATPase activity and macroergic phosphates depend on the amount of oestrogens, as progesterone has only a very slight additional effect. The same applies to the resting membrane potential which increases as a result of the action of oestrogens, while the action of progesterone is controversial.

## CERVICAL CYCLE

The cervix, similar to other parts of the uterus, undergoes periodic changes during the menstrual cycle which are important in preparation for reproduction. The changes are manifested in the (1) secretion of mucus, (2) function of the endocervical mucosa, (3) activity of the cervical and isthmic musculature.

**Cervical mucus.** The biophysical as well as biochemical properties of the cervical mucus change. The complex of biophysical properties is sometimes described as the cervical factor; it depends on the influence of ovarian hormones and is of importance for the penetration of sperm into the uterus and it is of diagnostic value as the basis for some ovulation tests (Fig. 24). The amount of mucus increases in the course of the cycle and during ovulation reaches a level of 200–700 mg//24 hours, while at other times the maximum is 60 mg/24 hours. The transparency is greatest at the time of ovulation and so is the index of refraction (1.33 compared with 0.01 at other periods), while its light dispersal is lowest. The index of consistence, which also depends on oestrogens, is lowest during ovulation. As far as

*Fig. 24.* Properties of cervical mucus throughout the menstrual cycle (n = 10, mean values ± SE) (339).

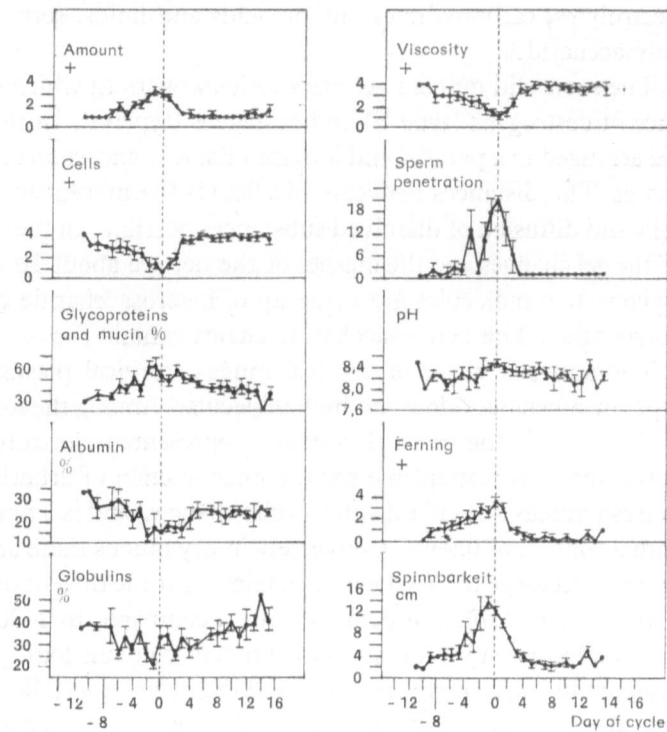

rheological properties are concerned, the viscosity of cervical mucus is lowest at the time of ovulation. This is associated with its high "Spinnbarkeit", 10–15 cm, as compared with 1–2 cm during the remainder of the cycle. Arborization (crystallization) of cervical mucus (ferning), i.e. the presence of crystallized fern-like patterns in the dried mucus, is positive, while in other stages only cellular structures or slight crystallization are apparent. The water content is 96–98%, and during the other phases 92–94%. The dry weight of mucus is, however, lowest during ovulation. The pH is usually alkaline, the values in the course of the cycle vary (6.5–8) and during ovulation they reach the maximum. The number of leucocytes in mucus is at its lowest during ovulation, while the rate of penetration of sperm cells is highest, 1.5–2.0 mm min, being only 0.1–0.5 mm/min during the remaining days of the cycle.

Cervical mucus is according to biochemical and ultracentrifugation studies made up of two main components. The first component is a semisolid mucoid gel consisting of glycoprotein macromolecules which are condensed into micelles, their pattern depending on the endocrine condition of the organism, while the second component is cervical plasma which contains low-molecular substances such as electrolytes, carbohydrates, amino acids and lipids, serum proteins, peptides and polysaccharides.

The semisolid mucoid gel has a reticular pattern which changes under the influence of oestrogens (type E) and gestagens (type G). In the mid-cycle the micelles are arranged in a parallel and longitudinal way and contain 100–1,000 glycoprotein chains. The distances between micelles (1–10 $\mu$m) render the movement of sperm cells and diffusion of dissolved substances possible. In the luteal phase the structure of the gel changes and the meshes of the net are about $10 \times$ smaller (0.3 $\mu$m). The glycoprotein molecules are made up of heterosaccharide chains attached to a long polypeptide. The heterosaccharide chains contain fucose and sialic acid.

The aqueous phase of cervical mucus (cervical plasma) is constituted of two types of substances: low and high molecular. Among the former the most important — NaCl — is the most abundantly represented electrolyte and is together with potassium ions responsible for the phenomenon of arborization. Sodium chloride in fresh mucus does not display cyclic changes, and is a practically isotonic solution with a content of 0.93°$_0$. Conversely in dry mucus there are marked cyclic changes in the percentage of NaCl with a maximum at the time of ovulation; the salt content at the time of ovulation being 40–70°$_0$, compared to 2–20% at other times. As to high-molecular substances, cervical mucus contains locally produced IgA and IgG proteins and lactoferrin, enzymes and their activators (alkaline phosphatase, aminopeptidase, esterase, amylase, muramidase or lysozyme, carbonic anhydrase). Their concentration has mostly a cyclic course with the minimum during the preovulation peak of oestrogens. As to serum proteins the following were detected: albumin, prealbumin, $\gamma$-globulin, orosomucoid, $\alpha_1$-antitrypsin, haptaglobin, transferrin which also have their minimum during the preovulatory period and reach their peak during the luteal phase (460). Biochemical findings thus explain the basis of many biophysical properties of mucus, they indicate the dependence on oestrogens and progesterone during the menstrual cycle and assist the reproductive process.

**Changes of the endocervical mucosa** also depend on ovarian hormones. Cyclic factors are, however, much less marked than in the endometrium; the changes are not morphological, and only changes in the intensity and nature of secretion are found. The cervical canal and branched endocervical glands are lined with a single-layer cylindrical epithelium which produces mucin. Among the secretory cells of the endocervix there is also a small number of ciliated cells. The cyclic changes are manifested by an increase in the height of secretory cells and accumulation of mucus in the apical end with the maximum at the time of the oestrogen peak. At that time the secretory cells contain the largest amount of glycogen, glycoprotein and mucopolysaccharides. After ovulation the secretion drains into the glands. Investigations of the ultrastructure confirmed that the peak of secretion of the glands corresponds to the time of ovulation.

**Changes in the cervical and isthmic musculature.** By means of manometric HSG hypotonia of the cervix was demonstrated in the first phase of the cycle and hypertonia during the secretory phase, while the body of the uterus showed the reverse. In the connective tissue of the cervix there is considerable deposition of $^{35}$S, which, however, declines during the early luteal phase but soon rises again to the preovulatory level. It serves for the synthesis of chondroitin sulphate in the collagen fibres of the cervix and participates in the formation of interfibrillar bridges which combine the fibrils into bundles. Chondroitin sulphate is probably responsible for the constriction of the cervix during proliferation and secretion and its reduced synthesis is associated with atonia of the cervix at the time of ovulation. Hypotonia and opening of the cervix resp. are used for diagnostic purposes in an ovulation test.

Ovarian hormones also induce cyclic changes in other organs, such as the vulva, oviduct, mammary gland, urinary bladder and stomach. Cytological changes can be also observed in the oral and nasal mucosa, while there are changes of the basal temperature, metabolic and haematological changes as well as changes in the psychosexual sphere.


# VAGINAL CYCLE

The vaginal epithelium is histologically defined as non-cornifying multilayer squamous epithelium which consists of five cell layers. Changes of the vaginal epithelium are mostly evaluated from desquamated cells, i.e. from exfoliative cytology. The three cytological types of cells (according to the nomenclature of the IAC) correspond therefore with the histological definition of layers. From the stratum corneum originate superficial cells, from the stratum spinosum superficiale intermediary cells, and from the stratum spinosum profundum parabasal cells.

The vaginal epithelium is very sensitive to stimulation by sex hormones and they alter their height (number of cells) and density (number of rows in different layers), in particular under the influence of oestrogens, but also to a certain extent under the influence of progesterone and androgens. The number of exfoliated cells in cytology depends on the maturity of the uppermost layers which are shed. Due to the work of Papanicolau and Traut who in 1943 made use of morphological and staining properties, the typical pictures in different periods of life in women and cyclic changes during the menstrual cycle were characterized. Later, using quantitative criteria (percentage of cells) and other typical signs, indices were elaborated which can to a certain extent quantify the effect of hormones. The limitation is obviously the receptivity of peripheral tissue and the impossibility of response above a certain limit.

The pictures in vaginal cytology during the menstrual cycle are as follows:

In the early proliferative phase there are mainly cyanophil large and small intermediary cells. Occasionally there are also leucocytes. In the medium proliferative phase large intermediary and

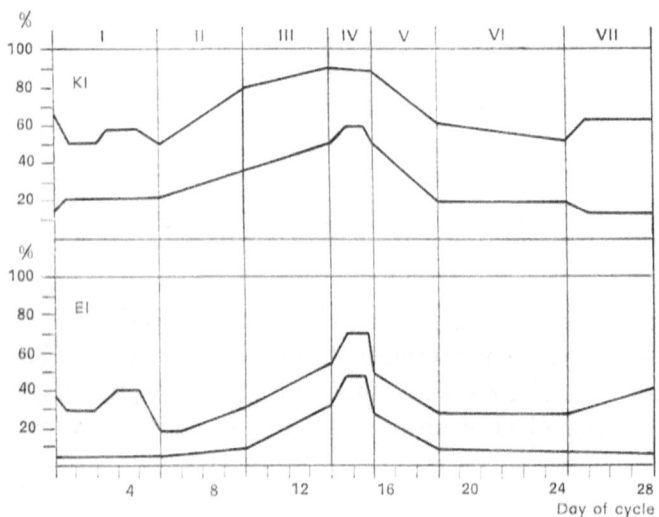

Fig. 25. Variations of the karyopyknotic (KI) and eosinophil (EI) index during the cycle (I — menstrual phase, II — early follicular phase, III — mid-follicular phase, IV — ovulatory phase, V — early luteal phase, VI — mid-luteal phase, VII — late luteal phase, n = 68, max.min. limits) (414a).

polyedric superficial cells increase in number and size; these are partly eosinophil, and partly cyanophil. The nuclei are partly pyknotic. In the late proliferative phase the large superficial cells with margins, which are occasionally folded, spread. They are eosinophil and have pyknotic nuclei. There are no leucocytes. In the postovulation phase massive shedding of cells begins with the formation of typical conglomerates where the cells are superimposed on each other. Superficial eosinophil cells with a pyknotic nucleus are found only rarely. As a rule we find intermediary cells with a vesicular nucleus and cyanophil cytoplasm with folded margins. The medium and late secretory phase is characterized by a predominance of typical clusters of intermediary cells with a vesicular nucleus, cyanophil plasma and folded margins. There are numerous leucocytes and Döderlein's lactobacilli. The cytological appearance of menstruation is characterized by numerous red blood cells, individual large and small intermediary cells with vesicular nuclei and medium numbers of leucocytes (see Fig. 24).

For quantitative description in particular the following indices are used: (1) karyopyknotic index — the ratio of all mature cells with a pyknotic nucleus to mature cells with an enlarged nucleus (Fig. 25); (2) eosinophil index — ratio of eosinophil to cyanophil cells; (3) maturation index — ratio of parabasal to intermediary and superficial cells, from which the so-called cytograms were developed.

For work with computers the so-called maturation value is used, i.e. figures suggested for different cell types. After revision the following values are used: superficial = 1, intermediary = 0.5, parabasal = 0.0.

Oestrogens cause proliferation of the vaginal epithelium up to the upper cell layer; in the cytogram they are manifested by the presence of only flat superficial cells with eosinophil plasma and a pyknotic nucleus. Androgens cause considerable proliferation but only to the intermediary cell layer and we thus record small and medium intermediary cells with cyanophil staining and large nuclei with a delicate chromatin net in the cytological picture. The picture has a faded appearance, but is clean without cell debris and leucocytes. Gestagens also cause proliferation up to the intermediary layer only, in the cytological picture we find in particular intermediary cells with cyanophil plasma which form clusters and have folded margins.

Cyclic changes occur also in the pH of the vaginal medium (pH 3–6). During menstruation it varies round neutral values, during major bleeding it reaches even alkaline values. In the proliferative phase the pH is acid (5.7), during ovulation the values rise to neutral, on the second day after ovulation they decline again to acid and only 1–2 days before menstruation they rise again to neutral levels. Changes in the pH are caused by lactic acid, which is formed by Lactobacillus acidophilus by the breakdown of glycogen. The latter is contained in intermediary cells of the vaginal epithelium in particular, while in superficial cells its content is small and the PAS positivity there is due to mucopolysaccharides. The amount of lactobacillus and vaginal glycogen displays similar cyclic changes as the pH.

# Climacteric and Menopause

The *climacteric* in women is the transitory period between the reproductive age and the onset of the senium. It is the period between 45 and 60 years of age. The menopause is the short period of the last bleeding still controlled by ovarian function which as a rule occurs in the first third of the climacteric and divides it into the pre- and postmenopausal period. The *premenopause* lasts about 4–5 years, gradually the ovulatory function and progesterone production recedes and frequent irregular bleeding occurs till menstruation ceases. The *postmenopausal period* is characterized by gradual extinction of ovarian function. The senium starts after the age of 60 by regression of anabolic steroid production in the adrenals. This classification was adopted by the International Federation of Gynaecologists FIGO (for review see 252). Previously the term climacteric and menopause were frequently used as synonyms.

The age at menopause is not the same for all women and depends on many factors. The period between 40 and 53 years is considered normal, and in the majority of women it is between 45 and 50 years. Cessation of menstruation before the age of 40 and its persistence after the age of 55 is considered abnormal and calls for examination. In the course of time the onset of the menopause has shifted to more advanced age. In Finland it shifted within a period of 60 years by two years, to the age of 49 years. The corresponding figure for Switzerland is 49.2 (Basle 51.4 years) with a shift of 4 years. In Germany the average is 49.3 years or 51.4 years, and in the USA the majority of workers quote the age of 48 years. The average of the menopause in Holland is 51.4 years. Partial data for the ČSSR give the mean age of menopause as 51.2 years (by the method of status quo) and 48.8 years resp. (weighted arithmetic mean). The decisive factors seem to be climatic and social conditions. In low altitudes and in rural areas the menopause occurs later than in the mountains and towns. In married women and multiparae the onset of the menopause is later. Smoking results in earlier onset of the menopause. Perhaps constitution also plays a part, as thin women have the menopause earlier than obese women. The relationship to the age of onset of menarche has not been elucidated so far: according to some authors late menarche is associated with a shorter period of maturity and an earlier onset of the menopause, while older data maintain that in women with late menarche the onset of the menopause is later; but according to other authors this relationship does not exist. Nevertheless the declining age of menarche and the later onset of the menopause lead to a prolongation of the fertile period in women. The shift of the menopause to more advanced age is, however, not as great as the shift of the mean life span of women. In civilized countries in the second half of the last century the mean age of the menopause coincided with the average life span of women, while today, when the mean life span is 75 years, women live for another 20 years after the fertile period, i.e. after the menopause. This state of affairs which developed gradually has a great social and medical impact as regards economic activity of women during the postmenopausal period, which represents a third of their life, and for clinical medicine which is increasingly more frequently faced with the necessity of treating some pathological conditions of the postmenopausal period or to prevent their development.

## ENDOCRINE REGULATORY MECHANISM DURING THE CLIMACTERIC

At present the view is adopted that the cause of the onset of the climacteric is the gradual exhaustion of ovarian follicles which leads to secondary hypergonadotropic insufficiency of the ovary. The generative and endocrine function of the ovary depends on the presence of follicles which are able to respond to gonadotropins. The number of these follicles is exhausted, in particular due to atresia of follicles, in the course of life. Only a small proportion of follicles (about 450) are used for ovulation. Gradual loss of follicular structures which produce hormones leads to a decline of oestrogen as well as progesterone production. The first clinical changes associated with this are described as manifestations of ovarian dysfunction. Disorders of the corpus luteum function frequently occur, and anovulatory cycles or dysfunctional bleeding due to varying oestrogen levels produced by non-ovulating and persisting tertiary follicles are seen. Only when oestrogen production declines below the threshold of endometrial bleeding, does the menopause set in. In the clinical manifestations of receding endocrine ovarian function there are, however, wide variations — from disorders of the cycle with excessive or insufficient bleeding as regards frequency and quantity, up to a sudden symptom-free onset of amenorrhoea.

# OESTROGENS IN THE POSTMENOPAUSE

From mean normal values during the cycle $30.1 \pm 6.7$ µg/24 hours total urinary oestrogens decline in the premenopause (41–45 years) to 22, one year before the menopause to 20, one year after the menopause to 13.2 and during the subsequent 5 years to 9.5 µg/24 hours (252). According to other data two years after the menopause the mean value of total urinary oestrogens is 8.3 (2.7–36.3 µg/24 hours) and the most abundant fraction is oestriol, 6 µg, followed by oestrone, 1.5 µg, oestradiol 0.8 µg/24 hours (414).

Recent methods of saturation analysis have confirmed reduced values of plasma oestrone and oestradiol in the postmenopausal period. The plasma oestrone level after the menopause varies round 30 pg/ml (25–40 pg/ml), the oestradiol level round 12 pg/ml (6–15 pg/ml) according to data reported by different authors. Oestradiol declines much more than oestrone. While oestradiol plasma levels decline according to some authors, as compared with normal levels by 80–90%, those of oestrone decline only by 50–70%.

The mean values of metabolic clearance assessed for oestradiol are $580 \pm 30$ l/d//sq.m, for oestrone 1,050 $\pm$ 70 l/d/sq.m. Both represent a diminution by cca 25%, compared with metabolic clearance during the period of normal cycles.

# OESTROGEN SOURCES IN WOMEN AFTER THE MENOPAUSE

From the above oestrogen levels it is obvious that in women after the menopause only a small amount of oestrogens is secreted, which may originate from three sources: extrafollicular structures of the ovary, adrenal cortex, and extraglandular formation from precursors in the periphery.

Despite the proceeding degeneration of functional structures of the ovary it was shown that stromal cells increase in number, sometimes even in the form of nodular or diffuse hyperplasia. Therefore the problem whether the ovary after the menopause is able to produce oestrogens or their precursors was investigated, in particular by histochemical methods. According to more recent data 61% of ovaries after the menopause have numerous active stromal cells, and 71% have active hilar cells. In these instances it was possible to detect by qualitative as well as quantitative methods a double activity of glycolytic enzymes and a tenfold increase of glucose-6-phosphate dehydrogenase, and in the ultramicroscopic picture an abundant endoplasmatic reticulum and numerous tubulovesical mitochondria as typical criteria of steroid biosynthesis in these active cells were observed. The activity of the ovaries was in 90% consistent with signs of oestrogenic stimulation of the endometrium, while an atrophic endometrium corresponded with inactivity (59). Incubation trials with labelled steroids confirm that the ovaries after the menopause are able, even without the follicular apparatus, to synthesize steroids from precursors, mainly androgens, but also from progesterone and acetate. Hilar cells which are found in 71% of the ovaries after the menopause also secrete androgens. Stromal and hilar cells thus secrete androgens and are at least partly responsible for the virilization frequently observed in women after the menopause. However, these ovaries do not secrete oestrogens primarily, or if so only rarely, as was confirmed by investigations *in vitro*, when in most instances biosynthesis terminated at $C_{19}$-steroids (androstenedione, testosterone, dehydroepiandro-sterone, androstenediol).

The second assumed source of oestrogen formation after the menopause is the adrenal cortex. By adrenalectomy the oestrogen production after castration can be reduced (65), while by means of ACTH it can be raised. In experiments *in vitro* after incubation of labelled testosterone with the microsomal fraction of human adrenal cortex 17$\beta$-oestradiol was detected. The 0.05 percentage of aromatization indicates, however, that direct oestrogen secretion from the adrenal cortex is minimal.

*Extraglandular conversion of androgens in peripheral tissues* is the main if not only source of oestrogen produced during the menopause. The main product is oestrone, which is formed by aromatization of androstenedione. Quantitative data on this formation of oestrogens are given in several publications (for review see 184, 316). From the percentage of aromatization (1.3%) in castrated, adrenalectomized and normal control females and from the plasma production of androstenedione (3.4 mg/24 hours) the peripheral conversion of oestrone was calculated as cca 44 $\mu$g/24 hours. If after injection of oestrone about 22% urinary oestrogens are excreted, then the amount of oestrogens obtained by conversion is about 10 $\mu$g/ /24 hours. The oestrogen values assessed in urine are consistent with these cal-culated values from androstenedione conversion. This provides evidence that the direct oestrogen secretion from the ovaries as well as adrenals is minimal.

The problem next investigated by ablation of organs was to what extent the ovaries and adrenals contribute towards the level of oestrogens or their precursors produced during the menopause. Older work which did not yet take into account the peripheral conversion of precursors, only provided evidence that the fractions of urinary oestrogens do not differ between women after the normal menopause and women after bilateral ovariectomy (65). Plasma values of oestrogens in more recent work also revealed no differences between the normal menopause and surgical or radiation castration. Castration after the menopause did not alter their level which suggests that these oestrogens do not originate from the postmeno-pausal ovary (65). However, some authors report reduced oestrogen values after castration during the menopause. It seems, however, that a decline occurred only in those cases where the preoperative values of oestrogens in the menopause were higher than those usually reported. More recent work has provided evidence that, as regards oestrogen precursors, testosterone and androstenedione decline in the plasma of premenopausal women to about one half, however, in the postmenopause testosterone declines only slightly, while postmenopausal androstenedione displays similar values as after castration. As a result of castration testosterone declines markedly, while androstenedione does not. Moreover when women after the menopause were operated a 15 times higher testosterone concentration and 5 times higher androstenedione concentration were found in the ovarian vein than in the periphery (249). After stimulation of the adrenal cortex after the menopause by means of ACTH in the adrenal vein, as compared with the periphery, the oestrone, androstenedione and dehydroepiandrosterone level increased, while the oestradiol and testosterone concentrations did not increase. It is therefore assumed that the majority of precursors of postmenopausal oestrogens originate from the adrenals in the form of androstenedione. The contribution of the ovary is smaller and is represented in particular by testosterone. The most recent publication which investigated the level of all sex steroids after the menopause under basal conditions after stimulation with ACTH, suppression with dexamethasone and after stimulation with hCG concludes that the ovary after the menopause contributes directly or indirectly by about 50% to the testosterone level and by 30% to the androstenedione plasma level (523).

The problem where the peripheral conversion of adrenal androstenedione to oestrone occurs has not been resolved unequivocally. According to some authors it takes place in the liver, according to others in adipose tissue or the brain, where in particular the hypothalamus and amygdala have the largest amount of aromatizing enzymes. Testosterone is converted there mainly to oestradiol and androstenedione to oestrone. Bone, hair follicles and fibroblasts in cultures also possess the capacity for conversion of androstenedione. Adipose tissue seems to be an important extragonadal source of oestrogens. For saturation of aromatizing enzymes a low concentration of androgens is sufficient.

Surprising results were obtained in investigations of *steroid excretion in ovariectomized and adrenalectomized women*. Contrary to assumptions that oestrogens after elimination of these two sources will disappear, in 16 of 49 thus investigated patients a mean urinary excretion of 3 $\mu$g/24 hours of oestrogens was found with an upper range of 59 $\mu$g/24 hours. The assumed sources were: dietary intake, substitution of cortisone or finally ectopic tissue of the adrenal cortex. Because in the investigated patients in addition to urinary oestrogens dehydroepiandrosterone, androsterone, etiocholanolone and pregnandiol were also found in small amounts, the presence of ectopic adrenal tissue seemed most probable. The frequent occurrence of this ectopic tissue was previously demonstrated by histological examination during necropsy in the area of the a. coeliaca and during gynaecological operations in the broad ligament.

# GONADOTROPINS IN THE CLIMACTERIC

Urinary excretion of gonadotropins or their plasma levels are markedly raised after the menopause. The increase is due to disinhibition of the tonic centre in the hypothalamus as a result of the reduced plasma oestrogen level. TGA rises according to older data from maximum mean values during the cycle (4 IU/24 hours) to 18.5 IU before the menopause, and the maximum of 25 IU, i.e. values six times higher are reached during the five-year-period after the menopause. Only after the age of 65 do the TGA values decline and become stabilized during old age at a level which is always higher than during the cycle but lower than after the menopause (252). FSH and LH values assessed in urine by RIA are on average $64.4 \pm 36.3$ IU/ 24 hours for FSH, and $52.8 - 35.5$ IU/24 hours for LH.

More recently radioimmunological methods revealed average values of 51 to 150 mIU/ml and average LH values between 47 and 96 mIU/ml in the postmenopausal plasma according to various papers. Plasma thus contains more FSH than LH, and as compared with values during the cycle, FSH increases more ($4-10 \times$) than LH ($3-7 \times$). The LH/FSH ratio in women after the menopause is 0.7 and is markedly lower than the ratio of their tonic secretion during the normal cycle when it is about 1.0, and during cyclic secretion at the time of ovulation when it is 2.0.

The change from the normal cycle to the premenopause was analyzed in detail for the whole spectrum of hormones. First the midcycle peak of LH declined during ovulatory cycles with progesterone while the basal FSH and LH levels were normal, then the cycles were anovulatory and first the basal FSH level rose, while LH and oestradiol were normal and only later both the FSH and LH level rose and the oestradiol level declined. Divergent changes of FSH and LH during the premenopause assumed an altered feedback mechanism at the adenohypophyseal level or participation of another regulating factor on FSH from the ovary of the inhibin type (253, 430, 475).

The variations of FSH as well as LH are considerable, towards the senium these variations diminish, however. Women after surgical castration very rapidly reach postmenopausal values. FSH rises to double the level as early as the subsequent day, but LH only after 6 days.

During the first three years after castration the FSH and LH levels remain higher than during the same period after a normal menopause and only later are the levels in both groups similar.

By radiation castration the first maximum is reached after about 3 months, then the gonadotropin levels rise slowly for several years, as in the postmenopausal period.

There exists no correlation between the gonadotropin level and climacteric symptoms (for review see 4), although older work maintained that it existed.

Changes of the gonadotropin levels caused by disinhibition of the hypothalamus are reversible after therapeutic administration of oestrogens and subsequent administration of gestagens respectively. The effect depends on the dose and the combination. During the postmenopause more oestrogens are needed to reduce gonadotropins than in eugonadal women (for review see 89). The hypothalamus is thus able to react during the menopause not only to a negative but also to a positive feedback even into old age; then with the decline of the basal level of circulating gonadotropins this ability declines.

The prolactin level in women after the menopause does not differ from the level before the menopause, according to others it declines and correlates with the oestradiol level.

## HYPOTHALAMIC NEUROHORMONES IN THE CLIMATERIC

It was reported by several authors that the LH-RH plasma level in women after the menopause is elevated. By some methods it was possible to detect LH-RH in particular in the peripheral plasma of women after the menopause, while during the cycle, except for the midcycle peak, it was below the borderline of detectability. The episodic character of the increased LH-RH output is probably the reason for the more marked variations of plasma gonadotropins after the menopause. The LH and FSH response in plasma after administration of LH-RH in women after the menopause is significantly elevated which is at variance with other data on a reduced sensitivity to gonadotropins.

## OTHER STEROIDS IN THE CLIMACTERIC

**Pregnandiol** excretion and the plasma **progesterone** level are very low after the menopause and correspond to values recorded in men. By chromatographic methods on average 0.63 (0.28–0.86) mg/24 hours pregnandiol are detected, and by gas chromatography even less — 0.17 (0.04–0.28) mg/24 hours. The progesterone values are, depending on the methods used, on average from 0.09–0.34 ng/ml, and those of $17\alpha$-hydroxyprogesterone are $0.24 \pm 0.1$ ng/ml. It is generally assumed that they are produced in the adrenal cortex.

The urinary **17-oxosteroid** excretion in women has a typical course which is not influenced by the menopause. It rises from zero values at birth and reaches the maximum at the age of about 25 years. During the period between 20 and 40 years the values vary from 7 to 12 mg/24 hours. From the age of 25 the excretion declines for a period of 10 years, from 35 to 55 incl. the climacteric; it does not change further and after the age of 60 it declines rapidly. 17-Hydroxycorticoids behave in a similar way. Both steroids thus do not change in conjunction with the climacteric.

The excretion of **androgens** and their sources were discussed in the chapter on the peripheral conversion to oestrogens. The urinary testosterone values in women after the menopause are 6.9 μg/24 hours, the plasma values $262 \pm 47$ pg/ml, and the plasma 5α-dihydrotestosterone values $168 \pm 27$ pg/ml. They do not differ from values recorded during the cycle. Dehydroepiandrosterone values, $1,800 \pm 930$ pg/ml, and androstenedione, $530 \pm 120$ to $920 \pm 38$ pg/ml, are half as compared with those during the cycle.

## ANATOMICAL CHANGES IN THE ORGANISM DURING THE CLIMACTERIC

The greatest changes occur in the **ovary.** The ovary atrophies first of all organs. The size of the ovary diminishes even after the age of 30 years and declines to half after the menopause.

The size is subject to great individual variations with different types of gradual atrophy and a different degree of reduction of structures, in particular in the cortex. In case of polycystic changes the ovary even enlarges temporarily. The follicular apparatus diminishes throughout life by a process of atresia, as has been mentioned before. The speed and extent of this degeneration depends on the phases of life and exogenous differences. With the onset of the menopause follicles with the ability to ovulate cease to be formed. Primary follicles are found in deeper layers even after the menopause and disappear without the formation of corpora fibrosa and hyalinization. The cortex of the ovary wrinkles, while the stroma is gradually replaced by fibrous connective tissue. This process is final and occurs as a rule in the senium. During the period between 40 and 60 years on the other hand, hyperplasia of the stroma in the shape of irregular groups of luteinized cells and hyperplasia of hilar cells, both of which bear signs of hormonal activity, is very frequent. Finally atrophy also affects the blood circulation by general degenerative changes in the vascular walls: fibrosis with hyaline transformation, muscular hyperplasia and calcification of the media. The cause of atrophic changes in the ovary is not known but it is obviously genetically programmed. Changes in the other genital organs are the consequence of declining levels of oestrogen whereby their proliferating action is eliminated.

The **oviducts** atrophy, become thinner, the walls lose their folds and the lumen becomes narrowed.

In the uterus the **myometrium** atrophies. The uterine wall becomes thinner, and loses fluid, while hyaline degeneration develops along with atherosclerosis. The musculature diminishes and is replaced by fibrous tissue.

During the premenopause the **endometrium** frequently displays signs of hyperproliferation or glandular cystic hyperplasia, but later it is usually atrophic.

The **uterine cervix** undergoes atrophic changes. The cervical glands atrophy, showing duct stenosis and formation of retention cysts, while the cervical canal becomes narrow and frequently obliterated.

The **vagina** loses its elastic tissue, and becomes reduced in size, in particular at the junction of the upper and middle third, while the mucosa becomes thin and smooth because the columnae rugarum disappear. The result is a short narrow vagina, easily vulnerable and irritable. The cytological maturation index (parabasal, intermediary and superficial cells) changes markedly. While during ovulation it is 0-40-60, shortly after the menopause it is 7–70–15, and three decades after the menopause the final ratio is 25-65-10. The acid vaginal pH changes after the menopause to neutral or alkaline, and Döderlein's lactobacillus disappears. The clinical consequence of these changes is a reduced resistance of the vaginal wall and frequent incidence of colpitis.

The flabbiness of the pelvic connective tissue, musculature of the pelvic base and ligaments leads to a more frequent incidence of prolapse of the genitalia and incontinence. Atrophic changes of the vulva are manifested by a reduced vascularization and reduction of subcutaneous fat; the clinical consequence of atrophic changes is frequent dyspareunia, sometimes kraurosis, pruritus and leukoplakia.

During the premenopause — perhaps due to an oestro-progestational disbalance — frequently irregularities develop in the proliferation of alveoli and ducts of the **breast** — mastopathia cystica fibrosa. After the menopause the glandular portion, skin and subcutaneous layer of the breast atrophy.

In addition to changes of the genital organs we also find important **extragenital changes** caused by oestrogen deficiency. The skin becomes more pigmented, the tonus declines, the skin on the neck becomes less elastic, and adipose tissue is often deposited in the lower half of the body with a typical localization. As to the locomotor system the muscular apparatus becomes hypotrophic, while in the skeleton so-called climacteric osteoarthropathies develop with a typical lumboileosacral localization, and osteoporosis is frequent. The secretory and motor activity of the digestive tract is frequently reduced and this leads to constipation.

# MAIN CLINICAL SYMPTOMS OF THE CLIMACTERIC

Climacteric complaints are those symptoms which are conditioned by a change of ovarian activity and which occur shortly before and after the menopause. They include disorders of bleeding, neurovegetative and psychic disorders. Trophic and somatic disorders resp. have already been discussed previously. If the climacteric complaints are potentiated or persist for very long, we speak of the climacteric syndrome as a pathological entity requiring treatment.

## CLIMACTERIC DYSFUNCTIONAL UTERINE BLEEDING

Climacteric dysfunctional bleeding caused by a disorder of ovarian function is most frequent before the menopause. In the differential diagnosis other causes must be considered: carcinoma of the uterus, endometrial polyps, submucosal myoma, incorrect hormonal therapy, abortion, a hormonally active ovarian tumour, and coagulopathies. Most important is the recognition of carcinoma which before the menopause is the cause of haemorrhage in 25%, but six months after the menopause in 50% of the cases. Dysfunctional bleeding is of the ovulatory and anovulatory type. In the former case it is due to corpus luteum insufficiency and irregular shedding of the endometrium which is manifested frequently as an irregular cycle or oligomenorrhoea and menorrhagia. The second anovulatory type is more frequent. It involves a simple anovulatory cycle, glandular cystic hyperplasia and haemorrhage from an atrophic endometrium.

## VEGETATIVE DISORDERS

Vegetative disorders are rare in the premenopause but their number increases during the postmenopausal period. About 75% of all women have these symptoms with different intensity and duration and in cca 10–15% they are so severe that they make them seek medical assistance. We do not know the cause of this wide variation. The development of these disorders is explained by the fact that deficiency of oestrogens which have a stabilizing effect on the vegetative nervous system, stimulates the parasympathetic nerve and this upsets the vegetative balance. Impairment of hypothalamic functions affects the cardiovascular system and all organs innervated by the autonomic nervous system. The organism tries to re-establish the equilibrium by hypersympathicotonic flushes. The relationship between oestrogens and catecholamines acts perhaps pathogenically. Thus hot flushes into the head develop as the most constant symptom of climacteric complaints. It is associated with reddening of the skin, of the chest, neck and a feeling of heat. Flushes are usually associated with perspiration and a rise in blood pressure. The frequency of hot flushes varies greatly. Often they occur 2–3 times a day, sometimes every hour, for several weeks. They may also occur during the night and repeatedly interrupt sleep being associated with unpleasant intensive perspiration. After months, sometimes years, the hot flushes eventually recede spontaneously or after treatment. Their relationship to oestrogen deficiency is not quite clear. In some women they do not occur at all, as in women with hypoestrogenic secondary amenorrhoea. Direct assessment of oestrogens in women after castration and check-up data after oestrogen treatment revealed that there is no correlation between the clinical climacteric symptoms and the total level of oestrogens, oestradiol, oestrone and the maturation index. No significant difference was found between oestrogen levels in women with and without symptoms (498). Other vegetative symptoms are palpitations, tinnitus, vertigo, migraine, meteorism, constipation, and diarrhoea or spasm of the biliary pathways.

## PSYCHIC DISORDERS

Psychic disorders in the climacteric must be differentiated from vegetative disturbances although they are associated because psychic disorders are not directly connected with reduced oestrogen levels. They are encountered frequently even during the premenopause when there is still an adequate oestrogen level. They are rather more due to exogenous factors which lead to the manifestation and deterioration of constitutional mental lability. They are manifested by insomnia, emotional lability, irritability, and depressions or even involutional psychosis. Exogenous factors which have an effect include interpersonal relations established even during childhood, but above all whole-life experience, the relationship with the partner and work. An adverse effect is exerted also by fear of a decline of sexual activity and ageing after the termination of ovarian function. It depends thus on the type of personality and the environment whether the woman becomes adapted easily to the newly created situation or not.

# ORGANIC DISEASES IN THE CLIMACTERIC

During the period of the climacteric some organic diseases occur the connection of which with the decline of the oestrogen level is accepted by some and denied by others. These diseases include: a higher incidence of cardiovascular disorders, in particular coronary sclerosis, osteoporosis and some forms of oesteoarthropaties.

## CORONARY DISEASE

The participation of the climacteric and oestrogen deficiency resp. in the development of coronary disease and atherosclerosis resp. has been investigated for some time, the conclusions are, however, frequently controversial. This applies to numerous experimental investigations, pathological studies, epidemiological retrospective and prospective surveys, clinical research of risk factors of coronary disease and preventive long-term oestrogen treatment, etc. Conclusions from pathological investigations revealed that comparison of ovariectomized women and controls does not provide a uniform answer to the question whether oestrogen deficiency affects the development and severity of coronary sclerosis. Statistical investigations confirmed that women develop coronary sclerosis 10 to 20 years later than men. Apparently this is due to some protective factor. For some time it was assumed that this protective action is exerted by oestrogens and that their inadequate secretion during the climacteric leads to a balanced ratio of this disease in men and women. The low ratio 1:19 in favour of women rises after the age of 50 years to 1:5 and after 70 years it is 1:1. Recently it was demonstrated that due to the higher mortality of men the rise of this disease in women depends above all on age. As to prospective investigations one of the most extensive was the so-called Framingham study which followed up more than 5,000 subjects for a period of 8 years. The sex-conditioned protective mechanism was confirmed. It was not conclusively

141

demonstrated, however, that it was due to oestrogens. This mechanism can, however, be overshadowed any time by a so-called risk factor. Some risk factors were assumed to be associated with oestrogen deficiency after the menopause: the lipid and carbohydrate metabolism and hypertension. Oestrogens influence serum lipids and lipoproteins. Some decline, others rise. Cholesterol and low density lipoproteins ($S_f$ 0–20) decline, triglycerides, phosphatides, free fatty acids and high density lipoproteins rise. Individual lipoproteins, however, may become mutually converted in plasma by the action of lipoprotein lipase. Furthermore oestrogens influence the carbohydrate metabolism, i.e. cause a reduced glucose tolerance. Preventive administration of oestrogens in the menopause did not provide satisfactory evidence that oestrogens were the cause of the protective effect. The mutual complex of relations between the menopause, atherosclerosis and oestrogens has not been resolved and further directed investigations are needed. Previous favourable conclusions were replaced by scepsis (for review see 269, 477). Oestrogens are not used for the treatment of atherosclerosis.


## OSTEOPOROSIS

The second serious problem which is associated by some with oestrogen deficiency after the menopause is postmenopausal osteoporosis. It may be defined as a reduction of bony tissue which qualitatively does not differ from the normal. Clinically it is associated with considerable lower back pain and back pain in general. It leads to enhanced kyphosis and thus reduction of height, and frequently spontaneous fractures also occur. On X-ray decalcification is apparent when it reaches about 30–50%. Osteoporosis is a biological process associated with ageing of the organism in both sexes. It was, however, shown that in 85% of patients it affects in particular women between 50 and 70 years of age. After the menopause about 25% of women suffer from marked osteroporosis. Premature osteoporosis is known to occur in hypofunction of the ovaries, after premature castration and in dysgenesis of the gonads. Consistent with this, investigations involving the long-term administration of oestrogens revealed regression of the disease in women after the menopause and prevention of the development of osteoporosis when oestrogens were administered preventively. Views on the pathogenesis of osteoporosis have, however, changed. According to the original idea oestrogen deficiency leads to a reduced osteoblast activity and androgen deficiency to reduced proteosynthesis, both thus inhibiting the building of bone matrix during its normal breakdown. Experimentally this view was refuted and another hypothesis was submitted according to which osteoporosis develops as a result of enhanced breakdown of calcium, while the building up of bone is normal. Oestrogens promote the calcium and phosphorus fixation in tissues and reduce calcium and hydroxyproline excretion in urine. There are, however, more factors which act in the pathogenesis of postmenopausal osteoporosis. Today we hold the view that it is not a specific disease produced by the onset of the menopause but the result of multifactorial action where the lack of oestrogens is only one of the pathogenetic agents (for review see 264). Partial factors are: diet with an inadequate protein and calcium intake, advanced age, female sex, and reduced physical activity. Not even the mechanism of oestrogen deficiency is clear. Oestrogen deficiency apparently sensitizes bony tissue to parathormone and reduces the somatotropin level which is actually lower in osteoporosis. Somatotropin is known to stimulate the formation of new bone. According to contemporary opinion it is thus necessary to provide comprehensive treatment of osteoporosis comprising physical therapy, a high-calcium diet (about 1 g/day), administered for a prolonged period, and long-term administration of oestrogens (for review asee 163).

# CLIMACTERIC SYNDROME AND ITS TREATMENT

As has already been mentioned, in about 25% of women the climacteric takes a completely symptom-free course. In the majority of women the symptoms are mild: only 10–15% of women have intensive complaints, described frequently as the climacteric syndrome and considered a disease. The climacteric is a physiological process and the borderline between physiology and pathology is only arbitrary. The extreme view based on physiology, does not treat climacteric symptoms at all, or restrict treatment only to sedatives, assuming that the symptoms are temporary, usually last six months to two years and then recede. The second extreme view, based on the assumed effect of oestrogen deficiency on the whole organism, recommends permanent oestrogen treatment regardless of the complaints, as prevention of climacteric symptoms, atherosclerosis, osteoporosis, arthropathies, etc. The intermediary way seems to be the view that treatment is indicated when the patient has complaints which make her seek medical advice.

The variety of objective and subjective complaints is great. Because it is essential to treat the main complaint, different approaches must be used. There are several possibilities: psychotherapy, treatment with sedatives and psychopharmaceutical preparations, vegetative treatment, physical and hormonal treatment.

## NON-HORMONAL TREATMENT

**Psychotherapy** is suitable in those patients where mental symptoms predominate which potentiate the climacteric complaints. This treatment involves an interview with the patient at which the doctor expresses understanding for the complaints and explains to her the causes of climacteric symptoms and explains that these are physiological phenomena which will recede. At the same time it is, however, necessary to detect the development of independent psychic disturbances precipitated by the climacteric which require psychiatric consultation or treatment. **Physical therapy** such as alternate hot and cold baths or showers, remedial exercise and swimming may also produce a very favourable effect as supplementary treatment. **Sedative and vegetative treatment** is very widespread and effective. Phenobarbital is used either alone or combined with radobeline, extractum valerianae, humuli lupuli etc. Sometimes parasympathomimetic and sympatholytic preparations are recommended of the reserpine and hydergine type, nowadays the α-sympatholytic preparation clonidin is recommended. When the psychic symptoms are very marked (emotional lability, irritation, tendency to develop depressions, anxiety neuroses), psychopharmaceutical preparations are administered in particular antidepressants such as meprobamate, derivatives of benzodiazepine, dibenzepine and tricyclic antidepressants. Among neuroleptic preparations chlorpromazine and chlorprothixene are suitable.

## HORMONAL TREATMENT

According to many authors the only causal treatment of climacteric complaints is to eliminate oestrogen deficiency by exogenous administration. The selection of preparations depends on the condition of the woman.

During the **premenopause** small doses of oestriol are administered, 1–2 tablets à 250 μg daily; this preparation does not interfere with the rhythm of the menstrual cycle and does not cause bleeding as it does not act on the endometrium. If during this period climacteric complaints are associated with irregular disorders of the cycle, oestroprogestational therapy may be used from the 5th to the 25th day of the cycle in the form of contraceptive preparations or similar mixtures. Oestroprogestational therapy may also be sequential. Some authors also recommend combined treatment with oestrogens and gestagens during the first two years after the menopause when oestrogens alone frequently cause bleeding.

**After the menopause** for treatment of the climacteric syndrome in general, oestrogens without gestagens are used. Treatment may be of three types: (1) oestrogens alone, (2) a combination of oestrogens and androgens, (3) a combination of oestrogens with sedatives and tranquillizers. Oral treatment predominates but depot preparations make it possible to restrict administration to one injection per 4–6 weeks. As far as the period of administration is concerned, short-term therapy is used, as long as the symptoms persist. More recently long-term therapy with oestrogens has been discussed for prevention of atrophic changes and organic diseases more or less associated with the postmenopause.

The oestrogens used for treatment are of different types. It must be said that they eliminate subjective complaints, and metabolic and atrophic changes of target organs most satisfactorily but at the same time they may cause side-effects, in particular bleeding. Those which have a central and peripheral action, a positive psychotropic effect and slight endometriotropic action are tolerated best. These comprise conjugated oestrogens, oestrone sulphate and oestriol. A considerable central effect and bleeding are produced by ethinyl oestradiol, mestranol, and stilboestrol. The proliferative action of different oestrogens is given in Table 11.

*Table 11* Daily substitution doses, endometrial threshold and proliferation doses (per 14 days) of commonly used oral oestrogens in climacteric women (290, 291)

|  | Daily substitution doses (mg) | Threshold dose (mg/14 days) | Full proliferation dose (mg/14 days) |
|---|---|---|---|
| Ethinyloestradiol | 0.02 –0.04 | 0.2 | 2 |
| Mestranol | 0.03 –0.05 | 0.3 | 3 |
| Quinoestrol | 0.025–0.05 | 0.3 | 2–4 |
| Diethyl stilboestrol | 0.5 –2.0 | 2.5 | 20–30 |
| Dienoestrol diacetate | 0.5 –4.0 | 3–5 | 40–60 |
| Oestradiol valerianate | 1.0 –2.0 | 6–10 | 60–80 |
| Conjugated oestrogens | 0.6 –1.25 | 5–12 | 60–80 |
| Oestriol | 1.0 –5.0 | 20 | 120–150*) |
| Oestriol succinate | 2.0 –6.0 |  |  |

*) Irregular, atypical proliferation, mostly in the basal layer.

An ideal, completely effective preparation without side-effect does not exist. The preparations are effective in 60 to 90%, bleeding develops in 2–10% of the patients.

(1) **Pure oestrogens**

A. *Classical*:
   a) oestradiol derivatives:
      oestradiol diproprionate (inj. 5 mg)
      oestradiol benzoate, oestradiol valerate (dragees à 2 mg, inj. à 5 mg to 10 mg)
      ethinyl oestradiol (perlingual tablets 0.05 mg)
      ethinyl oestradiol methyl ether (mestranol) (tablets à 0.05–0.15 mg)
   b) oestrone derivatives:
      oestrone piperazine, oestrone sulphate (tablets à 3 mg)
   c) oestriol (tablets à 250 μg)

B. *Synthetic non-steroid*:
   diethylstilboestrol (tablets à 0.5 mg) and its diproprionate
   chlortrianisen (capsules à 12 mg)
   hexoestrol

C. *Natural non-steroid*: zeranol (resorcylic acid lactone) (dragees à 75 mg)

D. *Conjugated equine oestrogens* (dragees à 1.25 mg)

(2) **Combination of oestrogens and androgens**

oestradiol benzoate 5 mg + testosterone isobutyrate 50 mg in inj. for a period of 4 weeks

oestradiol valerate 4 mg + dehydroepiandrosterone enanthate 200 g in injections for a 4-week period

ethinyl oestradiol 0.005 mg + methyl testosterone 2.5 mg per tablet (3 tablets per day)

(3) **Combination of oestrogens with sedatives and psychopharmaceutical preparations**

Combinations are used such as: oestrone and phenobarbital and theobromine, oestradiol benzoate with theobromine, caffeine, nitroglycerin, phenolphthalein, conjugated oestrogens with diazepam etc.


## SHORT-TERM TREATMENT

During short-term oestrogen treatment the preparation is administered as a rule by the oral route for 21–25 days per month with a one-week break. After several months treatment the doses are reduced and frequently supplemented by sedatives. Less frequently depot injections are used where the effect persists for 4–6 weeks. The uneven effect associated with this pattern of administration is subject to criticism. According to some authors this protracts the necessary therapeutic period.

A combination of oestrogens and androgens is also very effective and is used as a rule at a ratio of 1:20. Androgens have a psychotropic and anabolic effect with favourable action on libido. They also have, however, side-effects such as virilization, coarsening of the voice and acne. Therefore these combinations are restricted to patients where the favourable effects of androgens must be used. Recently for these combinations androgens are used which in the administered doses do not exert a virilizing effect. The latter include e.g. dehydroepiandrosterone enanthate.

The usually prescribed daily doses are 1–2 mg oestradiol valerate, 1.25 mg conjugated oestrogens (with a gradual reduction to 0.6 and 0.3 mg), 0.5–2.0 mg oestriol, 0.025–0.1 mg ethinyl oestradiol, 0.1–0.5 mg stilboestrol, 1.5 mg oestrone sulphate, 12 mg chlortrianisene.

The results of so-called short-term oestrogen and androgen therapy were evaluated in many comparative studies on the effect of different preparations (see Table 12) and in double blind trials with placebo. Double blind crossover experiments confirmed that the placebo effect is negligible (290), as compared with previous data which reported it in 30%. Comparative studies revealed clearly that oestrogens act most effectively on vegetative symptoms and less on psychic

146

symptoms. From this also ensues the expedience of combination with psychopharmaceutical preparations, mainly to suppress the remaining failures, especially when rudimentary mental symptoms have developed already before the climacteric and become more potentiated during the postmenopause. Contraindications for oestrogen treatment are disorders of the liver, thromboembolic disease, mastopathies, carcinoma of the mammary gland and genital organs.

## LONG-TERM SUBSTITUTION THERAPY

Contemporary ideas on oestrogen treatment during the climacteric are still based on the fact that it is a physiological process. Only women with climacteric complaints should be treated with minimum doses and for the period necessary to overcome the difficulties of adaptation to the new condition. In the fifties, however, recommendations were submitted for prophylactic long-term oestrogen treatment of all women after the menopause. Advocates of the prophylactic administration recommended above all conjugated oestrogens or a combination of oestrogens followed by gestagens, also expressed recently in the form of so-called graded sequential therapy. The reason for this treatment were: (1) to suppress climacteric syndromes, (2) to delay the development of somatic atrophic changes, (3) to delay atherosclerosis, (4) to prevent osteoporosis and its sequelae. The objection was that about one quarter of all women do not suffer from climacteric symptoms and that so far the effect of oestrogens on atherosclerosis has not been clearly demonstrated and in osteoporosis it is one of several factors, and finally that the prolonged administration of oestrogens may have a carcinogenic action.

The problem of the carcinogenic action of oestrogens has not been resolved conclusively

Table 12  Comparative effect of some medicaments on climacteric syndrome

| Preparation | Dose mg | Route of administration | Number of cases | Total effect (%) | Excellent | Good | Small | No change |
|---|---|---|---|---|---|---|---|---|
| Conjugated oestrogens | 1.25/d/20d | p.o. | 41 | 35 (85%) | 16 | 19 | 5 | 1 |
| Oestradiol benzoate + testosterone isobutyrate | 5.0 + 50.0 monthly | i.m. | 23 | 21 (91%) | 16 | 5 | 1 | 1 |
| Oestriol | 1.0/d/30d | p.o. | 41 | 22 (54%) | 13 | 9 | 4 | 15 |
| Chlorotrianisene | 12.0/d/30d | p.o. | 15 | 4 (27%) | 1 | 3 | 6 | 5 |
| Piperazine oestrone sulphate | 1.5/d/21d | p.o. | 53 | 45 (85%) | 18 | 27 | 8 | 0 |
| Oestradiol valerianate + dehydroepiandrosterone enanthate | 4.0 + 200.0 monthly | i.m. | 43 | 37 (86%) | 26 | 11 | 4 | 2 |

and is still the subject of controversial discussion. The probability that a woman after the menopause not using oestrogens will develop carcinoma of the endometrium is 1:100,000 per year, in women using oestrogens 4–8:100,000 per year (for review see 303, 477).

The problem whether to administer oestrogens on a long-term basis or not is even more serious because in some parts of the world the administration of oestrogens is becoming very widespread and according to a survey in the USA 15% of women after the menopause use oestrogens. Further studies are needed. The contemporary state of knowledge does not permit recommending or refuting this therapy. So far it seems advisable to use it only in some groups of women, e.g. after early castration, in osteoporosis, during treatment of some atrophic changes, etc.

# Symptomatic Classification of Disorders of the Menstrual Cycle

## NORMAL MENSTRUAL CYCLE

### DURATION OF MENSTRUAL CYCLE

Normal implies in clinical language the range of values which are found in healthy "normal" subjects. As far as parameters of the menstrual cycle are concerned, it is a statistical problem. To assess the range of normal values is not difficult, if their relative frequency displays a normal distribution the rate of which is illustrated by a Gaussian curve. It seems that this type is also characteristic for the length of the menstrual cycle of women (Fig. 26). According to generally accepted views 95 % of all possible values are within the defined normal range; this range is the interval of $\pm 1.96$ of the standard deviation $(s)$ from the arithmetic mean (within the interval of $\pm 2.0$ are 95.45% of all elements in the group).

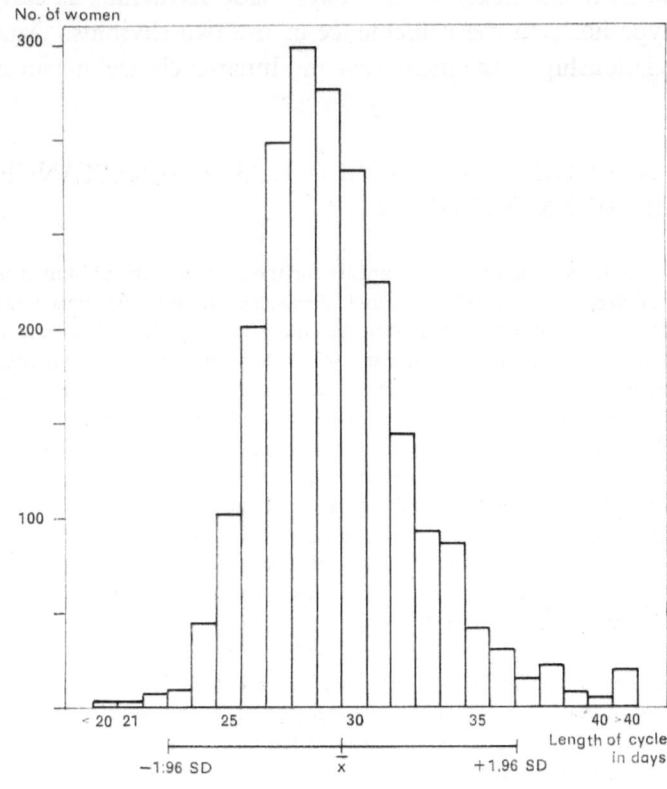

*Fig. 26.* Mean length of menstrual cycle (in 10 and more cycles) of 2,316 women aged 15–44 years (83).

The last investigation concerned with the length and variability of the human menstrual cycle (83) assessed from 30,655 recorded cycles in 2,316 women has shown that the average length from individual averages (evaluated in the course of 10 or more cycles) is 29.4 days ($s = 3.27$). According to the above definition of normality we may thus assume that any case will with a probability of 0.95 be within the interval of 23.0–35.8 ($\doteq 36$) days, i.e. beyond this interval with a probability of 0.05. An older survey of 13,500 cycles in 973 women comprising data recorded in the literature from 1889–1937 assessed in a similar way the length of the cycle as 29.3 days ($s = 3.24$).

This value of the average length of the menstrual cycle of women applies to all age groups. More detailed investigations revealed that the average length of the cycle depends on the woman's age. Between the age of 15–44 it shortens (from 30.5 days in women aged 15–19 years to 28.1 days at the age of 40–44 years) and its variability diminishes (the value of $s$ declines from 8.95 to a minimum of 6.61 in the group of 35–39-year-old women) (83).

The periodic uterine bleeding occurs roughly once per month, hence the term **menses, menstruation.** The similarity of the above average length of the menstrual cycle and the mean duration of the synodic lunar month (i.e. from one new moon to the next) — 29.5 days made Arrhenius as early as in 1898 express the hypothesis on the coincidence of the two rhythms. Data in the literature on the relationship of the menstrual and lunar cycle are, however, quite controversial.


## PHYLOGENY AND BIOLOGICAL IMPORTANCE OF MENSTRUATION

In phylogeny menstruation appears for the first time in subhuman primates, in monkeys from the Old World — *Catarrhini* – incl. *Pongidae*. In some flat-nosed monkeys from the New World (*Platyrrhini*) the observed cyclic bleeding from the genitals corresponds to the ovulatory haemorrhage which is due to a decline of the level of circulating oestrogen as e.g. in the bitch. These monkeys are on a lower level of evolution and in their endometrium spiral arterioles are lacking.

Menstruation is apparently associated with haemochorial placentation. The development of the placenta during phylogeny follows the path of a progressive erosion of maternal tissue by the trophoblast till finally in primates the syncitiotrophoblast is surrounded by maternal blood. The trophoblast becomes gradually thinner during phylogeny and eventually becomes the haemomonochorial placenta of primates. Concomitantly there is the development towards the endocrine specialization and autonomy of the placenta (e.g. the formation of chorial gonadotropin in primates which can be detected in the peripheral blood of women already eight days after ovulation, i.e. shortly after implantation).

According to an interesting hypothesis (56) menstruation is not merely a passive manifestation of the destruction of the endometrium prepared for nidation but an active process, a periodic preparation for haemochorial contact during implantation of the developing zygote. This is manifested in monkeys by implantation bleeding (so-called placental sign). In women it is manifested clinically only rarely as "menstruation" during pregnancy because it coincides with the time of the latter. [Slight bleeding is found in 3.75% of cases, with the same intensity as menstruation in about 1.0% of all pregnancies (272).] Much more frequently it is possible to detect erythrocytes in the vaginal smear and chemically detectable haemoglobin is always present in the vaginal secretion. The haemochorial contact is an impulse for the plasmodial reconstruction on the trophoplast, and for the differentiation of the plasmoditrophoblast. Blood surrounding the nidated zygote must not clot, as its circulation ensures the haemotrophic nutrition of the embryo and the immunological inhibition of the invasion of the cytotrophoblast into maternal tissue. Menstruation is considered (56) a preparation for this implantation haemorrhage, a certain culmination of the cycle.

## MECHANISM OF MENSTRUAL BLEEDING

The mechanism of menstrual bleeding, i.e. the mechanism of the haemorrhagic necrosis of the superficial portion of the endometrium, is still the subject of discussion.

During the last week of the menstrual cycle the endometrium (observed after transplantation into the anterior chamber of the eye of the monkey *Macaca mulatta*) becomes thinner and the spiral arterioles display rhythmical vasoconstriction lasting 1–2 minutes followed by a period of vasodilatation. Subsequently vasoconstriction extends over several hours. After the arrest of circulation and ischaemic necrosis haemorrhages develop which eventually affect the entire surface of the endometrium in an islet-like fashion till desquamation of the entire superficial layer occurs.

According to contemporary ideas (380), concurrently with the premenstrual decline of circulating ovarian steroids rapid absorption of the endometrial oedema occurs with retraction of the stroma and compression of the spiral arterioles. The alteration of the endothelium leads to haemorrhage *per diapedesim* with release of prostaglandins (in particular $F_{2\alpha}$). Prostaglandins stimulate the contractility of the uterus and cause vasoconstriction of the basal arteries. Thus almost complete ischaemic necrosis of the surface portion of the endometrium occurs. The subsequent vasodilatation, partly reflex in nature, and partly caused by histamine released in the necrotic tissue, leads to extravasation of blood between the basal and superficial spongious layer of the endometrium and its desquamation. However, the chief event of menstruation is regression rather than cell death. The vast majority of cells of the spongiosa remain viable and undergo remodelling to participate in the new cycle. The only cells which die or become detached are from the compact and upper spongious layers (146).

The participation of prostaglandins in the mechanism of menstruation is suggested by the rise in their concentration (in particular $F_{2\alpha}$) in the endometrium during the secretory stage of the menstrual cycle. In menstrual blood the concentration of prostaglandin $F_{2\alpha}$ is at least ten times higher which is explained by increased premenstrual synthesis and or inhibition of its metabolism (see p. 119).

**The trigger impulse of menstrual bleeding** is the breakdown of the level of circulating ovarian steroids, under physiological conditions of the ovulatory cycle, in particular a decline of the progesterone concentration; in an anovulatory cycle pseudomenstruation is induced by a decline in the level of circulating oestrogens. Ovarian steroids, however, are obviously not the only factor which decides on the onset of endometrial bleeding. During so-called irregular shedding (p. 301) uterine bleeding starts already during the period of hormonal activity of the corpus luteum; the raised basal temperature of the luteal phase declines only after several days bleeding. Conversely cases of amenorrhoea with ovulation are described with a biphasic basal temperature curve and secretory transformation of the endometrium. This stimulates the hypothesis on the participation of a vasomotor factor, perhaps of central nervous origin (225). A dissociation of the two factors, the hormonal and assumed neurogenic factor, which under physiological conditions are closely associated, might explain some pathological conditions. Clinical experience indicates that uterine bleeding may occur during any phase of the menstrual cycle even from an atrophic endometrium due to emotional disturbance ("Schreckblutung") (497). It seems that the assumed neurogenic factor is able by itself to induce haemorrhage from the uterine mucosa. Innervation of the endometrium in subhuman primates and humans is not restricted to the basal layer. It also penetrates into the functional zone, non-myelinated fibres form a reticulum round arterioles and small glands and terminate freely in the stroma. The extent of innervation in the functional zone probably also determines the depth of the shed endometrial portion. It is assumed that the innervation of the endometrium mediates not only vasomotor action but also trophic impulses (for review see 96). The relationship with the receptiveness of the endometrium to hormonal stimulation still remains open. Contrary to methods impregnating neurofibrils, the results of histochemical studies which demonstrate monoaminergic nerve fibres in the human uterine mucosa, are equivocal and controversial.


## CLOTTING DEFECT OF MENSTRUAL BLOOD

Menstrual blood does not clot under normal conditions — which is an advantage — as it must drain from the uterine cavity. On the other hand, e.g. after curettage, blood in the uterus clots, similarly as after conization. In uterine menstrual blood fibrinogen is lacking. From necrotic endometrial tissue an activator of plasminogen is released (present also in cervical mucus) which transforms practically all plasminogen in blood into effective plasmin and fibrinolysis occurs. "Clots" in menstrual blood are not true clots but merely red cell aggregates which are formed in the vagina. The concentration of endometrial plasminogen activators in the secretory phase is higher than in the proliferative phase and reaches its maximum on the first day of menstruation. In some cases of menorrhagia their concentration is significantly raised; perhaps they play there some pathogenetic role (for review see 444).

**Vicarious menstruation.** Vicarious menstruation is cyclic extragenital bleeding which occurs at the time of uterine menstrual bleeding either concomitantly or more rarely instead of it. Most frequently bleeding from the nose or other mucosal membranes is encountered, as the latter display certain cyclic changes in relation to the menstrual cycle. It is bleeding due to decrease of the level of circulating ovarian hormones (in particular oestrogens), or more frequently due to an existing lesion. A separate group is formed by vicarious menstruation based on extragenital endometriosis.

## DURATION OF MENSTRUATION

The duration of menstruation assessed on 5,307 women was on average 5 days ($s = 1.41$) (325). According to the above defined criterion of normality thus 95% of all possible values are within the range of 2.3 ($\doteq 2.0$) and 7.7 ($\doteq 8$) days. An older investigation which recorded 823 menstruations found an average duration of 4.6 days ($s = 1.07$).

## MAGNITUDE OF BLOOD LOSS DURING MENSTRUATION

Data in the literature display a great variability as regards blood losses during menstruation, however, individual values are remarkably constant. A blood loss not exceeding 1 ml/kg body weight (i.e. cca 1% of the total amount of circulating blood) which does not lead to a change in the haemoglobin concentration and plasma iron after menstruation is considered normal. In a group of almost 500 women after elimination of those with a Hb concentration below 12 g/100 ml and plasma iron below 80 µg/100 ml an average total blood loss of 33.2 ml during menstruation was found. Because of the asymmetric distribution of values (due to some individuals with a major blood loss), the normal range was not determined by using the standard deviation of the mean, but by using the 95th percentile = = 76.4 ml (i.e. 95% of women have menstrual blood loss smaller than 76.4 ml). As an arbitrary upper range of normal values therefore a total loss of 60–80 ml is taken; when the loss is greater than 80 ml, there is already a decline of the Hb and plasma iron concentration (444).

Subjective data of women on the magnitude of the blood loss and the intensity of menstrual bleeding respectively are extremely unreliable, some of them evaluate even massive bleeding still as "normal". More reliable are data referring to an obvious change of the former estimate. The use of more than 2–3 sanitary towels per day may be considered as indicating excessive blood losses. Further menstruation longer than seven days is often associated with excessive haemorrhage (444).

153

Under out-patient conditions we can in these instances evaluate the compensation of the menstrual blood loss by estimating the haemoglobin concentration and plasma iron before and after menstruation.

# DISORDERS OF THE RHYTHM OF THE MENSTRUAL CYCLE

## SHORTENED CYCLE (POLYMENORRHOEA, EPIMENORRHOEA)

The cycle is considered shortened when it is shorter than 23 days (see p. 150). In that case it is essential to follow the BBT in the course of 2–3 cycles. Only then is it possible to decide whether the shortening is at the expense of the luteal or follicular phase.

When the follicular phase of the menstrual cycle is shortened and the duration of the luteal phase is normal, therapy is not necessary, not even in case of desired pregnancy, if premenstrual biopsy of the endometrium (microabrasion) reveals its mature secretory transformation. This is so-called *polyovulation*.

When the luteal phase of the menstrual cycle is shortened to less than 9 or 10 days, frequently with a stepwise rise of the BBT curve, we usually find a defect of secretory transformation secondary to poor corpus luteum function in the pre-menstrual biopsy (see p. 256). Biopsy of the endometrium is in that case more important for the diagnosis than estimation of the level of circulating progesterone. Even when the progesterone secretion is normal, we may find inadequate transformation of the endometrium. This disorder is classified as pseudocorpus luteum insufficiency, i.e. a local defect of progesterone action on the endometrium (259a).

The BBT curve may also be monophasic. Suspected anovulation must be confirmed by endometrial biopsy. Cases of monophasic BBT are known with quite normal postovulatory progesterone secretion (244).

## OVULATION BLEEDING (CYCLIC INTERMENSTRUAL BLEEDING)

Ovulation bleeding may last several hours, or as much as 1–2 days. Usually it is only slight bleeding or a haemorrhagic discharge during the ovulation period in the middle of the menstrual cycle, usually between the 12th and 16th day. As a rule it occurs periodically ("pseudopolymenorrhoea"), with irregular spontaneous remissions. It may be associated with pain in the hypogastrium which, however, may also occur alone („*Mittelschmerz*"), in particular in case of inflammation of the uterine adnexa. The pain lasts as a rule only several hours, may, however, be quite intense. The mechanism of its genesis is not known. Perhaps it is peritoneal irritation by blood or follicular fluid or rupture of the follicle or tubal spasms.

Ovulation bleeding is oestrogen withdrawal-bleeding, it coincides with the brisk decline of the preovulatory peak of their secretion or the decline of oestrogen formation immediately after rupture of the Graafian follicle. Endometrial bleeding is in that case most frequently only bleeding *per diapedesim*. In approximately 90% of women during this period occult uterine bleeding can be detected by means of the benzidine reaction in the vaginal secretion; a positive reaction is indirect evidence of ovulation.

Ovulation bleeding is detected by means of the BBT curve. Endometrial biopsy corresponds to the end of the follicular or beginning of the luteal phase of the cycle. Treatment is not necessary. It is sufficient to inform the patient of the cause of this bleeding.


## PROLONGED CYCLE (OLIGOMENORRHOEA, RAROMENORRHOEA, OPSOMENORRHOEA, SPANIOMENORRHOEA)

A prolonged cycle implies a duration of more than 36 days (see p. 150). Clinical experience shows that if menstruation does not occur within 6 weeks, the probability of early spontaneous menstruation declines rapidly and usually there is a shorter or longer amenorrhoic phase. [In 99% of all cases the length of the menstrual cycle is within the interval of $\pm 2.58\,s$ from the mean, i.e. an interval of 21.0–37.8 $(= 38)$ days.] For the differential diagnosis of oligomenorrhoea it is again very important to follow the BBT curve during 2–3 cycles.

A prolonged menstrual cycle with a biphasic BBT curve and a normal duration of the hyperthermic phase does not call for treatment. There is less opportunity of impregnation as ovulation does not occur as frequently as under normal conditions (*oligoovulation*).

When the menstrual cycle is prolonged, we are more likely to encounter a shortened luteal phase of the BBT curve or a monophasic, anovulatory curve. For testing insufficiency of the corpus luteum or anovulation endometrial biopsy is again essential. Irregular alternation of ovulation and anovulation, more frequently associated with oligomenorrhoea than a regular menstrual cycle, is described as *subovulation*. Occasional spontaneous menstruations, interrupting the amenorrhoic interval are usually anovulatory pseudomenstruations; ovulation, however, cannot be ruled out. In the literature, pregnancies are recorded which followed immediately after a previous amenorrhoic period.

Prolongation of the menstrual cycle at the expense of the luteal phase (the hyperthermic phase of the BBT curve is longer than two weeks) is much rarer. A luteal phase longer than 16 or 18 days arouses suspicion that the uterine bleeding was not menstruation but a very early abortion. Ex post the diagnosis cannot be made — pregnancy could be confirmed only by premenstrual evidence of hCG in the blood or urine by a sufficiently sensitive method. The alternative is "persistence of the corpus luteum", probably caused by a small luteal cyst with hormonal activity.

# DISORDERS OF THE INTENSITY AND DURATION OF REGULAR MENSTRUAL BLEEDING

## EXCESSIVE AND PROLONGED BLEEDING (HYPERMENORRHOEA AND MENORRHAGIA)

Excessive menstrual bleeding (*hypermenorrhoea*) can be described as cyclic uterine bleeding exceeding the possibilities of compensatory mechanisms and is manifested by a postmenstrual decline of the Hb and plasma iron concentration — thus we can objectivize the subjective judgement of the patient. The total blood loss exceeds as a rule 60–80 ml, i.e. about 1 ml kg body weight (1% of the total amount of circulating blood — see p. 153).

If the excessive menstrual bleeding is moreover prolonged to more than 7 or 8 days, we speak of *menorrhagia*.

From the above described hypermenorrhoea and menorrhagia we must differentiate premenstrual bleeding (*premenstrual spotting, Vorblutung*) or postmenstrual bleeding (*Nachblutung*) which precedes or follows a relatively well defined menstruation. It is much weaker and sometimes it has the appearance of a brown discharge.

Recording of the BBT curve will show that hypermenorrhoea or menorrhagia may be associated with a biphasic type of curve. The most frequent cause is organic — an isolated submucous myoma, which cannot be detected by palpation, or submucous propagation of palpable uterine myomatosis. Endometrial polyps are much less common. An invaluable diagnostic aid in that case is hysterography. If uterine bleeding starts during the hyperthermic phase of BBT, most probably irregular shedding of secretory transformed endometrium is involved; the diagnosis can be confirmed by bioptic examination: premenstrual microabrasion will detect secretion; curettage on the fifth day of menstruation will reveal persisting secretory endometrium concurrent with areas of regeneration (see p. 301). Menorrhagia as an isolated manifestation of impaired blood clotting is extremely rare; increased capillary fragility is also described. One of the causes of ovulatory menorrhagia may be an isolated drop of plasma iron — before a reduced Hb concentration is manifested. A subsequent defect of cytochrome oxidase with an impaired contractility of the uterine musculature and the wall of spiral arterioles is assumed. Secondary anaemia with a decline of plasma iron thus causes further deterioration of the initial condition, whatever the cause of menorrhagia. Conversely a monophasic BBT curve and premenstrual endometrial biopsy provide evidence of the anovulatory character of excessive and prolonged cyclic uterine bleeding.

Of extreme interest is the finding that the concentration of endometrial $PGE_2$ and $PGF_{2\alpha}$ is raised not only in women suffering from dysmenorrhoea (see p. 162) but also in menorrhagia and metrorrhagia of the dysfunctional type and in myomatosis of the uterus.

Premenstrual bleeding is most frequently a manifestation of corpus luteum insufficiency (see p. 256). For detection of the cause again the BBT curve, premenstrual endometrial biopsy and assessment of the circulating progesterone or the concentration of excreted pregnanediol are decisive.

During postmenstrual bleeding we assume an inadequate intitial production of ovarian oestrogens. Evidence is difficult to provide: again endometrial biopsy is performed and possibly vaginal cytology.

## SPARSE BLEEDING (HYPOMENORRHOEA)

Symptomatic definition of hypomenorrhoea is difficult because an objective criterion is as a rule lacking. Anamnestic data are most reliable if a secondary change of the type of menstruation is involved — when the woman recorded a striking decline of the intensity of menstrual bleeding the former intensity of which she considered as normal.

When the menstrual cycle is regular, hypomenorrhoea occurs relatively rarely, in 1–4% of all cases. If it does not interfere with fertility, it is not necessary to make any therapeutic provisions (if there is a typical biphasic BBT curve and mature secretory transformation of the endometrium). The phenomenon is obviously still within the range of normal variability of menstrual bleeding and is a stage towards rare amenorrhoea with a preserved ovulatory cycle (so-called *sub-threshold cycle, amenorrhoea spuria*), when the secreting endometrium undergoes regression without haemorrhage and desquamation.

Alternation of hypomenorrhoea with menstruation of normal intensity and duration and a regular cycle arouses suspicion of interference by complete anovulatory cycles or cycles with corpus luteum insufficiency. The position can be elucidated by a BBT curve and premenstrual endometrial biopsy.

Hypomenorrhoea is most frequently associated with anovulatory oligomenorrhoea or prolonged menstrual cycles with corpus luteum insufficiency. The diagnosis causes no difficulties.

Organic causes of hypomenorrhoea are less frequent. The main ones are as follows: (1) tuberculosis of the endometrium, (2) intrauterine adhesions and (3) insufficiency of the endometrium (*endometrial sclerosis*). The first group is

157

usually the consequence of a specific lesion of the endometrium established during puberty, the two latter follow typically a previous pregnancy and curettage during the puerperium. Sclerosis of the endometrium is a condition when a considerable portion of the mucosa is replaced by ciccatrical tissue without formation of adhesions. Only a small amount of mucosa is obtained, it responds, however, always by secretory transformation. Hypomenorrhoea in tuberculous endometritis is typically associated with primary sterility, intrauterine synechiae (Asherman's syndrome) with abortion or secondary sterility, similarly as ciccatrical endometrial sclerosis. Hysterography and endometrial biopsy are essential for revealing the causes of organic hypomenorrhoea.

# IRREGULAR UTERINE BLEEDING (METRORRHAGIA)

Metrorrhagia is irregular uterine bleeding which lacks a cyclic character — the menstrual cycle is disturbed. Metrorrhagia is a symptom which has organic (anatomical) or functional causes.

The organic causes which we must seek above all are varied. The cause of uterine bleeding may be a malignant neoplasm of the uterine cervix or corpus, a submucous myoma, a mucosal polyp, endometritis, impaired blood coagulation, residues after incomplete abortion or extrauterine haemorrhage.

A disorder of physiological function controlling the menstrual cycle is the cause of so-called functional uterine bleeding. We prefer the term *dysfunctional haemorrhage* which was used first in 1930 by Graves (180). Although in the literature the two terms are still used promiscuously, we feel that the term dysfunctional haemorrhage expresses more pertinently the fact that it is uterine bleeding caused by a disorder of regulatory functions, i.e. dysfunction of mechanisms which under physiological conditions control the menstrual cycle in women.

Dysfunctional uterine bleeding in the wider sense of the word is a broad term which comprises a range of pathological conditions incl. some where the cyclic character of uterine bleeding is preserved and which are not manifested by metrorrhagia. Fundamentally we differentiate between two groups (10) (see p. 263):

A. dysfunctional ovulatory bleeding:
   a) with defect of follicular phase
   b) with defect of luteal phase
B. dysfunctional anovulatory bleeding:
   a) with persistence of follicle
   b) with insufficiency of follicle

The term dysfunctional uterine bleeding in the narrower sense of the word implies metrorrhagia with prolonged persistence of the follicle.

# ABSENCE OF UTERINE BLEEDING (AMENORRHOEA)

Amenorrhoea is defined as the absence of menstruation during reproductive life. If a woman has not started to menstruate by the age of 17 years (arbitrary border-line), we speak of primary amenorrhoea; if she ceased to menstruate after one (the first) or after several spontaneous menstruations it is secondary amenorrhoea. The borderline between the latter and oligomenorrhoea is arbitrary; an interval of more than three months is described as amenorrhoea. In the literature we encounter a protraction of this interval to six months as well as suggestions for abandoning the confusing borderline between oligomenorrhoea and secondary amenorrhoea by eliminating the term oligomenorrhoea and by describing every prolongation of the menstrual cycle above the upper bordeline of normal as amenorrhoea.

A special group is formed by so-called *cryptomenorrhoea* where an anatomical obstruction, occlusion of the uterine cervix, vagina or hymen, congenital or acquired, prevents the flow of menstrual blood from the genitalia.

Amenorrhoea is merely a symptom which has different causes, functional or organic. According to the localization of this lesion we differentiate the cause (102):

A. central:
  a) psychogenic
  b) hypothalamic
  c) hypophyseal
B. intermediary:
  a) exhaustive diseases
  b) metabolic disorders (endocrine glands — thyroid, adrenals, pancreas — and liver)
  c) nutritional disorders
C. peripheral:
  a) ovarian
  b) end-organ failure

The classical differentiation into amenorrhoea grade I and II by means of the progesterone test only expresses the degree of proliferation of the endometrium. The level of ovarian oestrogen production in grade I is sufficient for prolifer-ation essential for bleeding from the withdrawal of the circulating exogenous progesterone level (positive test), in grade II the oestrogenic preparation of the endometrium is inadequate (the test is negative). Both conditions have certain dynamics, in the same woman we can observe not only deterioration of the disorder but also spontaneous improvement, although this is as a rule only tem-porary.

## PHYSIOLOGICAL AMENORRHOEA

If we use the above definition as a basis, then only amenorrhoea associated with pregnancy and lactation is physiological.

The restoration of the menstrual cycle after childbirth displays great individual variability. 50% of non-lactating women menstruate already during the 9th week after childbirth, in the 20th week 50% of lactating multiparae and in the 26th week 50% of lactating primiparae. In Czechoslovakia at the end of the third month after parturition 57% of all women cease to breastfeed, between the 5th and 6th month 90% and after the 8th–11th women no longer breastfeed. The period of lactation and its intensity retard the restoration of the menstrual cycle and ovulation. Restoration of the menstrual cycle (RMC) during full breastfeeding (BF) is characterized by the equation $RMC = 1.5 + 0.6\,BF$, where BF is the duration of breastfeeding in months. If the woman does not breastfeed the first menstruation occurs roughly 1.5 month after childbirth. The first cycle is ovulatory in almost 80% of all cases; however, a relatively frequent insufficiency of the corpus luteum is reported.

Puerperal amenorrhoea is considered a manifestation of slow restitution of the activity of the hypothalamo-hypophyseal system which controls the ovarian cycle and is inhibited during pregnancy. Reports from the literature which suggest persistence of the cyclic function of hypothalamic regulating areas in pregnancy are rare and controversial. Despite this the duration of pregnancy was associated with a multiple of the "suppressed" menstrual cycle and along with it related to the lunar cycle — the average duration of pregnancy being characterized as corresponding to 9.5 lunar synodic months.

## PAINFUL SYNDROMES CONNECTED WITH THE MENSTRUAL CYCLE

### DYSMENORRHOEA

We may describe as dysmenorrhoea menstruation associated with pain (*algomeno-rrhoea*) or other complaints of an extent that the general condition of the woman is impaired. She cannot perform (for several hours or days) her activities in the usual way and as a rule seeks medical attendance. This stricter definition is at least an attempt at a certain objectivization of complaints.

The inaccurate definition of the term and the subjective criteria of complaints are the reason of the very variable data on the incidence of this syndrome in the literature. To summarize, no more can be said than that it varies within a range of tens of per cent. The number of cases needing bed rest is reported to be 3–15%.

For practical reasons it is important to differentiate dysmenorrhoea from the syndrome of premenstrual tension (see p. 163) and other painful syndromes, where the complaints start or end several days before or after menstruation and which have a different pathogenesis. Dysmenorrhoea is characterized in particular by pain in the hypogastrium and low back pain which start not sooner than one day before menstruation and end at the latest one day after menstruation. The variability even within this range is considerable. The pain may start at the onset of uterine bleeding or precede the latter by several hours or a day and sometimes it becomes milder at the onset of bleeding. The pain is intermittent, spasmodic, may be tolerable or call for bed rest and sometimes may lead to work incapacity. Sometimes it is associated with nausea and vomiting, diarrhoea or symptoms reminiscent of premenstrual tension.

We differentiate between primary and secondary dysmenorrhoea. As *primary dysmenorrhoea* we describe the syndrome which starts with menarche, or more frequently soon after menarche in the course of the first two years of gradual stabilization of the menstrual cycle. As *secondary dysmenorrhoea* we describe the syndrome which starts at any later time in the reproductive period of the female. We refute thus the term used sometimes in the literature, so-called early secondary dysmenorrhoea.

This classification with regard to the onset of complaints is usually consistent with the classification according to the local gynaecological finding. For primary dysmenorrhoea a normal finding on palpation is typical (therefore the term *idiopathic, essential or functional dysmenorrhoea*), while secondary dysmenorrhoea (*symptomatic or organic dysmenorrhoea*) is often associated with some organic pelvic diseases.


IDIOPATHIC DYSMENORRHOEA

The cause of functional dysmenorrhoea is not known. There exist a number of theories which try to explain its etiopathogenesis.

The contemporary literature abandons the old theory which related functional dysmenorrhoea with hypoplasia of the uterus. Hypoplasia is the most frequent organic finding in functional dysmenorrhoea (in as much as 12–60% of cases as compared with 8.6% in all women with gynaecological diseases although in another large group of dysmenorrhoeas only 3% hypoplasias were recorded). In women with uterine hypoplasia, however, dysmenorrhoic complaints are reported only in 29–40% of the cases.

The most widespread theory is based on the fact that functional dysmenorrhoea is manifested practically only in ovulatory cycles. A dysbalance between oestrogens and progesterone is assumed (however so far it was not conclusively confirmed by biochemical methods).

Spastic contractions of the uterine muscle and the increased gastrointestinal motility (and more frequent attacks of bronchial asthma during menstruation) are interpreted at present by the excessive action of endometrial prostaglandins (see p. 119). In dysmenorrhoic women the endometrial prostaglandin concentration is higher than that in healthy women (for review see 548).

Remarkable evidence of the endogenous predisposition is the observation that functional dysmenorrhoea is extremely rare in pyknosomic women; in some large series only in 2% complaints were reported, in others the percentage is higher.

A special part in the development of functional dysmenorrhoea is ascribed to psychogenic factors. Perception of pain has a general psychological aspect which is beyond the dimensions of the lesion and sensory signalization. Tolerance of pain depends on a great individual variability of the threshold of pain perception and is modified by the cultural background (ethnically), early experience from childhood and the attitude of the parents. Pain is a complex experience not only a subjective impression caused by a specific stimulus. Therefore, the intensity of pain is not always proportional to the stimulus which evokes it. Thus e.g. anticipation, increased attention, anxiety and tension enhance the painful experience. Some painful syndromes are therefore described as psychogenic with the implication that the primary cause of pain is psychological — the patient perceives pain because he unconsciously wants or needs it. Psychological causes are the domain of psychosomatic medicine which in functional dysmenorrhoea finds a whole range of psychological motivations (if we omit psychoanalytical phantasies) which differ, depending on the age of onset of dysmenorrhoic complaints. In general dysmenorrhoea is considered an expression of demonstrative and aggressive protest and defense. In this connection it is of interest that cases of membraneous dysmenorrhoea (where the endometrium is shed *in toto* as a cast of the uterine cavity) were observed also in the chimpanzee (*Pan troglodytes*).

Reports have been published that 40–100% of all cases of functional dysmenorrhoea are psychogenic. For the diagnosis of psychogenic dysmenorrhoea it is important that it is frequently combined with other neurotic symptoms. A raised index of neuroticism and anxiety is found and a tendency to transform intensive emotional experience into somatic reactions. There also exist, however, opposite findings which did not detect any correlation between functional dysmenorrhoea and neuroticism and it is therefore considered a psychosomatic syndrome. In neurotic women, however, the authors recorded dysmenorrhoic complaints more frequently than in healthy women.

A psychogenic origin of dysmenorrhoea may be assumed as most probable only after a failure of therapy with prostaglandin synthetase inhibitors or ovulation inhibitors.

## SYMPTOMATIC DYSMENORRHOEA

Organic dysmenorrhoea is by definition in a causal relationship with pelvic pathology; various pathological conditions are mentioned. Although in individual cases the causes of the relationship cannot be ruled out (e.g. myoma, inflammation), and it must be searched for — it is with the exception of endometriosis not statistically significant for the group.

The participation of endometriosis is beyond doubt. Typical for dysmenorrhoic complaints is that they precede uterine bleeding (complaints may already be caused by premenstrual oedema of the dystopic endometrium) and persist throughout the menstrual period. Endometriosis, however, cannot be ruled out even if palpation is negative, and then laparoscopic examination is essential. Conversely, cases are known when despite an extensive finding dysmenorrhoic complaints are absent. Only approximately one half of all patients with confirmed endometriosis suffer from dysmenorrhoea.

## SYNDROME OF PREMENSTRUAL TENSION

The syndrome of premenstrual tension is a recognized clinical entity since the early thirties. In 1931 it was the subject of two papers from apparently opposite angles — endocrinological and psychosomatic. In the literature we also encounter the term *premenstrual syndrome* or *premenstrual dysphoria*.

The cause of the syndrome is as vague as that of functional dysmenorrhoea. An important role is ascribed to premenstrual fluid retention, which may be excessive, values up to 1.5–4.0 l are reported. "Latent" oedema is also taken into consideration in cephalgia and abdominal complaints. The retention is associated with hyperoestrogenism. However, in a completely anovulatory cycle where production of ovarian progesterone is lacking, the syndrome of premenstrual tension does not seem to occur. The link of the syndrome with the ovulatory cycle suggests rather the participation of progesterone. Its action on electrolyte metabolism is considered, the action of progesterone being opposite to the action of aldosterone (progesterone stimulates urinary sodium and chloride excretion, while potassium is retained, and aldosterone exerts the opposite effect). The effectiveness of exogenous progesterone in the syndrome of premenstrual tension is, however, not conclusive; against the possible role of relative progesterone deficiency evidence is provided by the frequent absence of the syndrome in aluteal cycles. In this connection it is better to consider primarily elevated aldosterone secretion which can apparently be induced by psychogenic stimuli. We must not overestimate either the role of aldosterone and fluid retention — after elimination of oedema by diuretics in a considerable proportion of subjects the symptoms of premenstrual tension persist. The marked therapeutic effect of androgens is interesting, in particular on some symptoms, especially mastodynia.

The idea of an allergic mechanism of the development of the syndrome, in particular an allergy to endogenous oestrogens or progesterone is tempting as administration of progesterone sometimes leads to deterioration of the complaints.

The correlation of the syndrome of premenstrual tension with neuroticism is beyond doubt. If we omit psychoanalytic phantasies, it is probable that psychological factors play a similar role in the development of the syndrome as in functional dysmenorrhoea. A predisposing factor is obviously the premenstrual period, the influence exerted on the CNS by a changed level of circulating ovarian steroids (see p. 24). This background of increased excitability of the CNS predisposes not only to the perception of the described painful sensation and the development of cyclic emotional lability with the clinical picture of premenstrual tension, but in extreme cases it also leads to a breakdown of reactions of self-preservation (attempted suicide is three times more frequent during the premenstrual period and during menstruation) and the development of acute psychosis or deterioration of already existing psychotic symptoms. Provoking psychological factors again include experience from early childhood and defects of normal psychosexual development, impaired attitude to the role of the female and sexuality and neurotic defense mechanisms. If these factors are present, then they are present permanently, i.e. throughout the menstrual cycle. They may evoke, however, the typical symptomatology of the premenstrual syndrome only during the period when in quite normal women even physiological variations of ovarian secretion cause detectable changes of the general condition evaluated so far subjectively as "normal". The predominance of organ manifestation (manifest and "latent" oedema) in the premenstrual syndrome also suggest, in our opinion, a certain concurrent disorder of physiological regulatory mechanisms.

Dramatic relief of several types of premenstrual symptoms (breast symptoms, oedema, weight gain and mood) produced by administration of bromocryptine, a dopamine agonist suppressing PRL secretion (see p. 282) demonstrates that hypotheses about the psychobiology of premenstrual syndrome will need to be revised and take into account the role of PRL.


## OVULATION PAIN (CYCLIC INTERMENSTRUAL PAIN)

The term ovulation pain ("*Mittelschmerz*") is used to describe painful sensations, unilateral or bilateral, in the hypogastrium at the time of ovulation which are frequently associated with slight bleeding (see p. 154).


# DISORDERS OF THE MENSTRUAL CYCLE IN HIRSUTISM

*Hirsutism* implies excessive hair growth on the body with a typical male distribution. (*Hypertrichosis*, on the other hand, is excessive hair growth with a female distribution, as a rule conditioned by racial, constitutional and familial factors.) Hirsutism is usually encountered as an isolated phenomenon. Less frequently it is part of *virilization*, concomitantly with the absence or suppression of secondary female sex characteristics with male body build (development of skeleton and musculature, adipose tissue distribution, voice) and hypertrophy of the clitoris; in rare instances virilization without hirsutism is encountered.

Basically we differentiate — from the gynaecological point of view between two groups of hirsutism: (1) with disorders of the menstrual cycle and (2) without disorders of the menstrual cycle.

**Hirsutism with disorders of the menstrual cycle.** Disorders of the cycle in hirsutism are very variable. From amenorrhoea (secondary and sometimes also primary) via oligomenorrhoea to dysfunctional uterine bleeding of the metrorrhagic type. The common sign is anovulation or rare ovulation. The assumed cause is hyperandrogenism, androgenic hyperfunction of ovarian, adrenal or combined, or peripheral origin (see p. 271).

**Hirsutism without disorders of the menstrual cycle.** This is so-called idiopathic or constitutional hirsutism in the narrower sense of the word. The ability to ovulate is preserved, as has been repeatedly confirmed by the biphasic BBT curve, by biopsy of the endometrium and even fertility. In general, common biochemical examinations or functional clinical tests will detect only slight if any androgenic hyperfunction.

Data on the incidence of hirsutism vary between 10–28% of women. It is estimated that only 10% suffer from hirsutism of such a degree that it calls for examination by a specialist. In 50–60% of all cases the development of hirsutism has already started before the age of 20, usually during the period of sexual maturation.

In the wider sense of the word *idiopathic hirsutism* comprises cases with an unexplained cause which also include disorders of the menstrual cycle. The opposite is *symptomatic hirsutism* where the source of hyperandrogenism is known, while with regard to the causes we differentiate between the adrenal form (congenital AGS, acquired AGS, "borderline" AGS, hypercortisolism, adrenocortical masculinizing tumours), ovarian form [follicular hyperthecosis (Stein-Leventhal syndrome), stromal hyperthecosis (thecomatosis), hyperplasia of Leydig's hilar cells, ovarian masculinizing tumours] and the combined form, whereby peripheral transformation of prehormones to testosterone cannot be neglected.

Sometimes *ACTH-dependent hirsutism* (excretion of 17-oxosteroids excretion and testosterone secretion is inhibited by glucocorticoids) and *gonadotropin-dependent hirsutism* (17-oxosteroid excretion and testosterone secretion is stimulated by the action of hCG and inhibited by ovarian steroids) is differentiated. The effect of steroids and gonadotropins is, however, not sufficiently selective and therefore does not prove that the ovarian or adrenal cause of hirsutism is involved (see p. 275).

According to contemporary knowledge we need not assume in idiopathic hirsutism with a normal level of plasma testosterone that the sensitivity of target tissues is increased (contrary to the known inborn defect of sensitivity of testosterone target tissues and the lack of sexual hair in the syndrome of testicular feminization). In eumenorrhoic women with hirsutism the binding capacity of TEBG is markedly reduced. It cannot be ruled out that in these cases a primary lesion may be involved and not a secondary change caused by a raised androgen level. In hirsute women with menstrual dysfunction the binding capacity of TEBG is even lower although the level of circulating testosterone may be practically unaltered.

165

# ABNORMAL PUBERTAL DEVELOPMENT

The borderline of the physiological onset of development of characteristics of sexual maturation varies in the literature. It is recommended to define as normal the range $\pm 3$ standard deviations ($s$) from the arithmetic mean (within this interval are 99.73% of all members of a group; 99% of possible values are within the range of 2.58 $s$) (84). The recommendation to use the interval $\pm 4\,s$ is in our opinion exaggerated. For the urban (Prague) population of girls, Luksch and Reisenauer in 1966 (311) characterized the onset of the development of signs of sexual maturation by mathematical and statistical methods as the age when 99% of the investigated girls display a zero value of a certain sign and 1% the maximum value. They defined the termination of development as the age when 99% of the girls display a maximum value and 1% a zero value (see Table 1). These data are used in our own practice.

We differentiate disorders of sexual maturation into two groups: (1) disorders due to acceleration and (2) disorders due to retardation of the sexual development.

## PREMATURE PUBERTAL DEVELOPMENT (SEXUAL PRECOCITY)

Disorders of pubertal development due to acceleration are classified as follows:
A. Complete form of sexual precocity
  a) true precocious puberty
  b) pseudoprecocious puberty
    aa) isosexual
    bb) heterosexual
B. Incomplete form of sexual precocity
  a) premature thelarche (gynarche)
  b) premature pubarche (adrenarche)
  c) premature menarche

## TRUE PRECOCIOUS PUBERTY

"True" precocious puberty is the manifestation of an abnormally early onset of ovarian function as a result of adequate stimulation by pituitary gonadotropins. The basis is early function of hypothalamic regulatory mechanisms.

Symptoms may appear even during the first year of life. An extreme case is a regular menstrual cycle from the age of 8 months in a girl who gave birth to a baby at the age of less than 6 years (184). Premature development of the reproductive endocrine system, in addition to the development of sex signs in the typical

166

sequence, also causes an accelerated somatic growth, rapid bone ageing and premature disappearance of the epiphyseal plates with arrest of skeletal growth. This results in small stature.

With regard to the cause we differentiate between the following groups:

**Idiopathic (cryptogenic) form.** This form comprises about 90 % of all cases. The diagnosis can be made only *per exclusionem*, by eliminating organic causes. It is difficult to define marginal cases from the extreme variants of normal, e.g. early menarche in so-called frühnormale Pubertät.

Till recently the disorder was ascribed to an abnormality of genetic factors which determine the time of maturation of the regulatory mechanism of the genital cycle. Therefore constitutional precocious puberty was considered an extreme variant of the normal (so-called scatter phenomenon), a "physiological anomaly" of development. In a large group, however, only in less than 10% of all cases was a heredofamilial incidence found (incl. twice in monozygotic twins). In 80% of the girls marked though non-specific abnormalities of the EEG were found, while in normal children and adolescents they are found according to data in the literature in 6–16%, and more frequently in children than in adolescents (306). It seems thus that in the majority of cases the idiopathic form is not constitutional but cryptogenic although these terms are used promiscuously. Probably only a variant of the cerebral form is involved. As such, this form has already been anticipated. An unidentified disorder of the CNS is assumed, probably as a consequence of prenatal damage or birth trauma which directly or indirectly affects areas associated with the regulation of the gonadotropic activity of the adenohypophysis. (In model experiments on animals it is possible by inducing certain lesions in the hypothalamus or amygdala to hasten sexual maturing.) The hypothesis, however, does not explain why in the female this form of disorder of sexual maturation is encountered about 7.5 times more frequently than in males.

The affected girl is threatened in particular by premature arrest of growth. Moreover, there is the danger of sexual abuse and pregnancy, psychosexual problems and traumas. The purpose of treatment is effective inhibition of secretion of pituitary gonadotropins.

The use of medroxyprogesterone acetate has been suggested which being a so-called pure gestagen lacks a complicating accessory oestrogenic or androgenic effect which in this case is quite undesirable. A depot preparation for injection is used — 100 to 200 mg are injected after 1-, 2- or even 4-week intervals. The criteria of action which determine the individual dosage are mainly clinical: eumenorrhoea, diminution of the breasts, decline of oestrogenic activity in the colpocytogram and possibly a decline of gonadotropin secretion. Subsequent experience revealed that in some instances the level of circulating gonadotropins does not decline (but if so, then as a rule the concentration of LH declines more than that of FSH), and thus the possibility of a hypothalamic disorder of the mechanism of the inhibitory progesterone feedback is considered. Further the arrest of enhanced bone maturation is not always successful.

Apparently a more favourable effect on the prognosis for height in adult life in girls is attained by the administration of the gestagenic anti-androgen cyproterone acetate. The daily dose 50 mg or 100 mg/m$^2$ during long-term administration does not reduce the concentration of plasma LH and FSH (it significantly inhibits, however, the release of LH in the LH-RH test) and reduces the testosterone concentration only insignificantly but normalizes the concentration of circulating oestradiol and causes the disappearance of karyopyknotic superficial cells in vaginal smears and regression of clinical signs of premature puberty, while cyclic uterine bleeding ceases, the growth of the breasts and sexual hair not only fails to proceed but there is even regression of the changes which have already occurred. Treatment prevents accelerated bone growth (i.e. acceleration of osseous age). Under physiological conditions only six months after the first menstruation growth slows down significantly: the mechanism of the final disappearance of epiphyseal plates is obviously very complicated, with participation of androgens, oestrogens and growth hormone. Reduction of the responsiveness of the adenohypophysis to LH-RH by the action of cyproterone acetate is ascribed to the direct action on the anterior pituitary lobe either by the gestagenic activity of the steroid or the effect of a secondarily reduced level of plasma oestradiol. The possibility of inhibited ovarian steroidogenesis by the action of cyproterone acetate on the ovaries cannot be excluded.

**Cerebral (hypothalamic) form.** This form differs from the idiopathic form by the presence of neurological symptoms. The latter may, however, develop only secondarily, whille in an early phase this form may simulate the idiopathic one.

In the development of organic affections of the CNS the following are involved:

a) **Intracranial tumours.** Precocious puberty has been described in tumours with varying localization and different origin from astrocytoma of the cerebellum to glioma of the optic chiasma, however, never in pituitary tumours. Very frequently it is encountered along with inborn hyperplastic malformation of the base of the hypothalamus (hamartoma). A special position is held by tumours of the pineal body. It is remarkable that in girls they are not associated with impaired sexual development. This fact along with the observation that in boys with pineal tumours there may exist hypogonadism along with precocious puberty rather suggests that between tumours of the pineal and premature sexual development no direct relationship exists. The specific symptomatology of some intracranial tumours depends obviously on the pressure they exert or on their destructive action on the environment which affects directly or indirectly areas regulating the gonadotropic activity of the adenohypophysis.

b) **Inflammatory lesions of the central nervous system.** Conditions after encephalitis, less frequently after meningitis of different origin (in particular morbilli and tuberculosis) may be complicated by premature sexual development.

c) **Different neurological diseases.** Various diseases are mentioned, congenital and acquired, which may be associated with premature sexual development: microcephaly, craniostenosis, porencephalic cysts, cerebral atrophy, tuberculous sclerosis, mongolism, hydrocephalus and head injuries, where the interval between the injury and the initial symptoms is as a rule relatively short (4–8 weeks).

The differential diagnosis of the idiopathic and cerebral form is difficult in hamartoma, unless other symptoms of associated disorders of the development of the CNS are also present. Because a congenital malformation is involved, it is typical that manifestations of premature sexual development develop very early, usually during the first year of life. Sometimes clinical diagnosis is not possible and the cause of some cases of the apparently idiopathic form of pubertas praecox may be actually a hamartoma.

The treatment of the cerebral form differs, depending on the cause which also determines the prognosis.

**Dysplasia polyostotica fibrosa (Albright-McCune-Sternberg syndrome).** Albright's syndrome which is found almost solely in girls is characterized by segmental hypostotic and hyperostotic affection of the skeleton, pigmented light brown spots on the skin at sites corresponding to the osseous lesions and premature sexual and somatic development. The cause of precocious puberty is probably hyperostosis of the skull base and the secondary effect of hypothalamic areas regulating the pituitary gonadotropic activity by pressure, as in other expansive intracranial processes. According to this concept it would be a variant of the cerebral form of precocious sexual development.

In Albright's syndrome the skeletal development is impaired. The segmental character indicates the participation of the CNS. Causal therapy is not known.

Reports on teenage pregnancies in Albright's syndrome are lacking and the absence of luteinization of the ovaries is also common to the majority of cases with the cerebral form. In the idiopathic form of pubertas praecox there is premature function of intact physiological mechanisms which regulate sexual maturation (the level of circulating immunoreactive FSH and LH is markedly raised, compared with age matched controls), and thus the only abnormality is the reduction of the infantile period before the onset of pubertal acceleration. In the cerebral form and in Albright's syndrome, however, these regulatory mechanisms are impaired and thus the LH secretion may be defective and ovulation does not occur.

**Rare forms with an obscure aetiopathogenesis.**

a) **Pubertas praecox in juvenile hypothyroidism.** The majority of cases of juvenile hypothyroidism are associated with retarded but normal sexual maturation and a very small stature. (In cases of very small stature with developed secondary sex signs and retarded skeletal maturation hypothyroidism must always be suspected.) Sometimes, however, untreated cases develop pubertas praecox (237, 522, 540a), frequently with galactorrhoea, but usually without acceleration of hair growth. An enlarged sella turcica is often found. According to the original pathogenetic concept primary thyroid insufficiency leads through a mechanism of inhibitory (negative) feedback not only to an increased production of pituitary TSH but for obscure reasons also to an increased production of gonadotropins and possibly other tropic hormones of the adenohypophysis. (Hypothalamic TRH also has a certain stimulating effect on the release of PRL, and this may explain the frequently associated galactorrhoea.) An alternative is the decline of the basal metabolism below the critical range already mentioned (see p. 17) and according to Ruf's hypothesis the hastened maturation of catecholaminergic neurons of the CNS mediated by pancreatic proinsulin with subsequent elevated gonadotropin secretion. Causal treatment is normalization of thyroid function by suitable substitution (445).

b) **Pubertas praecox associated with Silver's syndrome.** Russel-Silver's syndrome is characterized among other features by congenital lateral asymmetry, small stature and premature sexual maturation without acceleration of skeletal development.


## PSEUDOPUBERTAS PRAECOX

"False" premature sexual maturation comprises cases with premature development of the genitalia and secondary sex characteristics without a primary effect on the maturation of the hypothalamo-hypophyseal system. The premature development of sex characteristics is the result of the action of gonadal hormones — homologous in the isosexual form and heterologous in the heterosexual form, where the source is not the hormonal activity of the gonads.

**Isosexual form.** Because adequate gonadotropic stimulation of the gonads is lacking, the ovaries do not initiate cyclic function, ovulation does not occur and the premature development of sex characteristics is not associated with fertility, as is the case in true pubertas praecox. According to the site of pathological oestrogen formation we differentiate between:

a) the ovarian type:
aa) oestrogen producing tumours
bb) hCG producing tumours
b) adrenal type
c) iatrogenic type

The most frequent source of oestrogens is a granulosocellular ovarian tumour, or rarely a thecocellular tumour (thecoma) or teratoma. Follicular ovarian cysts are usually the manifestation of a central regulatory disorder and premature development of sex characteristics proceeds even after their extirpation. In some instances they are, however, functionally autonomous and removal leads to arrest and regression of the impaired development.

Cases where the cause is a chorioepithelioma growing in an ovarian teratoma are rare. hCG stimulates oestrogen production in the contralateral ovary.

The adrenal type of isosexual pseudopubertas praecox is extremely rare. In congenital hyperplasia of the adrenal cortex the increased oestrogen production is masked by the action of androgens. Several cases have been reported where the masculinizing action of androgens was also associated with premature uterine bleeding and sometimes also development of the breasts as a sign of oestrogenic stimulation. Only in exceptional instances do symptoms of isosexual pseudopuberty precede manifestations of the heterosexual effect of adrenal androgens. Adrenal tumours, adenomas or carcinomas produce oestrogens only exceptionally and thus cause isosexual pseudopuberty. More frequently premature menarche only precedes virilization. Cases were also described where the source of oestrogens in isosexual premature pseudopuberty was aberrant adrenal tissue in the vicinity of the ovaries.

The iatrogenic isosexual type caused by administration of oestrogens may be manifested not only by pigmentation of the areolas, development of the breasts and sexual hair but also by uterine bleeding and may also affect skeletal maturation. The development of pubic and axillary hair and skeletal growth are ascribed to the stimulating action of oestrogens on the production of adrenal androgens. It is of interest that the breasts also develop under the influence of androgens and anabolic steroids. It is not known whether androgens act directly or only after conversion into oestrogens. The changes are completely reversible.

Diagnosis should determine the cause of isosexual precocious pseudopuberty. In addition to X-ray techniques which can reveal an ovarian or adrenal tumour (pneumopelvigraphy and retroperitoneal pneumoperitoneum) a functional test can be also applied. In the presence of an oestrogenically active tumour or adrenal hyperplasia a sufficiently effective dose of gestagen causes in the hitherto purely oestrogenic colpocytogram changes typical for the luteal phase of the menstrual cycle. In true precocious puberty it leads to inhibition of hypophyseal gonadotropic secretion, to a decline of ovarian oestrogens and typical hypoestrogenic or even atrophic changes in vaginal smears.

The purpose of treatment is to eliminate the sources of pathological oestrogen secretion or rarely hCG secretion also. In congenital adrenogenital syndrome with an enzyme defect of steroid biosynthesis specific corticoid treatment is indicated to suppress ACTH hyperproduction. Not only androgen but also oestrogen production becomes normal.

**Heterosexual form.** The heterosexual form of precocious pseudopuberty in girls is a manifestation of the action of adrenal or ovarian androgens. It is not merely an accelerated development of the genitals and sex characteristics but in particular abnormal masculine development. This problem is already beyond the scope of our work and we refer therefore to special literature on the subject (for review see 239, 382).


## PRECOCIOUS THELARCHE

The pure form of precocious thelarche implies cases of isolated premature development of the breasts without manifestations of oestrogenic activity in the colpocytogram. The condition is usually transient and regresses spontaneously. The pathogenesis is obscure. It may be due to primary premature maturation of the target organ with abnormal sensitivity to the physiological oestrogen level in the organism.

In about two thirds of cases of precocious thelarche, however, there are also manifestations of oestrogenic activity in the colpocytogram, accelerated bone ageing and increased 17-oxosteroid excretion. Thelarche praecox is then only the clinically most marked manifestation of sometimes only temporary, idiopathic true precocious puberty and may be associated with precocious puberty. The levels of circulating FSH and LH are slightly elevated in precocious thelarche.

In the first form of precocious thelarche treatment is not necessary, in the second one the same treatment is indicated as in the idiopathic form of true precocious puberty. In both long-term follow-up is essential.


## PRECOCIOUS ADRENARCHE (PREMATURE PUBARCHE)

The pure form is characterized by the isolated premature growth of pubic hair without other signs of premature sexual development. In most cases the production of adrenal androgens is increased, as reflected by plasma DHEA and DHEA--sulphate concentrations. At the same time there is also an elevated plasma oestradiol concentration, and 17-oxosteroid excretion is usually elevated. Sometimes there are signs of cerebral damage (epilepsy, spastic pareses, mental retardation, abnormality in the EEG and PEG).

The differential diagnosis from true precocious puberty is difficult because the onset of the development of other signs of sexual maturity may start after an interval of several years. The classification therefore depends on age and the condition calls for systematic follow-up. The pathogenesis is obscure.


## PRECOCIOUS MENARCHE

Cases were described where premature menarche preceded the onset of pubarche or thelarche or both, as well as cases where premature menarche remained isolated and usually after some time receded spontaneously. Precocious menarche is usually associated with oestrogenic manifestations in the colpocytogram and accelerated bone age. It is thus transient incomplete idiopathic true precocious puberty. The condition calls for systematic follow-up. Treatment is the same as in the idiopathic form of precocious puberty.


## DELAYED PUBERTAL DEVELOPMENT

Pathological retardation of sexual development may be complete if the infantile condition persists in the sexual sphere. We speak of *sexual infantilism* (502). Sometimes there is a late but normal onset of development. This is called *pubertas tarda*. Retardation may be incomplete, i.e. the development of one of the sex characteristics does not start at all or is significantly delayed. Disorders of sexual maturation, i.e. retardation can be classified approximately as follows:

A. Complete form:
    a) sexual infantilism
    b) delayed puberty
B. Incomplete form:
    a) primary amenorrhoea
    b) delayed menarche

## SEXUAL INFANTILISM

Sexual infantilism implies persistence in the infantile anatomical and physiological stage of development, i.e. in the prepubertal condition. In complete sexual infantilism there is only partial development of sex characteristics or their development does not start at all because the impulse for sexual maturation is lacking or is incomplete. In incomplete or so-called partial sexual infantilism some sex characteristics develop normally, others persist in the infantile stage. Here, along with other causes, an impaired reactivity of certain target structures is assumed (e.g. genital hypoplasia, sparse sexual hair, hypoplasia of the breasts), while the impulse for sexual maturation is intact.

The causes of complete sexual infantilism (in hypothalamic, hypophyseal, thyreogenic, diabetic, hepatogenic and hypometabolic forms) make these patients seek in particular paediatric care, as the affection in the sexual sphere is in the background of the general picture of the disorder. For gynaecological practice sexual infantilism associated with gonadal dysgenesis is most important.

## DELAYED PUBERTY

The term delayed puberty implies a markedly retarded onset of sexual maturation which, however, takes the typical normal course of development of sex characteristics and culminates in menarche. It may, but need not, be the beginning of primary menstrual dysfunction. The onset of puberty may be considered delayed if breast development has not begun by the age of 13 years.

The cause is a delayed release of hypothalamic regulatory mechanisms. Unless there is a marked influence of the socio-economic environment, delayed puberty is most frequently an expression of the constitutional type. It displays familial incidence and has a dominant autosomal type of heredity. The incidence is estimated to be $3\%$.

# PRIMARY AMENORRHOEA

As an arbitrary upper range of physiological menarche in the literature usually the age of 17 is given which is consistent with the age at which in Prague urban population the development of this sign of sexual maturation is completed (see Table 1). If by that age menarche does not occur, we speak of primary amenorrhoea. If by that time the development of sex characteristics has not started, which under normal conditions precede the first menstruation, primary amenorrhoea is the manifestation of complete sexual retardation, part of general sexual infantilism. Primary amenorrhoea may be only an isolated manifestation of incomplete sexual retardation if preceded by the development of other signs of sexual maturation.

Primary amenorrhoea is a symptom affecting different parts of the reproductive system, its regulatory mechanisms or its organ effectors. The disorder originates during fertilization or shortly after, or in the course of organogenesis or even later postnatally at any time before the onset of menarche. According to the localization of the disorder in the reproductive system we can differentiate between several basic groups which are also the groups of the pathogenetic classification:

A. Chromosomal (gonosomal) disorders:
   gonadal dysgenesis with abnormal karyotype
B. Gonadal disorders:
   a) true gonadal agenesis
   b) pure gonadal dysgenesis
   c) gonadal dysgenesis in 46,XX
   d) ovarian "dysgenesis" (ovarian dysplasia, syndrome of rudimentary ovary)
   e) premature ovarian failure
C. Central disorders:
   a) psychogenic disorders
   b) hypothalamic disorders
      aa) hypogonadotropic hypogonadism (eunuchoidism)
      bb) primary syndrome of polycystic ovaries
   c) hypophyseal
D. Disorders of internal genitalia:
   a) congenital (gynatresia)
   b) acquired
E. Disorders of the receptivity of target organs:
   a) normogonadotropic hypogonadism
   b) syndrome of resistant ovaries (follicular "dysgenesis")
   c) testicular feminization

The differential diagnostic approach must be comprehensive. It comprises findings obtained by clinical description (height, breast development and sexual hair, development of the external and internal genitalia, extragenital anomalies), by visualization of the internal genitalia (pneumopelvigraphy or laparoscopy), biopsy of the gonads, assessment of the karyotype, X-ray of skull, examination of the sense of smell, estimation of the plasma concentration of FSH, LH, oestradiol and progesterone. Further investigations are — if necessary — the progesterone withdrawal-bleeding test, the oestrogen stimulation test, the gonadotropin stimulation test, and the LH-RH test. A stepwise flow chart of the diagnostic approach (decision tree) to delayed pubertal development is shown in Fig. 38.

Reflections on the incidence of different disorders are premature — clinical series of cases of primary amenorrhoea are too small and involve therefore the error of small numbers. Thus e.g. the incidence of chromosomal aberrations varies from 20 to 40%.

Therapy of primary amenorrhoea depends on the cause which also determines the prognosis *quoad fertilitatem*.


## DELAYED MENARCHE

The term delayed menarche implies the absence of spontaneous menarche by the age of 17 years, although the development of other signs of sexual maturation have taken a normal course or if more than five years have elapsed from the onset of breast changes and there have been no menses. It is recommended to follow-up preventively all girls who do no start to menstruate by the age of 16 years.

An extreme case reported in the literature is that of a woman with normal development of secondary sex characteristics except menarche who began to menstruate spontaneously at the age of 38 years; a regular menstrual cycle with a monophasic BBT curve followed. Ovarian biopsy revealed, however, a mature corpus luteum and several corpora albicantia (39).

The most frequent cause is an assumed hypothalamic disorder. (Delayed menarche was found more frequently in prematurely born girls.) In female transmitters of testicular feminization menarche is often delayed. The observation is explained by the effect that the appropriate gene under heterozygous conditions causes delayed menarche, while in 45,XY individuals it leads to male pseudohermaphroditism. Also in rare cases of juvenile hyperthyroidism (see p. 17) and juvenile diabetes (see p. 191) menarche is usually delayed.

# Pathogenetic Classification of Disorders of the Menstrual Cycle

## PSYCHOGENIC DISORDERS

Psychogenic disorders of the menstrual cycle are a sphere of psychosomatic medicine in gynaecology (as has already been mentioned in the case of dysmenorrhoea and the syndrome of premenstrual tension). Its basis is *corticovisceral pathology* (for a competent review see 285).

Corticovisceral pathology uses as a basis the Pavlovian concept on the cerebral cortex, the phylogenetically and ontogenetically highest department of the CNS which is concerned with the analysis and synthesis of all external and internal stimuli, and which integrates and coordinates all somatic and vegetative visceral functions of the organism, i.e. also the ovarian cycle in females, via subcortical centres and the endocrine system. (The term *cerebrovisceral pathology*, used sometimes, comprises also all mediating central nervous structures, however, it does not emphasize the leading role of the cerebral cortex.)

According to the basic corticovisceral concept the cortex of the cerebral hemispheres has a trigger and correcting effect not only on the most complex reflexes but also on all autonomic visceral systemic, organ, cellular and subcellular functions. In the control of autonomic visceral functions a decisive part is played in particular by limbic, premotor and orbital areas of the cerebral cortex.

### CAUSES AND MECHANISM OF THE DEVELOPMENT OF CORTICOVISCERAL DISORDERS

The cause of corticovisceral disorders is psychogenic. *"Psychic trauma"*, a broad and general term, is in the Pavlovian terminology an excessively intensive stimulus or collision of excitation and inhibition which causes excessive straining of nervous processes not only in the cortex but also in the subcortical area, in regions regulating autonomic visceral functions and the activity of the endocrine glands. This results in a "breakdown" of higher nervous activity (HNA), neurosis and a corticovisceral disorder (organ neurosis, vegetative neurosis). According to

177

contemporary ideas neurotization may develop not only in the cortex but also in subcortical regions (experimental neurosis and "cortico"-visceral disorders develop also in decorticated animals).

The initial trigger mechanism is psychic trauma. In the Pavlovian terminology we may differentiate, depending on its nature, between exhaustive, conflict and stereotype neurosis.

The depth and duration of corticovisceral disorders depend on the degree of impairment of compensating defense mechanisms of the cerebral cortex and of the cortico-subcortical integration, as well as on the extent of involvement of sub-cortical autonomic visceral regulating areas in the neurotic process. The extreme is a lethal disorganization of regulation mechanisms and psychogenic death (e.g. "voodoo" death or death from total despair known in concentration and prisoner of war camps).

The effect of psychic trauma may be immediate (*mental shock*) or it may be manifested after several months latency. In those instances everyday general stimuli act on a weakened background and finally lead to the brakdown of HNA.

Since depression is probably associated with disorders of turnover or metabolism of central biogenic amines, it is tempting to postulate that an alteration of central catecholamine function may be causative in the development of neuroendocrine aberrations. In socially subordinated female monkeys not only plasma cortisol but also PRL is raised and fertility is reduced concomitantly with inhibition of LH surge which is normally induced by giving oestrogen. Behavioural interactions are thus capable of altering the primate female brain dopaminergic system con-trolling hypophyseal gonadotropin and PRL secretion (57). Similarly, in some women with amenorrhoea-galactorrhoea syndrome psychometric tests and elevated plasma noradrenaline level demonstrate the role of psychic stress in inducing an alteration of brain catecholamine-dependent regulatory mechanisms (549).

Neurosis and corticovisceral disorders develop most frequently in the two extremes of the four basic types of HNA [types of nervous activity: strong unbalanced type (choleric), strong balanced inert type (phlegmatic), strong balanced excitable type (sanguinic) and weak type (melancholic)]. Both extreme types have a low level of adaptive defense mechanisms in cortical and subcortical structures.

## PROBLEM OF ORGAN SPECIFICITY OF CORTICOVISCERAL DISORDERS

The key problem of psychosomatic medicine is the problem of specific affection of an organ or system of organs. From clinical practice it is known that psychic trauma causes in one subject a cardiovascular corticovisceral disorder, in another a gastrointestinal and in a third an endocrinopathy, etc. The explanation of these facts is so far only speculative.

178

It is known from clinical experience that in psychogenic corticovisceral pathology the psyche is not always affected. Similarly, in a neurosis the vegetative resonance may be lacking.

In the interaction of man and the external environment the social factor is in the foreground the biological action of which plays a part in particular via the neocortex. A specifically human stimulus is the verbal stimulus, "the signal of the signal". The morphological substrate of the specifically human so-called second signal system of the CNS are in particular the speech areas of the cerebral cortex. There are reports on the induction of amenorrhoea and the induction of menstruation by hypnotic suggestion (126). Injection of a placebo with a strong suggestive explanation causes endometrial haemorrhage in one third of amenorrhoic women with adequate production of endogenous oestrogens (407).

# HYPOTHALAMIC DISORDERS

The group of hypothalamic disorders of the menstrual cycle comprises — as opposed to corticovisceral disorders with secondary affection of the hypothalamic function — dysfunctions where the noxious factor has primarily damaged the hypothalamus. As regards differential diagnosis we must thus consider the possibility of psychosomatic disease without clinically manifested affection of the psyche, i.e. without neurosis. The symptomatology is the same, the difference is only in the absence of detectable psychic traumatization.

Lesions in primarily hypothalamic dysfunction are only rarely the consequence of classical organic damage (tumour, injury or inflammation). In the great majority idiopathic disorders are involved. This is the case in the majority of common menstrual dysfunctions where we are faced most frequently with a disorder at the level of hypothalamic regulation. In a random sample of 300 women with menstrual dysfunction a 70.3% incidence of hypothalamo-hypophyseal disorders was established (95% confidence limit 64.8–75.4%) (405). Disorders of the hypophyseal reactivity to hypothalamic trigger hormones (LH-RH test), i.e. true hypophyseal insufficiency, accounts only for a fraction of "hypothalamo-hypophyseal" disorders.

This classification, however, also comprised psychogenic corticovisceral disorders and thus the actual incidence of primarily hypothalamic menstrual dysfunction is somewhat lower than the percentage given above. The group of hypothalamic disorders also contains *post-partum so-called partial hypophyseal insufficiency* where the LH-RH test provides evidence of a sufficient functional reserve of gonadotropic secretion of the pituitary.

Schematically we can differentiate between **three pathogenetic groups of disorders of hypothalamic regulatory mechanisms:** (1) isolated disorder of the rhythm with preserved ovulation, (2) disorder of the cyclic control of the secretion of hypophyseal gonadotropins, where the cyclic release of LH and FSH (and ovulation) are lacking but the tonic secretion of gonadotropins is sufficient to maintain the formation of ovarian oestrogens adequate for the proliferation of the endometrium and (3) disorder of the control of tonic secretion of hypophyseal gonadotropins, the ovarian oestrogen production being inadequate (monosymptomatic gonadotropic hypopituitarism). The clinical manifestation of the first type of dysfunction of regulatory mechanisms is ovulatory oligomenorrhoea, of the second type e.g. a complete anovulatory cycle or anovulatory oligomenorrhoea — amenorrhoea with a positive progesterone withdrawal bleeding test or dysfunctional bleeding respectively, and of the third type amenorrhoea with a negative progesterone test.

In addition to secretion of LH-RH/FSH-RH the production of PIF may also be affected and menstrual dysfunction is associated with hyperprolactinaemia and possibly galactorrhoea (see p. 280). Sometimes other hypothalamic regulatory mechanisms are also impaired: in disorders of the menstrual cycle, in particular in oligomenorrhoea or amenorrhoea very frequently (in about one third) obesity is encountered. Postpartal menstrual dysfunction of the hypothalamic type is associated with obesity in about one half of the cases. Clinical experience shows that weight reduction leads also to normalization of the menstrual cycle. Here too we must consider the possibility of corticovisceral pathogenesis and concurrent hypofunctional thyropathy.


## HYPOPHYSEAL DISORDERS

Hypophyseal as compared with hypothalamic disorders of regulation of ovarian activity are very rare. This finding was possible only after using the LH-RH test in menstrual dysfunction.

It seems that direct hypophyseal damage is *post-partum panhypopituitarism* (Sheehan's syndrome) where the LH-RH test is negative, and some other primary hypophyseal disorders which are of minor importance. Idiopathic (essential) hypofunction may include also *autoimmune affection of the adenohypophysis* ("hypophysitis"), most frequently as part of a pluriglandular insufficiency (see p. 200).

The causes of hypophyseal insufficiency may be summarized as follows:
A. primary (idiopathic, essential)
B. secondary
    a) injury or surgical operation
    b) tumours
        aa) primary
        bb) metastatic
    c) vascular disorders

180

aa) Sheehan's syndrome
bb) aneurysm
 d) infectious diseases
   aa) abscess
   bb) granulomatous diseases
   cc) meningitis
 e) systemic diseases
   aa) sarcoidosis
   bb) xanthomatosis
   c) leukaemia, lymphoma

The pathological process may be directly in the pituitary (intrasellar) or in its vicinity (extrasellar).

# GONADAL DISORDERS

In these menstrual dysfunctions the disorder affects primarily, i.e. directly, the ovary. The ovary may be affected at any stage of development or after its completion. Biopsy is decisive for the classification of gonadal disorders.

In disorders of ovarian development we differentiate between the following series: defect — rudiment — hypoplasia (490).

*Defect*, i.e. extremely rare complete absence of ovary (**agonadism**) may result from aplasia (due to the absence of primordial germ cells), agenesis [due to destruction of primordial germ cells, to their inadequate number or poor functional quality when similarly as in aplasia their inducing action on the development of the gonad is lacking (see p. 1–2)] or degeneration (due to disappearance of already existing gonads).

*Rudiment* is in this classification a product of inhibition of prenatal development of the ovary (during the indifferent stage, before differentiation of the rete ovarii, after differentiation of the rete ovarii or later during intrauterine life) where follicles are lacking and only the stroma, indifferent epithelial elements, hilar cells and possibly the rete ovarii are present. This group also comprises dysgenetic gonads.

Absence or morphological alteration with functional insufficieny of the second X-heterochromosome does not prevent migration of primordial germ cells and the transformation of the gonadal primordium, the genital fold, into the ovary. Atresia of the germ cells begins only after three months, as in normal 46,XX foetuses. The amount of ovarian stroma increases, the gradual destruction of germ cells culminates about six months after birth and they disappear only during the period corresponding to puberty. The reason seems to be the inadequacy of follicular cells with following failure of formation of primordial follicles (follicles, however, can rarely be found in the ovary even after birth). The second gonosome (active portion of the heteropyknotic X chromosome) is obviously essential for the development of the normal ovary, for the regulation of atresia of germ cells and oestrogen biosynthesis. The result of this chromosomal aberration is a stripe of fibrous tissue instead of the ovary, so-called **streak gonad** or **dysgenetic gonad.**

*Ovarian hypoplasia* is divided into two groups. In both postnatal inhibition of ovarian growth occurred before sexual maturity was reached; they differ by the lack or presence of primordial and primary follicles:

a) In the first group the ovary is formed above all by the stroma which contains occasional atretic follicles; intact primordial and primary follicles are lacking, but thecal cells, hilar cells and rete ovarii are present.

b) In the second group the ovary contains rare primordial and primary follicles and small growing follicles, while a corpus luteum is always lacking. This ovary is described as **rudimentary anovulatory ovary** (239) or **dysgenetic ovary** (183). We find it in sex chromatin-positive subjects with a karyotype 46,XX or mixoploid subjects with mosaicism which contains the cell line 46,XX (or with one structurally altered chromosome) or 47,XXX.

Sometimes two forms of **ovarian hypoplasia** are differentiated (489) which differ as to the assumed period when the disorder of gonadal development took place:

a) *primary hypoplasia* with a poor germinal parenchyma (a disorder of the gonadal primordium is assumed),

b) *secondary hypoplasia* with a relatively ample germinal parenchyma (a developmental disorder is assumed while the gonadal primordium is normal).

Primary hypoplasia of the ovary is the connecting link with the dysgenetic gonad, its morphological picture corresponds to the rudimentary or dysgenetic ovary described above. Secondary hypoplasia is a transition to the normal ovary.

We assume that some noxious agent can also affect the ovary during the postnatal period, during the whole period from birth to menarche, as well as after sexual maturity has been reached or at any time during adult life. We suggest the possibility of toxiinfectious lesions (see p. 199) and do not rule out a corticovisceral parahypophyseal pathogenesis (see p. 177). However, so far, we know little about the importance of the innervation of the ovary from the physiological and pathophysiological point of view (see p. 25).

A special group of primarily ovarian disorders is formed by autoimmune gonadal damage (see p. 200).

The diagnosis of **primary ovarian disorders** is made possible by the compensatory hypersecretion of hypophyseal gonadotropins induced by the mechanism of inhibitory feedback of oestrogens and the gonadotropin test which will establish the incapacity of the ovary to respond to stimulation by exogenous gonadotropins by increasing oestrogen production. Examination of sex chromatin and assessment of the karyotype is essential.

An objective diagnosis and differentiation of the ovarian defect — rudiment — and hypoplasia is made possible by visualization of the organ (pneumopelvigraphy, pelvic endoscopy or explorative laparotomy) and biopsy of the gonad.

Clinically the primary ovarian disorder is manifested by menstrual dysfunction of the hypofunctional type: primary amenorrhoea or oligomenorrhoea starting at menarche or after a certain period of regular menstrual cycles, changing into secondary amenorrhoea with the symptoms of premature ovarian failure (syndrome of early climacteric and menopause respectively). The degree of affection of the gonad is decisive; extremes are on the one hand dysgenetic gonads and on the other hand hypoplastic ovaries with a relatively ample germinal parenchyma. Either the ovary does not even start the biosynthesis of oestrogens or the germinal epithelium becomes "exhausted" and the ovarian secretory function fails only after a relatively long time, sometimes even after regular menstrual cycles.

## UTERINE DISORDERS

The uterus, its mucosal lining and musculature is the target organ of ovarian hormones *par excellence*. Uterine causes of menstrual dysfunction may be the following:

A. organic:
   a) absence of uterus
   b) occlusion of uterus
   c) absence of endometrium
   d) inflammation of endometrium
   e) submucosal myomas or endometrial polyps

B. functional:
   a) disorders of endometrial sensitivity to ovarian steroids
   b) disorders of endometrial haemocoagulation mechanisms
   c) disorders of myometrial contractility
   d) disorders of postnatal development of the uterus

In rare instances the endometrium is refractory to oestrogens. A reduced sensitivity of the uterine mucosa to oestrogens is observed as a rule in prolonged hypooestrogenic amenorrhoea. It is interpreted as a disorder of the subcellular mechanism of oestrogen action; probably a decline of the concentration of the specific cytoplasmic receptor is involved due to impaired protein synthesis in target cells. Similarly, the sensitivity to progesterone also varies. Obviously a decline in the concentration of the specific cytoplasmic receptor protein is also involved the synthesis of which is stimulated by oestrogens (see p. 113). Most frequently disorders of the reactivity of the endometrium to endogenous ovarian steroids are encountered in **uterine hypoplasia.**

183

Some uterine types physiological in childhood may persist (so-called **hypotrophic uterus**) or a pathological type develops which is described by the term **dystrophic uterus** (395), the typical sign of which is in addition to small size also hyperanteflexion or hyperretroflexion. If complete proportional development of the uterus takes place but the uterus is substantially smaller than that of an adult nulligravida, we speak of hypoplasia.

Most frequently a hypoplastic uterus is diagnosed. The objective criterion, also for uterine hypotrophy and dystrophy, is the result of sounding (to assess the length and ratio between the body and cervix) and hysterography. A hypotrophic uterus is described in the clinical literature most frequently as an **infantile uterus** or uterus of the **intermediate type** (Übergangsuterus) which expresses the intermediate position between a qualitatively normally developed uterus and abnormalities ensuing from fusion of the paired base. In an intermediate uterus the muscular coat of the organ fused, on the hysterogram the uterine cavity has, however, the typical shape of a tricuspid star which corresponds to the two cornus and the corpus; thus, the shape of the uterine cavity of the foetus and neonate persists and it would be more apt to use the term foetal uterus. In the majority of cases this uterus is at the same time quantitatively underdeveloped, markedly smaller than a normal uterus. It is not possible to differentiate by palpation an intermediate uterus from a merely hypoplastic one and hysterography is essential. In addition to the shape of the cavity of the uterine body for the intermediate uterus the ratio of the length of the cervix and body is typical: the cervix predominates over the body, as in the infantile uterus (infantile in the physiological sense), the ratio being at least 1:1. For the characteristic of this disproportion between the uterine body and cervix the so-called uterine index is used (ratio of the length of the uterine body and cervix divided by two); the index is abnormal when it is smaller than 0.75.

Hypoplasia of the uterus is frequently associated with hypoplasia of the ovaries along with the other disorders of uterine development and sterility (according to data reported in 17–34% cases).

The cause of the reduced fertility of women with a hypoplastic uterus even in the presence of an ovulatory cycle is probably the simultaneous developmental defect of the endometrium. In some of these uteri the hyporeactive endometrium of the so-called isthmic type extends much further into the corporal cavity. In the hypotrophic uterus this defect is even more marked and it is quite common in the dystrophic uterus. This functional defect of the endometrium may be the cause of impaired nidation. Imperfect and uneven secretory transformations are typical and in about 3/4 of the cases impaired reactivity of the endometrium during therapeutic pseudopregnancy was demonstrated.

In Germany after the Second World War hypoplasia of the uterus was recorded in as much as 6% of the population of large cities.

A quite exceptional case of impaired endometrial reactivity is so-called **amenorrhoea spuria** where all indicators of ovarian function are normal (the woman is fertile) and the uterine mucosa undergoes typical cyclic changes but menstruation does not occur. The endometrium which undergoes secretory transformation does not desquamate, it is eliminated by regression without bleeding, as in lower primates. This is obviously an isolated disorder of the mechanism of menstruation (see p. 151) and is perhaps an atavism.

# DISORDERS DUE TO DYSFUNCTION
# OF OTHER SYSTEMS

Disorders interfering with the activity of the reproductive system may be summarized as follows:
A. metabolic disorders:
    a) disorders of endocrine function;
        aa) adrenal
        bb) thyroid
        cc) pancreatic
    b) disorders of hepatic function;
B. nutritional disorders:
    a) obesity
    b) malnutrition
C. exhaustive diseases

## DISORDERS OF THE MENSTRUAL CYCLE IN DYSFUNCTION
## OF THE ADRENAL CORTEX

Menstrual dysfunction is associated with hyperfunctional and hypofunctional syndromes of the adrenal cortex. According to Bleha and Küchel (47) we differentiate between:
A. hyperfunctional syndromes of the adrenal cortex:
    a) hypercortisolism:
        aa) primarily adrenal (peripheral)
        bb) secondary:
            $\alpha$) hypothalamo-hypophyseal (central)
            $\beta$) syndrome of ectopic ACTH overproduction
    b) hyperandrogenism (adrenogenital syndrome — AGS):
        aa) prenatal (congenital) AGS
        bb) acquired AGS
    c) hyperoestrogenism
    d) hyperaldosteronism*)
        aa) primary (autonomic) (Conn's syndrome)
        bb) secondary (adaptational)
B. hypofunctional syndromes of adrenal cortex:
    a) acute adrenal insufficiency*)

---

*) Disorders are not associated with menstrual dysfunction.

b) chronic adrenal insufficiency
   aa) primarily adrenal hypocorticalism (Addison's disease)
   bb) secondary hypocorticalism

## MENSTRUAL DYSFUNCTION IN ADRENAL HYPERFUNCTION

**Hypercortisolism.** Hypercortisolism was formerly divided into *Cushing's disease* (in so-called basophil adenoma of the pituitary found in 30–40% of all cases of excessive cortisol secretion) and *Cushing's syndrome* (in adrenal tumours in about 30% of cases of hypercortisolism). The clinical symptomatology includes in addition to typical obesity of the trunk a moon-shaped face, hypertension, adynamia with atrophy and weakness of the muscles, reddish violet striae of the skin, osteoporosis, steroid diabetes and sometimes also hirsutism, and in 30 to 60% of the patients also menstrual dysfunction, i.e. oligomenorrhoea to amenorrhoea. As opposed to hirsutism, the menstrual dysfunction is probably not due to the concomitantly raised production of adrenal androgens. It seems that it is not caused by the formerly assumed concomitant decrease in secretion of hypophyseal gonadotropins. Most probably, it is due to the direct inhibitory action of cortisol on the ovary. [Glucocorticoid receptor protein has been demonstrated recently in rat ovaries (310).]

The basic laboratory examination is the assessment of 17-hydroxycorticoids in urine which is an indirect indicator of cortisol secretion and of its metabolites. The most reliable criterion of cortisol activity is estimation of the free cortisol fraction in urine which reflects the raised levels of circulating free biologically active cortisol. For the differentiation of different types of hypercortisolism dynamic tests with dexamethasone, methopyrapone and ACTH are used (for review see 286, 537a). Retroperitoneal pneumography and an X-ray of the sella turcica are indispensable.

In the case of a confirmed adrenal or pituitary tumour surgical treatment is indicated. In bilateral adrenal hyperplasia the following treatment should be considered: a) with anabolics, b) adrenostatics, c) irradiation of the pituitary, and d) adrenalectomy (for details see special literature).

**Congenital adrenal hyperandrogenism.** The cause of prenatal (congenital) AGS is an inborn, recessive, autosomal adrenal enzymopathy, a defect of cortisol biosynthesis due to enzyme insufficiency: a) of 21-hydroxylase [the conversion of 17α-hydroxyprogesterone into cortexolone is impaired and that of progesterone into cortexone (DOC)], b) of 11β-hydroxylase (the conversion of cortexolone into cortisol and of cortexone into corticosterone is impaired) or c) of 3β-dehydrogenase (the conversion of dehydroepiandrosterone into androstenedione is impaired, and that of 17α-hydroxypregnenolone into 17α-hydroxyprogesterone and pregnenolone into progesterone is also impaired). As a result of a mechanism of inhibitory (negative) feedback hypersecretion of ACTH thus takes place and excessive stimulation of the adrenal cortex which is therefore hyperplastic and produces increased amounts of 17α-hydroxyprogesterone and abnormal steroids, a metabolite of which is, among others, pregnantriol and pregnantriolone excreted in major amounts in the urine. At the same time excessive amounts of androgens are formed (in particular of androstenedione and dehydroepiandrosterone); testosterone is formed mainly by the peripheral conversion of androstenedione. The result is an increased excretion of 17-oxosteroids in urine.

The excessive formation of adrenal androgens and the inadequate production of ovarian oestrogens are decisive for the clinical symptomatology, i.e. primary amenorrhoea and masculinization of the genitalia (pseudohermaphroditismus masculinus externus), its degree depends on the foetal period when androgen hyperproduction began and on its intensity.

**Acquired adrenal hyperandrogenism.** The cause of acquired AGS where the androgenization due to adrenal hyperplasia develops postnatally, usually in adult life, is not so far clear. In the majority of cases an enzyme defect, as encountered in the congenital syndrome, cannot be shown, nor is the biosynthesis of cortisol impaired. The excretion of 17-hydroxycorticoids and pregnantriol is frequently within the normal range or only slightly elevated, as is the excretion of 17-oxosteroids. Pregnantriolone is lacking. An increased sensitivity of the adrenal cortex is assumed, in particular for the biosynthesis of adrenal androgens, to ACTH. A marked reactivity of 17-hydroxycorticoid and pregnantriol excretion to exogenous ACTH is described. A second possibility can, however, not be ruled out, i.e. that hyperplasia of the partially defective adrenal cortex can ensure cortisol production but only along with excessive production of other steroids, i.e. androgens also responsible for the clinical symptomatology.

The symptomatology depends on the degree of adrenal androgenic hyperfunction; it comprises hirsutism, hypertrophy of the clitoris, virile changes of the hair growth, acne, a deeper voice, virilization of body build and oligomenorrhoea to amenorrhoea. From typical virilization a continuous range of stages exists — via so-called mild adrenal hyperplasia ("borderline" AGS) which is difficult to differentiate from the syndrome of polycystic ovaries — to idiopathic hirsutism with a normal menstrual cycle (see p. 165).

*Table 13* Relative antiinflammatory effect of corticoids

| Cortisone | 25 mg | 1 |
|---|---|---|
| Cortisol (hydrocortisone) | 20 mg | 1.25 |
| Prednisone | 5 mg | 5 |
| Prednisolone | 5 mg | 5 |
| Methylprednisolone | 4 mg | 6.25 |
| Triamcinolone | 4 mg | 6.25 |
| Paramethasone | 2 mg | 12.5 |
| Betamethasone | 0.75 mg | 33.3 |
| Dexamethasone | 0.75 mg | 33.3 |

Acquired AGS also comprises androgenization in patients with androgen producing adenomas or malignomas of the adrenal cortex. Virilization then develops rapidly and is intensive. 17–Oxosteroids in urine are markedly raised, as distinct from so-called mild adrenal hyperplasia, where they are only slightly elevated or are at the upper borderline of normal values.

AGS caused by hyperplasia of the adrenal cortex is treated by cortisol substitution. In normal children the daily cortisol production is $12 \pm 3$ mg/sq.m/24 hours, in adults it is estimated to amount to 15–40 mg/24 hours. The initial dose as a rule must be higher for several days or weeks, usually about double. In order to imitate the 24-hour variation of the circulating cortisol level, it should be divided in such a way that 3/4 of the dose are administered in the morning and 1/4 in the afternoon. It is essential to check the 17-oxosteroid excretion, at first always after a few days and later permanently after several weeks. The relative effectiveness of glucocorticoids is given in Table 13. Dexamethasone is suitable because it does not cause sodium retention. (For the total suppression of hypophyseal ACTH secretion a dose of 75 mg/24 hours of cortisone is sufficient. A daily dose higher than 60–75 mg cortisol administered longer than one week causes always adrenal insufficiency lasting several days.)

The criterion of treatment in the congenital form of AGS is feminization, development of female secondary sex characteristics and menarche, in the acquired form of AGS refeminization with restitution of the menstrual cycle. Fertility is preserved even in cases with serious virilizing malformations of the external genitalia, incl. the vagina, which may require surgical correction. When assessing the minimal still effective substitution dose of glucocorticoid, the menstrual cycle again serves as an indicator. Excessive doses involve the danger of the development of a cushingoid habitus, gastroduodenal ulcers, diabetes, osteoporosis and reduced resistance to infections and surgical stress.

For the treatment of borderline AGS it is recommended to administer 2.5 to 10 mg prednisone per day to suppress the urinary 17-oxosteroid values to that between 5 and 10 mg/24 hours. The criterion of effective treatment is a regular ovulatory menstrual cycle. During pregnancy the prednisone dosage has to be adjusted to maintain the 17-oxosteroid excretion within the expected range.

Treatment of adrenal hyperandrogenism (and hyperoestrogenism) caused by a hormonally active benign or malignant adrenal tumour is surgical.

**Adrenal hyperoestrogenism.** Adrenal hyperoestrogenism is extremely rare. The cause is most frequently a hormonally active, oestrogen producing carcinoma of the adrenal cortex. In childhood it causes isosexual pseudopubertas praecox, in adult women irregular and excessive uterine bleeding. The urinary level of total oestrogens is usually markedly raised.


## MENSTRUAL DYSFUNCTION IN ADRENAL HYPOFUNCTION

In chronic adrenal insufficiency with typical adynamia, pigmentation and wasting, and loss to complete disappearance of sexual (in particular axillary) hair the menstrual cycle usually persists; even pregnancy has been described. Oligomenorrhoea and amenorrhoea are usually encountered only in rather advanced forms of the disease.


## DISORDERS OF THE MENSTRUAL CYCLE IN DYSFUNCTION OF THE THYROID GLAND

It is known that between ovarian activity and thyroid function complicated mutual relations exist.

Oestrogens increase the binding capacity of thyroid hormones [triiodothyronine and tetraiodothyronine (thyroxin)] with plasma proteins, stimulate the synthesis of binding globulin, increase the level of protein-bound iodine (PBI) in blood but not the level of circulating free, i.e. biologically effective thyroid hormones (while androgens have the reverse action). The PBI level displays therefore a characteristic relationship with the menstrual cycle and resembles the BBT curve, it is higher during the luteal stage and reaches the maximum during the periovulatory period. During the menstrual cycle, however, the level of circulating thyroxin also changes significantly; during the luteal phase the concentration of total and free plasma thyroxin is lower than in the follicular phase although the concentration of plasma TSH does not vary in the course of the cycle. Some authors therefore speak of the *thyroid cycle*.

Thyroid hormones perhaps also influence the sensitivity of the ovary to gonadotropins. Data are not uniform in this respect; an increased as well as reduced sensitivity of the ovary to gonadotropins has been described. The peripheral oestrogen metabolism in women also changes in relation to thyroid function. In hypothyroidism the ratio of urinary oestriol rises, while it declines in hyperthyroidism. Hyperthyroidism, on the contrary, is associated with a rise in the formation of catecholoestrogens. Administration of thyroid hormones reduces oestriol excretion.


## MENSTRUAL DYSFUNCTION IN HYPOTHYROIDISM

Disorders of the menstrual cycle are reported in as many as 20% of all cases of hypometabolism, and a similar percentage is reported for sterility. Some authors found a predominantly hypofunctional symptomatology, in particular oligomenorrhoea and amenorrhoea, others, on the other hand, emphasize hyperfunctional disorders, menorrhagia and metrorrhagia. In patients with primary hypothyroidism galactorrhoea is frequently present; PRL elevation is highly variable.

Recognition of the pathogenetic role of the thyroid gland is made difficult by the fact that in addition to *thyroid hypometabolism (hypothyroidism)* there exist also cases of so-called *peripheral hypometabolism* where the production of thyroid hormones is normal but "utilization" in target tissues lags behind. In those cases common tests of thyroid function have normal values. Differentiation is based mainly on clinical symptomatology (in the following order by the incidence of symptoms: chronic fatigue, dry and brittle hair, possibly loss of hair, nervousness and irritability, dry skin, distension of the abdomen, hypersensitivity to cold, etc.) and assessment of BM.

In juvenile hypothyroidism precocious puberty is described (see p. 169).

Recently the empirical treatment of anovulation, in particular in sterility, was greatly expanded by the administration of thyroid hormones. The results are, however, not statistically conclusive (for review see 278). Unless confirmed hypothyroidism or peripheral hypometabolism are involved, this treatment is not justified.

For treatment of hypothyroidism thyroxin, triiodothyronine and dried thyroid

*Table 14*  Substitution therapy in hypothyroidism (67)

| | Mean daily complete substitution dose | Latency of clinical effect after onset of administration | Persistence of effect after discontinued administration |
|---|---|---|---|
| Thyroxin | 0.10–0.20 mg | 4 days | 10 days |
| Triiodothyronine | 0.06–0.12 mg | 1/4–3 days | 5 days |
| Dried thyroid | 60–180 mg | 4 days | 10 days |

preparations are suitable. Average complete substitution doses, the latency of the effect and its persistence after discontinued medication are summarized in Table 14. In menstrual dysfunction we usually start with one quarter doses which are gradually increased till a clinical effect is obtained which also takes the patient's reaction into account. The aim is the total suppression of the mentioned symptoms; signs of overdosage are tachycardia, palpitations, tremor, nervousness, insomnia, diarrhoea and loss of weight. Thyroid replacement therapy improves also secondary endocrine abnormities as above-mentioned galactorrhoea and hyperprolactinaemia.

## MENSTRUAL DYSFUNCTION IN HYPERTHYROIDISM

If hyperthyroidism is associated with menstrual dysfunction, it is most frequently oligomenorrhoea and amenorrhoea; sterility has also been recorded as well as a tendency to abort.

In juvenile hyperthyroidism, which is extremely rare, delayed menarche is described (see p. 17 and 175).

Treatment of hyperthyroidism must be supervised by a specialist.

## DISORDERS OF THE MENSTRUAL CYCLE IN DISEASES OF THE PANCREAS

Pancreatic functions also display a certain relationship with the menstrual cycle. The glucose tolerance of healthy women declines before menstruation; in diabetic women this change is even more marked, therefore decompensation is more frequent in the premenstrual period. It seems that oestrogens have a certain hypoglycaemic effect, an increased peripheral glucose utilization is assumed. It depends on intact liver function (for review see 550).

Premenstrual exacerbations of symptoms of pancreatitis are described. In compensated diabetes nowadays menstrual dysfunction is not one of the common symptoms of the disease and the ability to become pregnant is also not impaired in these women. (It is of interest that formerly menstrual dysfunction was found in as many as 40% of diabetic women.)

In diabetic women with amenorrhoea we must also consider secondary extrapancreatic diabetes. The combination with hirsutism and obesity is described as *Achard-Thiers syndrome*. It is a variant of acquired AGS with hyperandrogenism and concomitant hypercortisolism, caused by adenoma or hyperplasia of the adrenal cortex. Evidence of the secondary character of diabetes is the disappearance of the diabetic syndrome after cure of the basic disease.

In juvenile diabetes delayed menarche is found (40, 87, 541) and in extreme cases of inadequate insulin treatment of diabetes in childhood also sexual retardation may be a feature of diabetic infantilism (see p. 15 and 173).

## DISORDERS OF THE MENSTRUAL CYCLE IN LIVER DISEASES

The liver breaks down and inactivates oestrogens and in the liver conjugation of oestrogens with glucuronic and sulphuric acid takes place as well as protein binding; oestrogens are secreted by the bile as part of their enterohepatic circulation (for review see 110, 286, 537a). In chronic liver diseases this hepatic activity lags behind and therefore in the organism the active oestrogen concentration rises. A raised total oestrogen excretion in the urine and hyperoestrogenic disorders of the menstrual cycle were found. However, in the same way as no constant relationship exists between bilirubinaemia and the concentration of total oestrogens in urine, there is no unequivocal symptomatology of disorders: in chronic liver diseases manifestations of oestrogenic insufficiency are sometimes also described. Obviously not only the extent but also the type of damage of the hepatic parenchyma plays a part (for review see 550).

## DISORDERS OF THE MENSTRUAL CYCLE IN NUTRITIONAL DISORDERS

According to recent reports there probably exists an interrelation between energy homeostasis and the reproductive function of females.

The amount of energy stored in the organism as fat at the age corresponding to the period of completed adolescence corresponds roughly to 100,000 cal (418,700 J) and is a reserve for about one month of starvation. It is, no doubt, a certain atavism, an adaptation to long intervals of starvation between periods with excess food and increased energy output during intensive muscular work. Under contemporary living conditions with sufficient food and minimal muscular strain this adaptation is not needed. It seems, however, that impairment of this energy balance, in particular a diminution of the fat depot, or the reverse, is often the cause of menstrual dysfunction. Restoration of the equilibrium is the prerequisite of normalization of the menstrual cycle and ovulation.


## MENSTRUAL DYSFUNCTION IN MALNUTRITION

From experiments with laboratory rodents it is known that malnutrition leads to arrest of the ovarian cycle and atrophy of the ovaries. The same occurs on a protein deficient diet. The ovaries, however, do not lose the ability to respond to exogenous gonadotropins. Because the gonadotropin content of the pituitary in these animals does not decline, obviously their secretion is diminished. Malnutrition interferes thus with the production of hypothalamic trigger hormones. In primates malnutrition probably also damages the hypothalamo-hypophyseal trigger mechanism. In malnourished children with cystic fibrosis typical release of STH after insulin-induced hypoglycaemia and after arginine infusion does not occur; the reaction is restored after treatment leading to a weight increment.

Secondary amenorrhoea is one of the main symptoms in anorexia nervosa (see p. 251). Amenorrhoea also develops, however, after a less drastic body weight loss achieved on purpose by an exaggerated reducing diet in women who do not suffer from anorexia (295). Amenorrhoea as a rule persists for a certain period even after discontinuation of the diet and after normal body weight has been regained. Similarly as in anorexia nervosa the cause of the impaired menstrual cycle is probably the weight loss itself. It is reported (160) that already a loss of 10–15% body weight, i.e. in particular loss of body fat, is usually associated with amenorrhoea. It is therefore assumed that for normal ovulatory function of the female a certain minimum reserve of readily mobilized energy is needed. Moreover, the decline of body weight is associated with a change in the oestrogen metabolism: the 2-hydroxylation of oestradiol, i.e. the formation of catechol-oestrogens which probably act as endogenous antioestrogens rises (see p. 18).

A surprising finding is that in women with mental anorexia after a decline of the body weight below 46 kg the gonadotropin release after administration of LH-RH is minimal or altogether absent (387). Thus, reduction of body weight beneath a certain critical borderline interferes with the gonadotropin reserve of pituitary cells. It is very interesting that this critical weight is close to the critical weight for attaining menarche (see p. 17).

There are two basic types of obesity (adiposity), depending on the predominating manner of fat deposition in adipose tissue. Either it involves an increase in the number of fat cells in adipose tissue or an increase in the storage capacity of fat cells and their subsequent enlargement (for review see 43).

The number of fat cells depends on genetic factors (constitution) and epigenetic ones, i.e. the action of nutritional factors (chronic overeating) during a certain critical period, probably even during early childhood, and may be, also during the prenatal period (e.g. "overfeeding" of the foetus in diabetic foetopathy with embryomegaly). The number of fat cells becomes stabilized only after the age of 20 years. In women it is about 40 billions. An increased number of fat cells, no doubt, involves an increased hazard of the development of obesity.

The size of fat cells depends on the content of accumulated triglycerides and is determined by the caloric balance of the organism. The size of fat cells is a variable factor which in adults conditions changes in body weight and the amount of fat rather than the number of fat cells. An important pathogenetic factor is overeating caused by impaired hypothalamic regulation of appetite.

The sex-specific distribution of subcutaneous fat in women is in particular due to an increased number of fat cells in certain areas, especially in the abdominal and femoral area and enlarged fat cells in particular in the femorogluteal area. The specific action of oestrogens and androgens is obviously also associated with the described gynoid and android type of female obesity. Glucocorticoids also influence fat distribution (typical obesity in hypercortisolism).

In developed obesity the fat cells are enlarged and at the same time their number is increased. In the initial stage of obesity in particular the size of fat cells is altered, and with the advancing development of obesity their number steadily increases. We can therefore differentiate between a) *hypertrophic obesity* where enlargement of the fat cells is in the foreground and b) *hyperplastic obesity* where as a rule their number is increased and c) *the mixed type of obesity* which is probably most frequent.

Another classification of obesity differentiates between two basic types: a) *regulatory obesity* and b) *metabolic obesity*. While regulatory obesity develops as a result of dysfunction of regulatory mechanisms, e.g. hypothalamic, psychogenic, etc., metabolic obesity is due to an inborn error of fat metabolism. This form of obesity is called triglyceridosis (triglyceride-storage disease) (166).

Metabolic aspects of the genesis of obesity, in particular the role of insulin (secondary hyperinsulinism with a decline of the concentration of tissue receptors for insulin and raised proinsulin levels), hyperphagia and physical load are the subject of many investigations. A disorder of the dynamic balance between lipolysis in fat cells and their antagonists, prostaglandins, is also blamed, as insulin inhibits

193

their formation in adipose tissue. Obesity is probably a mixture of different syndromes. The number of fat cells in adults is a static factor which forms a non--metabolic basis for the action of metabolic (pathological) factors which decide on the replenishment of the stable "reserve". Although a negative caloric balance under strictly controlled conditions is always effective, the problem of obesity cannot be reduced only to the question of "strong will" (43).

A relatively large proportion of obese women suffer from menstrual dysfunction, in particular oligomenorrhoea and amenorrhoea (as much as 46% according to data reported). In women with extreme obesity we may even find marked ovarian changes: thickening of the tunica albuginea, increased luteinization of atretic follicles, a reduced number of maturing normal follicles and corpora lutea, an increase of atypically maturing follicles and corpora albicantia. A tendency to declining FSH secretion and a rise in LH was observed.

The enzymes of subcutaneous adipose tissue participate in the peripheral metabolism of androgens and oestrogens. The extent of extraglandular aromatization of plasma androstenedione to oestrone is greater in obese than in both young and postmenopausal women with normal weight. The increase of extraglandular androgen aromatase activity found in obese women contributes towards the increased rate of peripheral oestrone formation. Also the oestrogen metabolism changes with a rise of body weight (see p. 18). The urinary androsterone and androsterone/etiocholanolone ratio is significantly higher in obese women. The above findings may be related to frequent cases of menstrual dysfunction and/or slight hirsutism observed in these women.

The above-mentioned facts explain the clinical experience that reduction of body weight leads to normalization of the menstrual cycle without treatment with ovarian steroids in practically half of the obese women.


## DISORDERS OF THE MENSTRUAL CYCLE
## IN EXHAUSTIVE DISEASES

Serious diseases with alteration of the general condition are as a rule associated with hypofunctional menstrual dysfunction. We assume that a part is played by the marked decline in body weight and diminished fat reserves, as in malnutrition. In bacterial infectious diseases (e.g. typhoid fever or tuberculosis before the period of chemotherapy and antibiotics) or in virus diseases (e.g. influenza) toxiinfectious impairment of the function of hypothalamic regulatory areas may also play a part, if we can rule out — in tuberculosis — direct damage of the endometrium or ovaries. Impairment of the hypothalamic regulatory function is more probable than the direct action of bacterial enzymes or the influenza virus on gonadotropins.

# DISORDERS OF THE MENSTRUAL CYCLE WITH NORMAL OVARIAN FUNCTION

Ovulation and normal function of the corpus luteum as a criterion of ovarian function and the regulatory hypothalamo-hypophyseal system may be preserved in some menstrual dysfunctions of the hypo- and hyperfunctional type.

In these instances a central disorder of the ovarian cycle is most probably involved with shortening or protraction of the follicular phase followed by a normal luteal phase. The clinical manifestation is polymenorrhoea or conversely oligomenorrhoea with preserved ovulation. Or the cause of the impaired menstrual cycle is peripheral hypomenorrhoea or hypermenorrhoea, again with preserved ovulation and normal function of the corpus luteum. The extreme finding is the formerly mentioned amenorrhoea spuria where regression of the endometrium with secretory transformation without menstruation occurs.

A transient group are cases where ovulation, however, is preserved, the function of the corpus luteum is impaired and this disorder can be detected only by detailed examination. This occurs e.g. in luteal insufficiency in functional sterility (see p. 256) or irregular shedding of the transformed endometrium in menorrhagia (see p. 301).

Menstrual dysfunction with preserved ovarian activity also comprises ovulatory haemorrhage, dysmenorrhoea and the syndrome of premenstrual tension which are discussed separately.

# Aetiological Classification of Disorders of the Menstrual Cycle

## ESSENTIAL DISORDERS

In the majority of menstrual dysfunctions the aetiological factor, i.e. the primary factor which triggers the pathogenetic process manifested finally by clinical symptomatology, unfortunately escapes our recognition so far. We speak therefore of essential (idiopathic) disorders.

This applies in particular to hypothalamic disorders of the control of the menstrual cycle which are most frequent. In our clinical material we recorded about 60% of so-called hypothalamo-hypophyseal dysfunctions (405). After introduction of the LH-RH test into clinical practice we know that disorders of the hypophyseal reactivity to RH account only for a fraction of the cases. Although the above percentage also included all possible corticovisceral and suprahypothalamic disorders resp., the real frequency of which is not known, we assume that dysfunctions of the hypothalamic regulation of ovarian activity are most frequent among other pathogenetic mechanisms of disorders of the menstrual cycle.

These so-called hypothalamo-hypophyseal dysfunctions comprise a remarkable group of primary disorders which start shortly after menarche and follow immediately after the period of physiological variability of the menstrual cycle. They account for 40%, i.e. about 25% of all disorders of the menstrual cycle altogether (405).

We assume therefore that in these most frequent menstrual dysfunctions the role of aetiological factor is played by the complication of a certain pathological process (or rather processes) which affects a large proportion of the female population. The high incidence of primary menstrual dysfunctions suggests that the noxious agent frequently affects the hypothalamic regulatory area even before the menarche. We expressed the hypothesis (405) on the interference of the aetiological factor either during the prenatal period within the critical period of sexual differentiation of the hypothalamus (see p. 9) or during the postnatal period before mechanisms of the stimulatory (positive) oestrogen feedback start to act.

It is assumed that in the aetiopathogenesis of some disorders of the menstrual cycle the following may participate:

(1) Failure of mechanisms which protect the foetal CNS against the action of high oestrogen concentrations circulating in the foetus (428) and these oestrogens are able to masculinize paradoxically the female hypothalamus during the period of foetal neuronal competence:

a) pathological situations which interfere with progesterone production during pregnancy;

b) disorders of the specific oestrogen binding in foetal plasma (in man TEBG); in contrast to rat, human α-foetoprotein lacks the ability to bind oestrogens;

c) disorders of the foetal oestrogen metabolism (liver production of oestetrol, acting as physiological antioestrogen).

(2) Pathological situations which increase hCG production and/or disorders of hypothetical mechanisms which protect the foetus and its CNS against the action of hCG.

(3) So-called trivial virus infections of childhood which as a rule inapparently affect also the CNS.

Not even secondary menstrual dysfunctions which start at different intervals after regular menstrual cycles or pregnancy do not rule out the aetiopathogenetic role of a harmful interference even with the very early development of hypothalamic regulatory mechanisms. Experiments on laboratory rodents proved the existence of a so-called delayed anovulatory syndrome, which develops only after a certain period of regular ovarian cycles and fertility.

If the concept governing the sexual differentiation of the hypothalamus (see p. 9) found in laboratory rodents is generally valid and thus also decisive in primates, then some essential (idiopathic) menstrual dysfunctions and cases of anovulatory sterility could be the late consequence of a harmful interference with the early development of hypothalamic mechanisms and/or morphofunctional structures controlling the ovarian cycle.

# GENETIC DISORDERS

Some of the most severe disorders of the menstrual cycle are the manifestation of *chromosomal or genome mutation* affecting the pair of X gonosomes. It is an intra-chromosomal structural mutation, i.e. a chromosomal aberration of the deletion type (46,Xx), of the isochromosome (46,Xi), ring chromosome (46,Xr) or fragmentation (46,Xf) or aneuplodia in monosomia 45,XO or polysomia (triple--tetra- or penta-) X (47,XXX, 48,XXXX, 49,XXXXX). The abnormal karyotype may be pure or a chromosomal mosaic is present.

The finding of autosomal aberrations (deletion type) in autosomes No. 1, 2 and 3 in some menstrual dysfunctions calls for confirmation.

Chromosomal and genome mutations develop most frequently as gametic mutations, i.e. in gametes, in particular during meiosis (non-disjunction of homologous chromosomes, etc.). The karyotype of the individual is then uniform. When they develop only during mitotic division in the blastomere as somatic mutations, then a mosaic is formed with the mutated cell line and the normal cell line. In mutations of one blastomere during the first division the ratio of the two lines is 1:1. The later during development of the zygote mitotic non-disjunction occurs, the smaller the ratio of the mutated cell line to the normal line and the smaller the phenotypic effect of this genome mutation.

The causes of these mutations, i.e. the aetiological factors proper, are not clear. The presence of "spontaneous" mutations without a detectable external cause and mutations caused by radiation or chemical mutagens is assumed. From the heuristic aspect observations on the infectious, and in particular the viral agent, causing chromosomal changes in cellular infections are very useful. Isolated fragments of chromosomes and changes in the number of chromosomes were described. Such a foetal affection is particularly serious during the organogenetic period of embryogenesis. The mutagenic action of viruses may affect the gamete cells as well as somatic cells.

*Gene mutation* causes lack of sensitivity of peripheral target tissues of the 46,XY individual to testicular androgens; this causes the syndrome of testicular feminization (see p. 297). The appropriate gene locus is on the gonosome X (376); the disorder is inherited as X-gonosomal recessive or rather as autosomal dominating, bound to the male sex if the locus is on the autosome.

In the classification of inborn menstrual dysfunctions in phenotypic women with developed female genitalia we adhere to Jirásek (239):

A. pathological combination of gonosomes without disorders of the intrauterine development of gonads and efferent pathways (polysomia X);

B. defective development of gonads and efferent pathways
   a) with disorders of gonosomes (gonadal dysgenesis),
   b) without disorders of gonosomes (pure gonadal dysgenesis);

C. defective differentiation of efferent pathways in enzyme blocks
   a) with inadequate peripheral sensitivity to androgens (testicular feminization),
   b) with inadequate secretion of foetal androgens (androgen-sensitive male pseudohermaphroditism);

D. isolated disorders of the development of gonads and efferent pathways without disorders of gonosomes (gonadal dysgenesis, aplasia of vagina and uterus).


# TOXIINFECTIOUS DISORDERS

The aetiopathogenetic action of an infectious agent in the development of some disorders of the menstrual cycle is probable. We found e.g. a significantly higher incidence of epidemic parotitis during the period before menarche in women with future menstrual dysfunction than in the control group of pregnant women (406). Similarly, the anamnestic prevalence of this disease was significantly higher in infertile women than in pregnant women. The significantly greater accumulation of primary hypothalamo-hypophyseal disorders of regulation in women who suffered as children from epidemic parotitis as compared with women with menstrual dysfunction who did not contract the disease, is of interest (406). We assume therefore that inapparent affection of the hypothalamus (latent viral encephalitis) associated with this disease of childhood is more important in the pathogenesis of future menstrual dysfunction than e.g. concomitant oophoritis. We fear that not only infections with the parotitis myxovirus but also other so-called trivial virus infections of childhood may play the part of an aetiological agent of future disorders of the menstrual cycle.

The mechanism of action of the infectious agent is, no doubt, extremely complicated and obviously may differ from one case to another. We assume that in infectious diseases (in particular virus infections) the following may theoretically play a part:

a) primary affection of the hypothalamus
b) primary affection of the ovary
c) impaired energy balance of the organism due to a marked reduction of body weight and sub-cutaneous fat reserves (see p. 192)
d) impaired autotolerance and development of autoimmune disease
e) chromosomal or genome mutation (see p. 198)
f) gonadotropin inactivation (see p. 194).

# DISORDERS OF IMMUNOLOGICAL AUTOTOLERANCE

There are two basic groups of impaired autotolerance which result in autoimmunization, i.e. an immune reaction against antigens of the organism itself when the pathological immune reaction (autoimmune or autoaggressive reaction) damages various organs and tissues (for review see 370). These groups comprise the following:

A. primary pathological changes of a tissue- or organ-specific antigen ("*disturbed--antigen*" *disease*):

   a) protein altered by virus, specific antigen (e.g. a proteohormone) penetrates into the internal environment of the organism and causes an immune reaction; crossed immunity then damages organs or tissues;
   b) antigenic components of some species of bacteria are identical with components present in some normal tissues; crossed immunity damages organs or tissues of the organism;

B. primary pathological change of lymphoid system and immunoreactivity ("*disturbed-tolerance*" *disease*):

   a) heredo-familial tendency to develop clones of immunocytes which interfere with the immunological tolerance by creating an immune reaction against its own organ or tissue;
   b) autotolerance of T-cells (thymus dependent lymphocytes) impaired by viral or bacterial infection; under normal conditions these cells implement the cell-mediated immune reactions.

## AUTOIMMUNE DAMAGE OF THE OVARY AND ADENOHYPOPHYSIS

Among autoaggressive diseases for gynaecological endocrinology *autoimmune polyendocrinopathy* (pluriglandular insufficiency, Schmidt's syndrome) is of importance. It involves damage of two or more endocrine glands. In particular Hashimoto's thyroiditis and so-called primary (idiopathic) non-tuberculous cytotoxic insufficiency of the adrenal cortex may be associated with an ovarian lesion. Of particular interest are cases where "hypophysitis" was also described and we may thus consider primary as well as secondary failure of ovarian function.

Amenorrhoea may be primary or secondary, as a rule it is clinically manifested as a premature ovarian failure. Contemporary opportunities for the differentiation of circulating antibodies from steroid producing cells are imperfect. Antibodies react not only with cells of the internal theca and corpus luteum of the ovary but also with Leydig cells of the testes, and with cells of the trophoblast and adrenal cortex. Isolated autoimmune damage of the ovary is perhaps rare, although such cases were described. In some women with the syndrome of premature ovarian failure in addition to an antinuclear factor in particular antibodies against the cytoplasm of the ovum were detected. Conversely, only circulating antithyroid antibodies and antibodies against the gastric mucosa were also detected in some women with a pure premature ovarian failure without detectable autoimmune disease. Recently, however, it has been also possible in these instances to detect antiovarian antibodies (90a). It is assumed that in some cases the syndrome of premature menopause may be due to an altered immunoreactivity. The hypothesis was expressed that also the physiological (normal) menopause is an autoimmune process.

## AUTOIMMUNE DAMAGE OF MEIOSIS OR MITOSIS

It is remarkable that in some women with gonadal dysgenesis in addition to the most frequently detectable, i.e. antithyroid antibodies, antibodies against the cytoplasm of oocytes are also found. Antithyroid antibodies are found more frequently in cases with monosomia 45,X0 than in cases with a normal karyotype.

The fact that the titre of organ specific antibodies is not directly proportional to the severity of the disorder and that antibodies are also found in clinically healthy parents, in particular mothers and siblings, suggests that the cause is rather genetic, a heredo-familial disposition to impaired autotolerance where antibodies are a secondary manifestation.

Therefore among the three theoretical possibilities:
a) autoimmunity induces chromosomal aberration
b) chromosomal aberration is the cause of autoimmunity
c) an unknown aetiological factor is the cause of both autoimmunity and chromosomal aberration, we can probably rule out the second alternative. The hypothesis of the autoimmune mechanism of the development of defective meiosis or mitosis seems most plausible.

# PSYCHOGENIC DISORDERS

In psychogenic disorders of the menstrual cycle and in sterility the following sexual and non-sexual factors play an aetiological role:
a) new social situation
b) dramatic events (i.e. acute traumatization)
c) complicated emotional situations (i.e. chronic traumatizations).

This includes e.g. a) changes of the environment (in particular in adolescents), b) fear of unwanted pregnancy, loss of the beloved partner (refusal or death), mental "shock", c) desire for a child, erotic conflict (sexual maladjustment), conflict in family — divorce, illness etc.

Psychic trauma (see p. 177) has not only an emotional aspect but in humans an intellectual component also, which on the background of the development of personality conditions the trend of the emotion, its intensity and possibly also its elimination. Decisive is thus the individual experience of the provoking situation, its intellectual processing and perception.

# NUTRITIONAL AND METABOLIC DISORDERS

Under our living conditions probably only in exceptional instances isolated qualitative deficiencies of food composition are encountered and thus disorders of the menstrual cycle due to hypophyseal or gonadal dysfunction caused by deficiency of ascorbic acid, vitamin A, vitamin B complex and vitamin E are of little practical importance. It is, however, beyond doubt that vitamin deficiencies may be involved as part of the adverse action of malnutrition (see p. 192). In the majority of cases, however, the volitional factor (see p. 192) or psychic trauma inducing mental anorexia plays the aetiological part (see p. 251). Factors causing severe chronic diseases with exhaustion are involved less frequently (see p. 194).

# FUNCTIONAL DISORDERS OF OTHER ENDOCRINE GLANDS

In the pathogenesis of menstrual dysfunctions disorders of the adrenals, thyroid and pancreas are involved (see p. 185, 188 and 190). The aetiology of these disorders which in some instances exert an adverse secondary effect on the function of the system hypothalamus–pituitary–ovary is equally complicated as in primary disorders of the reproductive system and equally obscure. We refer therefore to special literature (for review see 286, 537a).

# Clinical Diagnosis of Disorders
# of the Menstrual Cycle

## BASAL BODY TEMPERATURE

Assessment of the basal temperature curve is one of the fundamental dynamic tests of ovarian function. It provides information on the presence or absence of corpus luteum function and thus also on the time of ovulation. Its experimental and clinical value is extensive (for review see 117).

The rectal temperature is considered most accurate, while least accurate and thus least suitable is the axillary temperature. With increasing frequency the oral temperature is assessed, sometimes by special thermometers. The basal temperature in the morning reveals the most marked differences, however, the temperature in the evening is also useful. The body temperature in the afternoon is less suited for the investigation of the biphasic phenomenon.

The standard of curves depends on the knowledge, and cooperation of the patients and on the recording of all intercurrent factors which influence the temperature. 2–10% of the curves cannot be evaluated according to experience reported in the literature. A curve recorded for six months has full diagnostic value, the minimum time of assessment is three months, and the preferable period eight months, depending on the purpose.

It is assumed that the cause of the biphasic shape of the basal temperature is the thermogenetic action of progesterone as in amenorrhoic women and in women after the menopause as well as in animals it is possible to induce its rise by progesterone or new synthetic gestagens. Conversely by administration of oestrogens the basal temperature declines. The thermogenetic action of progesterone is, however, most probably not direct and is mediated via the hypothalamus, as after the concomitant administration of 0.3 g phenobarbital and 20 mg progesterone per day the basal temperature did not rise. The impaired interaction at the hypothalamic level where the centre for thermoregulation is located may explain the low basal temperature during the secretory action of progesterone on the endometrium. Conversely there are observations of a raised basal temperature during a zero or inadequate secretory response of the endometrium. To raise the basal temperature a smaller amount of progesterone suffices (10 mg/day for a period of 5 days) than for the secretory action on the endometrium. Recently a hypothesis was expressed on the mediated effect of progesterone by means of amines (552).

Norepinephrine is known as a thermogenetic factor from animal experiments and humans. Its investigation in the course of seven cycles revealed significant differences of values between the phase of a low and high basal temperature (7.5–18.3 μg/24 hours, as compared with 14.7–51.5 μg//24 hours). In anovulatory cycles these differences were not found. It may be assumed that oestrogens stimulate the accumulation of norepinephrine on synapses, progesterone causes its release into the blood stream, acts on the thermoregulatory centre in the hypothalamus and raises the basal temperature. This hypothesis needs confirmation.

## EVALUATION OF THE BASAL BODY TEMPERATURE CURVE

The normal basal temperature curve during the cycle is biphasic (Fig. 27). The mean during the proliferation phase is 36.7°C, during the secretory phase 37.1°C; the mean rise during the ovulation period is 0.4°C (0.3–0.7°C), when the rectal temperature is measured. Oral and vaginal readings are by 0.2–0.3°C lower. The period of the raised basal temperature is described as the hyperthermic phase and lasts on average 13 days (10–16). It is much more stable than the period of low temperature during the proliferative phase which, depending on the length of the cycle, persists for seven days to several weeks. If the raised basal temperature persists for more than 16 or 18 days, it is probably due to pregnancy. The rise of temperature during the cycle should take place within two days, there are, however, great variations. The Expert Committee of WHO defined in 1967 as significant a rise of at least 0.2°C which takes place within 48 hours and persists for at least three days, as compared with the previous six-day lower temperature. A decline before the rise which originally determined the day of ovulation occurs only in 9–33% of all cases. The classical rise within 1–3 days from a low to a high temperature was recorded in 38%, a step-wise rise taking more than two days in 39%, and the rise could not be precisely assessed in 14%. In the normal population of healthy young women we found 83% biphasic and 17% monophasic curves.

## RELATIONSHIP OF BASAL BODY TEMPERATURE TO OTHER CRITERIA

The correlation of the rise of basal temperature with parameters related to ovulation is very important for the assessment of the day of ovulation. Most important was the comparison with the condition of the ovary on operation, i.e. **histological dating of the corpus luteum.** Older data report ovulation 0–4 days or 2–3 days after the rise of temperature. However, in 10 women where on operation a corpus luteum younger than 24 hours was found, no constant relationship with the basal

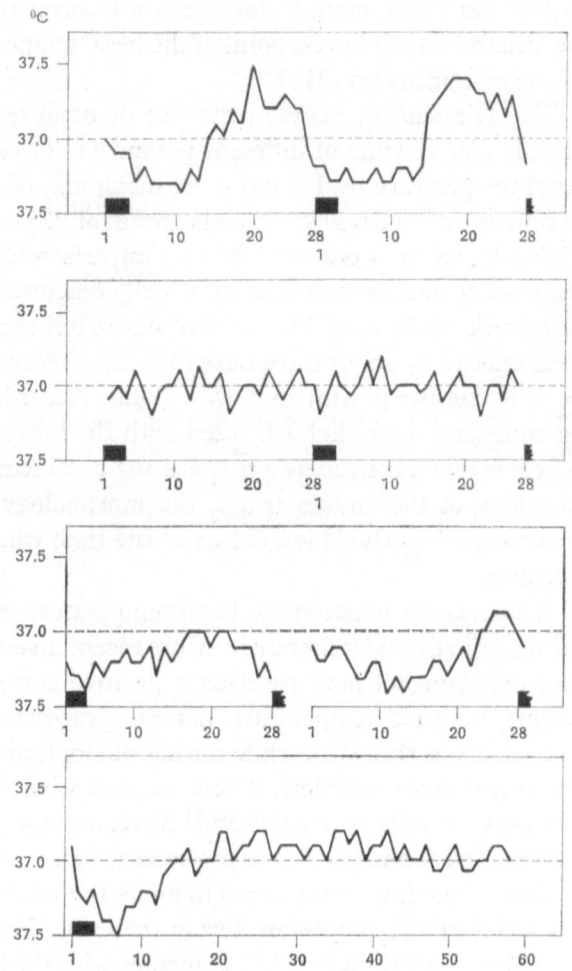

*Fig. 27.* Basal body temperature curves (normal biphasic, monophasic, inadequate or short luteal phase, pregnancy).

temperature was established. Conversely in eight other women a close correlation was recorded between the dated corpus luteum and the distance from the lowest point of basal temperature (r = 0.96); the mean distance of this point from the corpus luteum on the day of ovulation, dated according to Corner, was —0.75 days (313).

The majority of authors evaluated comparisons of the basal temperature with the **histology of the endometrium.** With the hyperthermic phase correspond signs of secretion and a positive response to glycogen, unless interference of the hypothalamus is involved. The onset of the secretory phase with the lowest point of the basal temperature was consistent within a range of ±2 days in 81% of cases. Similarly in other investigation (38) on the first day of the rise of basal temperature onset of secretion was observed in more than half the women and on the fourth day

205

in 100% of 179 women. A close statistical correlation (r = 0.93) was found between the distance of the lowest point of the basal temperature from biopsy and the dating of the endometrium (313).

The relationship between the rise of basal temperature and **cervical mucus** reveals that maxima of different parameters of cervical mucus precede the rise of basal temperature by 1–3 days, the maximum of mucus and minimum dry weight of mucus by 2–3 days (38), the maximum of "Spinnbarkeit" on average by 2.5 days.

Similar results were obtained by comparison of the rise of basal temperature and the peak of **oestrogens** in urine which coincided or preceded the maximum values of cervical indicators. The peak of oestrogen excretion preceded the rise of basal temperature by about three days (38). More recently it has been reported that this peak is consistent with its lowest point. According to more recent work plasma oestrone and oestradiol coincided with the lowest point of the basal temperature. There is thus a coincidence between the basal temperature, the oestradiol level, the histology of the endometrium, the morphology of the corpus luteum and LH secretion (313). Ovulation occurs at the time when the preovulatory peak of LH declines.

A correlation between the basal temperature with **pregnanediol** is reported in paricular in the older literature. More recent investigations of plasma **progesterone** and pregnanediol have revealed a positive correlation with phases of the cycle: during biphasic temperature normal progesterone secretion and pregnanediol excretion was recorded, while during monophasic temperature curves the levels of the two steroids were low. There are data where in ovulatory cycles confirmed by the peak of LH, oestradiol and correponding progesterone values monophasic curves were found in 20% of the cases (337).

One of the important correlations is the relationship of basal temperature and the **peak of LH secretion** during the cycle. From numerous recent publications we know that the peak of LH coincides with the lowest point before the rise of the basal temperature, sometimes quite variably (344), in other instances relatively accurately (313). As by comparison of LH secretion after 8- to 12-hour intervals with dating of the corpus luteum after laparotomy the peak of LH was determined to be 12 to 24 hours before ovulation (140), the coincidence of the lowest point of the basal temperature before its rise with the peak of LH secretion implies a time corresponding to one day before ovulation.

As is apparent, there is no uniformity in this respect and it is not possible to assess accurately the relationship of the basal temperature curve and ovulation. Some assume that ovulation occurs two days before the rise of the basal temperature, others one day before the rise, i.e. at the time of the lowest point of the basal temperature, while the majority assume that it occurs on the first day of the rise of basal temperature. This reflects the obvious variability of this criterion.

# CLINICAL IMPORTANCE OF BASAL BODY TEMPERATURE

The clinical importance of the basal temperature curve is extensive.

(1) We use it to assess approximately the **day of ovulation in healthy women** in order a) to determine the optimum time of conception, b) to prevent conception, c) to select the suitable time for insemination, d) to assess the time of delivery.

ad a) The *optimum for conception* is according to clinical experience about two days before the rise of basal temperature. Based on 91 conceptions after a single cohabitation in the cycle, this optimum was assessed as 2.7 days, other authors shift it, however, with regard to ovulation to one day preceding the rise of the basal temperature, to the time of maximum "Spinnbarkeit" of the cervical mucus and the oestrogen maximum resp. Use of the thus assessed optimum eliminates a part of the so-called unexplained sterility of otherwise healthy women.

ad b) *Prevention of conception.* The assessed optimum is used to determine the so-called infertile days (thermometer method — see p. 349). The first infertile period starts two days after the rise of the basal temperature and is terminated by menstruation, and the second lasts from the end of menstruation to the period of 6 days before the earliest assessed rise of the basal temperature.

ad c) *The time of insemination* is selected according to the conception optimum.

ad d) By assessing the fertilizing cohabitation and onset of pregnancy by means of basal temperatures it is much easier to calculate the *time of delivery* and duration of pregnancy resp. This is usually the case in pregnancies after clomiphene or gonadotropin treatment.

(2) In **disorders of the cycle** or in sterile women we diagnose: a) normal ovarian activity, b) disorders of the secretory stage, c) anovulation. By assessing the normal hyperthermic phase, lasting 10 or more days, we confirm normal ovarian activity with ovulation with great probability and avoid unnecessary treatment, e.g. in oligomenorrhoea, in some irregular cycles and hypomenorrhoea. A low temperature during the hyperthermic phase or a short duration of less than 10 days may suggest progesterone deficiency, but the presence of luteal deficiency calls for further confirmation. A monophasic temperature assessed for a period of six months suggests the diagnosis of anovulatory cycles or anovulatory oligomenorrhoea.

(3) The basal temperature curve helps us to **check therapy.** During clomiphene treatment the basal temperature rises typically, while after discontinuation it declines for several days and then rises again as evidence of induced ovulation, or pregnancy. After gestagen administration it rises and it can be used as a criterion of the action of depot preparations. During gonadotropin treatment the rise of basal temperature may, in addition to other symptoms, be a signal of hyperstimulation of the ovaries, and treatment is then discontinued.

(4) **During pregnancy** the basal temperature is maintained in the hyperthermic phase for a period of four months and then it declines for so far unknown

reasons. Hyperthermia persisting for more than 16 days can be recommended as a simple pregnancy test with a 97% reliability. In practice we found it very useful and we use it in all short-term amenorrhoeas before we perform a pregnancy test.

The basal temperature curve is thus a very dynamic test, which provides information on the action of progesterone and secondarily on ovulation with certain limitations which ensue from incorrect technique or hypothalamic mediation. The greatest number of impaired curves were recorded in neurotic women and in hypothalamic disorders. It must be supplemented by further tests of different peripheral hormonal effects.

## PROGESTERONE TEST

Withdrawal-bleeding from the endometrium caused by a sudden decline of circulating exogenous progesterone provides information on adequate or inadequate oestrogenic stimulation of the endometrium. If the haemorrhage commences later

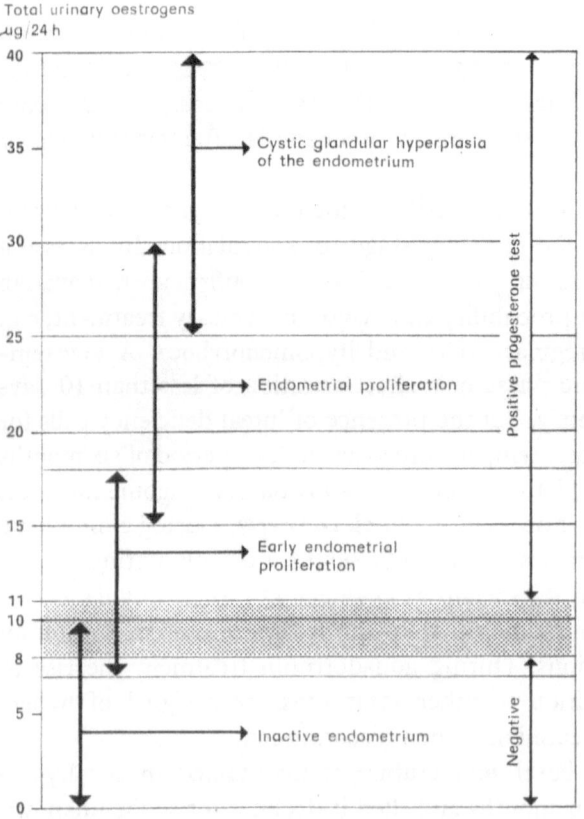

*Fig. 28.* Physiological and pathological conditions of the endometrium with a relatively constant urinary oestrogen excretion in relation to the progesterone test. (Hatched area indicates zone where test may be positive and negative.)

than seven days after a single i.m. dose of progesterone (which we prefer), or after termination of the oral administration of pure gestagen, it is probable that the production of endogenous progesterone has interfered.

A positive progesterone test provides information that the proliferation of the endometrium (formation of ovarian oestrogens) was sufficient for the development of the typical effect of a rapid decline of the plasma progesterone concentration, i.e.

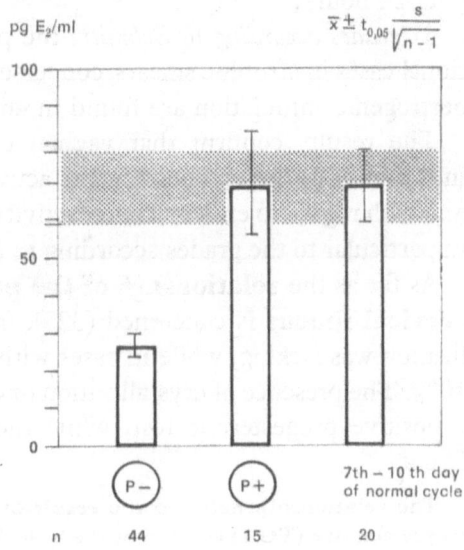

Fig. 29. Plasma oestradiol (E₂) in amenorrhoic women with negative (P−) or positive (P+) progesterone test. (Hatched area — 95 % confidence limit for mean concentration of circulating oestradiol in postmenstrual period in normal women) (217)

for bleeding from the uterine mucosa, although the amount of exogenous progesterone did not suffice to cause the typical secretory transformation of the endometrium. The prerequisite of a positive test is not mature proliferation, as is also demonstrated by the fact that positivity or negativity of the test depends on the urinary excretion of total oestrogens (the critical borderline is 10 μg/24 hours; within the range from 8–11 μg/24 hours the result of the test cannot be foreseen). Similarly close is the relationship between the excretion of total oestrogens and the degree of proliferation of the endometrium; when the values are lower than 10 μg/24 hours, the endometrium is atrophic, and an excretion of 7–8 μg/24 hours corresponds to incipient proliferation (Fig. 28).

In women with a negative progesterone test assessment of the plasma oestradiol level revealed a mean value of 27.1 pg/ml, while when the test was positive the mean value was 68.8 pg/ml which does not differ from the concentration of circulating oestradiol on the 7th–10th day of the menstrual cycle in healthy women (68.7 pg/ml) (Fig. 29) (217).

**Correlation of the progesterone test with vaginal cytology** depends probably on the criterion of oestrogenic activity in the vaginal cytogram:

a) *karyopyknotic index*: the progesterone test is usually positive when the values are higher than 20%, negative when values are lower than 20%;

b) *eosinophil index*: the progesterone test is usually positive when values are higher than 20%, negative when values are lower than 10%;

c) *cornification index*: the progesterone test is positive when there are more than 10% cornified cells, negative when there are less than 10%. A cornification index higher than 10% is associated with values of total oestrogen excretion higher than 8 μg/24 hours;

d) *grades according to Schmitt*: the progesterone test is positive only in exceptional cases in atrophic smears, conversely when it is negative, smears with a normal oestrogenic stimulation are found in 46.4% of all cases.

The results confirm that vaginal cytology is a substantially more sensitive indicator of peripheral oestrogenic activity than the histology of the endometrium and with regard to endometrial reactivity it gives too optimistic results. This applies in particular to the grades according to Schmitt.

As far as the **relationship of the progesterone test and crystallization of cervical mucus** is concerned (325), in 25% the test was positive when crystallization was lacking, while in cases with crystallization it was negative in less than 10%. The presence of crystallization of cervical mucus thus indicates very probably a positive progesterone test, while the absence of crystallization does not rule it out.

The relationship between the result of the progesterone test and the total gonadotropic activity (TGA) assessed by the biological method in urine resembles strikingly the correlation with the grades according to Schmitt used in vaginal cytology. When the test was positive, the TGA excretion was only very rarely subnormal and abnormally raised values were never recorded. When the progesterone test was negative, however, in 44.6% TGA excretion was normal. We assume that the cause of this discrepancy is the extremely variable amount of human hypophyseal gonadotropins which are needed for the stimulation of ovarian oestrogen secretion in the female; according to data in the literature it varies between 400 and 4,300 IU FSH. A positive progesterone test thus practically rules out a primary ovarian menstrual dysfunction, i.e. premature ovarian failure (syndrome of premature menopause).

For the progesterone test we use a single i.m. injection of 50–100 mg progesterone in oil. After injection of 50 mg the concentration of plasma progesterone reaches values usually recorded during the luteal phase of the menstrual cycle, and after administration of 100 mg the peak of the plasma progesterone level approaches values of the second trimester of pregnancy (363). After an i.m. dose of 50 mg progesterone the plasma level reaches its peak during the first 8 hours after injection and declines relatively slowly. The slow decline of the concentration of circulating progesterone after i.m. injection of the oily solution is explained by the diffusion of the steroid into adipose tissue during the rise and peak of its blood level, while during the period of declining concentration of the circulating hormones progesterone diffuses back into plasma. Therefore in the majority of subjects detectable plasma progesterone values were still found 48 hours after the i.m. injection of 50 and 100 mg in oil (363). Bleeding from the endometrium thus starts as a rule only 72–96 hours after injection.

The carry-over effect of the progesterone test observed in some instances where after endometrial bleeding induced by progesterone administration one or several spontaneous menstruations follow is remarkable. We observed spontaneous uterine bleeding after a positive progesterone test in 34.8% women. So far the mechanism of the stimulatory action of progesterone on the menstrual cycle is not clear. It is surprising that on the second day after an i.m. injection of 100 mg progesterone in 14 of 15 amenorrhoic women with a positive result a marked rise of plasma LH occurred which declined within 24–48 hours to the initial value (Fig. 30). A similar rise of LH was observed, on the other hand, only in one of 13 women with a negative

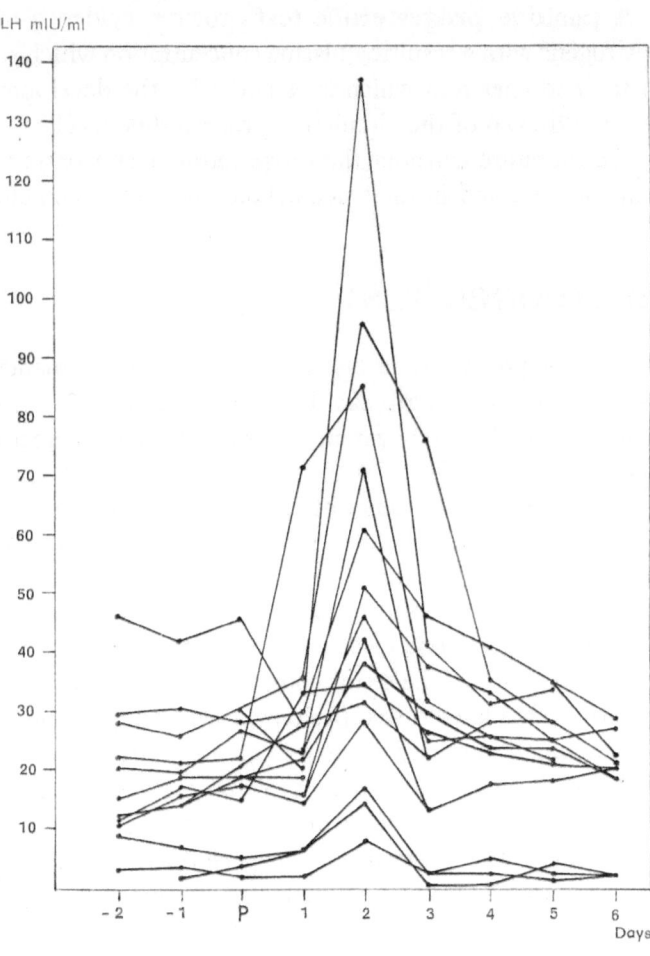

*Fig. 30.* Plasma LH in amenorrhoic women with positive progesterone test before and after i.m. injection of 100 mg (indicated on y-axis as P) (170).

progesterone test. It is assumed that the antioestrogenic action of progesterone is involved, similar to the competitive inhibition of the hypothalamic binding of oestradiol in the mechanism of the action of clomiphene.

The informative value of the progesterone test is increased by the fact that its positivity is not influenced in a major way by the placebo effect if the test is presented to the patient as a diagnostic test with two possible responses, depending on the hormonal situation of the organism (408).

**A negative progesterone test** thus suggests three possibilities:

a) secretory transformation of the endometrium in high concentrations of circulating progesterone (pregnancy or persistence of the corpus luteum),

b) inadequate proliferation or atrophy of the endometrium due to an inadequate production of ovarian oestrogens,

c) inadequate reactivity of the endometrium to ovarian oestrogens or more frequently destruction or absence of the uterine mucosa.

**A positive progesterone test** provides evidence of the secretion of ovarian oestrogens with a resulting plasma concentration which suffices for the proliferation of the endometrium which is essential for the development of haemorrhage from the withdrawal of the circulating progesterone level.

We therefore consider the progesterone test a basic out-patient examination in amenorrhoea and in the amenorrhoic phase of oligomenorrhoea respectively.


## OESTROGEN TEST

When the progesterone test is negative and pregnancy or possible persistence of the corpus luteum can be ruled out, we have to decide between two remaining possibilities: ovarian hypofunction and a defect or lack of reactivity of the endometrium.

Evidence of the presence of a reactive endometrium is uterine bleeding from the withdrawal of exogenous oestrogens. Oestrogen has to be administered in an amount sufficient for the proliferation of the atrophic endometrium. The oestrogen test is positive if bleeding occurs within two weeks after discontinued administration or if the progesterone test becomes positive in cases where bleeding did not start "spontaneously". The test is considered negative only when it remained repeatedly negative. It is known that prolonged deficiency of endogenous oestrogens reduces the endometrial sensitivity to exogenous oestrogens (see p. 115).

We administer mestranol, 0.15 mg per day, by mouth, for a period of three weeks; if within one week after completed administration uterine bleeding does not occur, the progesterone test is performed; if it remains negative, the oestrogen test is repeated. Instead of mestranol diethylstilboestrol may be administered — 1.0 mg — or ethinyloestradiol — 0.05 mg per day by mouth. The oral administration can be replaced by i.m. injections of oestradiol valerate, 10 mg per week for 3–4 weeks.

**A negative oestrogen test** thus suggests two possibilities:

a) the endometrium is lacking or destroyed by a pathological process,

b) the reactivity of the endometrium to oestrogens is inadequate.

The absence or presence and condition of the uterine mucosa may also be ascertained directly (by microabrasion); the sensitivity to oestrogens can, however, be tested only by means of the oestrogen test. For differentiation of the two possibilities endometrial biopsy is essential. An indispensible supplementary examination is X-ray hysterography.

**A positive oestrogen test** provides evidence of the presence of an endometrium which responds to ovarian oestrogens.

## GONADOTROPIN TEST

If the oestrogen test is positive, a decision must be made whether the deficiency of endogenous oestrogens is due to primary ovarian failure or whether it is a secondary phenomenon caused by inadequate stimulation of the ovary by gonadotropins.

For differentiation we may use the administration of exogenous gonadotropins and investigate directly the eventual rise of ovarian oestrogen production in peripheral blood or urine or indirectly by assessing typical changes in the vaginal cytology, cervical mucus and the endometrium. An unequivocal clinical positive reaction is uterine bleeding from the withdrawal of the circulating oestrogen level. An increased production of ovarian oestrogens suggests a preserved reactivity of the ovaries as well as inadequate secretion of pituitary gonadotropins.

Depending on the availability of gonadotropic preparations, we may use some listed in Fig. 31:

a) PMSG is injected i.m. daily, 500–1,000 IU and changes in vaginal smears and cervical mucus are concurrently investigated. If after three injections no response is obtained, then starting with the 4th day the dose of PMSG is doubled. If even after the following six injections no manifestations of oestrogenic stimulation are detected in the investigated indicators, the ovary is considered non-reactive.

In another variant of the test PMSG is injected i.m. daily — 5,000 IU — for three days only, and on the subsequent eight days urinary oestrone excretion is followed up. There are three possible types of oestrone excretion: (1) the basal level is lower than 5 $\mu$g/24 hours and does not increase after stimulation (the ovaries do not respond); (2) the basal level is lower than 5 $\mu$g/24 hours; gonadotropic stimulation leads, however, to a slight increase of oestrone excretion by more than 100% of the initial value (hypogonadotropic amenorrhoea); (3) oestrone excretion is at least 50 μg/24 hours and frequently more than 100 μg/24 hours (syndrome of polycystic ovaries).

In another variant of the test a single dose of 18,000 IU PMSG is injected i.m. Urinary oestrone excretion is assessed before administration and on the 7th day after injection of gonadotropin when the maximum is usually reached. A resulting value of oestrone excretion lower than 15 μg/24 hours indicates a subnormal

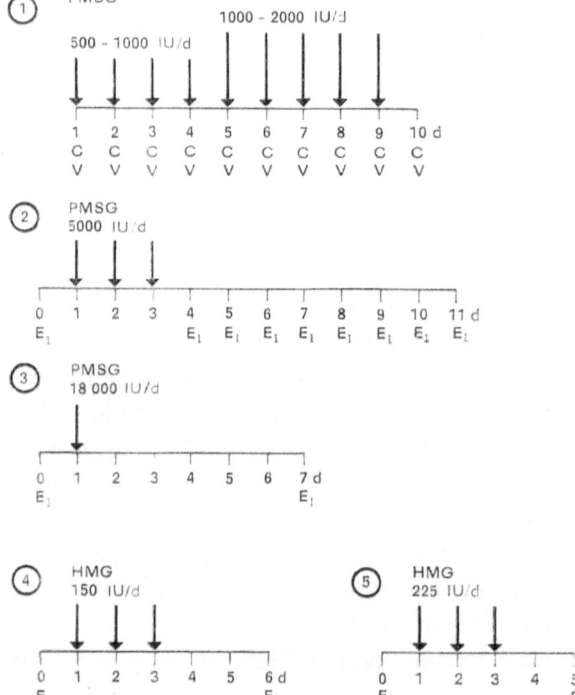

Fig. 31. Different variants of gonadotropin stimulation test. On time axis (days) administration of gonadotropin and its doses and criteria of evaluation of the effect are indicated. (C — "Spinnbarkeit" and ferning of the cervical mucus, V — vaginal cytology, $E_1$ — urinary oestrone excretion/24h, $E_T$ — urinary excretion of total oestrogens//24hours).

response of the ovaries: 15–80 μg/24 hours is the normal value; an excretion of more than 100 μg/24 hours is the manifestation of hypersensitivity of the ovaries and suggests the syndrome of polycystic ovaries.

It is recommended to perform an intradermal test in every woman before the first diagnostic administration of PMSG; usually a 0.1 ml solution containing 400 IU/ml is injected into the skin on the volar side of the forearm and a possible reaction is looked for within 15 min.

b) HMG is injected i.m. in a daily dose of 150 IU FSH + 150 IU LH for three days; total urinary oestrogens are assessed before the onset of administration and on the 6th day after the first injection. The normal reaction corresponds to a value of 40–150 μg/24 hours; while a level above 150 μg/24 hours is an excessive response, a concentration lower than 40 μg/24 hours is an inadequate reaction; sometimes the ovary may not respond at all. It is an advantage to investigate vaginal smears and cervical mucus concurrently. A normal reaction is encountered as a rule in normo-oestrogenic disorders of ovulation. It suggests the capacity of the ovary to ovulate after adequate gonadotropic stimulation. An excessive reaction occurs as a rule in the syndrome of polycystic ovaries.

HMG may be injected i.m. daily also in larger amounts: 225 IU FSH + 225 IU LH, also for three days; before the test is started and on the 5th day after the first injection the initial and final urinary oestrone concentration is assessed. There are three groups of possible responses: (1) a rise of oestrone excretion by less than 5 μg/24 hours (inadequate response); (2) a rise by 6–40 μg/24 hours (satisfactory reaction); (3) a rise by 41 and more μg per 24 hours (hyperstimulation, usually in the syndrome of polycystic ovaries).

In another variant of the test HMG is also injected i.m. three times on every third day (1st, 4th and 7th day), however, the daily dose is 375 IU FSH + + 375 IU LH. Before the beginning of the test and then on the 3rd, 6th and 9th day after the first injection "Spinnbarkeit" and crystallization of the cervical mucus are assessed and the vaginal cytology is evaluated. Before the test and on the 9th day after the first injection total urinary oestrogens are estimated. There are three possible responses: (1) a negative reaction (without manifestations of oestrogenic stimulation), (2) a weak positive reaction (positive reaction of cervical mucus, in the vaginal cytology a shift towards surface cells, total oestrogen excretion 10–20 μg//24 hours) and (3) a positive reaction (strongly positive reaction of cervical mucus, with mainly surface cells in the vaginal smear, total oestrogen excretion about 20 μg/24 hours. A simplification has since been recommended, i.e. daily administration of the above dose of HMG on three consecutive days without intervals, whereby the resulting reactions of the investigated parameters are evaluated on the 6th and 7th day after the first injection. This variant is suited to the assessment of the reactivity of the ovaries in hypogonadotropic amenorrhoic women.

An attempt to replace HMG in the above tests may be a combination of heterologous FSH, the biological activity of which is expressed in IU of HMG-IRP-2, together with the same number of IU of hCG instead of LH.

Gonadotropic stimulation tests comprise also the *test of gestagenic and oestrogenic (thecal) function of the corpus luteum* (Fig. 32). hCG is administered i.m. in amounts of 5,000 IU on the 3rd, 5th and 7th day after the rise of BT above 37°C; on the 8th day pregnanediol and total oestrogens in urine are assessed. A pregnanediol concentration lower than 5 mg/24 hours is the manifestation of gestagenic insufficiency of the corpus luteum. The normal range of total oestrogen excretion after stimulation is 55–85 μg/24 hours, a lower level suggests oestrogenic (thecal) insufficiency of the corpus luteum. The functional insufficiency of the corpus luteum can manifest itself isolated in one or both components of luteal steroid biosynthesis.

**A negative gonadotropin stimulation test** suggests the inability of the ovary to respond to the gonadotropic stimulus by an increased oestrogen biosynthesis. It is thus a primarily ovarian disorder of reactivity to gonadotropins (see p. 66).

**A positive gonadotropin stimulation test** indicates that the reactivity of the ovary to gonadotropins is preserved and the disorder of ovarian function develops as a result of primary inadequate production of hypohyseal gonadotropins; a pathologically raised reactivity is probably again a primarily ovarian disorder.

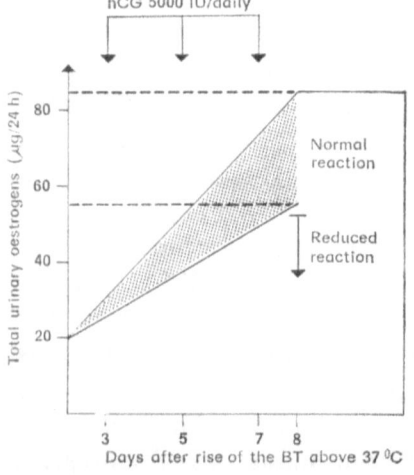

*Fig. 32.* Test of thecal (oestrogen) corpus luteum function (235).

A risk of the gonadotropin test is ovarian hyperstimulation in women with the syndrome of polycystic ovaries. When the test is performed in the out-patient department, the woman must be properly informed on the risk and the necessity of examination if she develops any complaints. When the syndrome of polycystic ovaries is suspected, we prefer not to use the gonadotropin test.

## VAGINAL CYTOLOGY

Evaluation of functional vaginal cytology should correspond to the basic clinical problems:

(1) Are oestrogens present in clinically significant concentrations, i.e. is the endometrium proliferated?

(2) How should the effectiveness of the dose and period of administration of oestrogen or gonadotropin which stimulates endogenous oestrogen secretion be compared quantitatively?

(3) How should the ovulation period be determined?

(4) Is progesterone present in clinically significant concentrations, i.e. was the cycle ovulatory and did the endometrium undergo secretory transformation?

216

## VAGINAL CYTOLOGY AND OESTROGENIZATION OF THE FEMALE ORGANISM (COMPARISON WITH THE ENDOMETRIAL HISTOLOGY)

A single assessment of the oestrogenization of the female organism is rendered possible by the semiquantitative diagram of grades elaborated by Schmitt (1953) which expresses the degree of proliferation of the vaginal epithelium with an accuracy sufficient for clinical practice. It is only of preliminary value and cannot replace dynamic investigations.

The value of urinary excretion of total oestrogens and in particular of oestriol correlates practically not only with all quantitative parameters (indices) of vaginal cytology but equally well also with the qualitative visual assessment. The correlation with oestrone excretion is poorer and there is no correlation with oestradiol excretion.

**Comparison of vaginal cytology and histology of the endometrium** is important (305):

in proliferation and hyperplasia of the endometrium we encounter a very different percentage of surface cells, however, in 95% of all cases there are fewer than 10% parabasal and basal cells;

in atrophy of the endometrium there were in 20% of the cases more than 30% surface cells in the vaginal smear and in almost 70% of all cases there were fewer than 10% deep cells.

Conversely, in smears with more than 60% surface cells in 16% of all cases an atrophic endometrium was detected. On the other hand, with more than 60% of parabasal cells proliferation of the uterine mucosa was never found. It seems that only the presence of parabasal and basal cells respectively in the vaginal smear provides certain information about the state of the endometrium; thus an "atrophic" smear correlates very well with atrophy of the endometrium. We observed that under these conditions the progesterone test is positive only in exceptional instances.

Evaluation of the vaginal mucosa colonization with Döderlein's lactobacillus is beyond the scope of vaginal cytology proper. This criterion of initial oestrogenic stimulation of the vagina at the onset of puberty in girls serves as indirect evidence of the presence of intermediary cells containing glycogen (311).

The frequency of discrepancies between the histology of the endometrium and a single assessment of the vaginal cytology varies in about 20% (531). In women with a disturbed autonomic nervous system it was found even more frequently, in as many as 40% of all cases. While we prefer therefore biopsy of the endometrium, vaginal cytology is indispensable where biopsy cannot be performed or where it would involve a risk.

# VAGINAL CYTOLOGY AND QUANTITATIVE EVALUATION OF THE OESTROGENIC EFFECT ON THE VAGINAL MUCOSA

For the quantitative evaluation of the oestrogenic action on the vaginal mucosa various cytological indices may be used (see p. 128).

The value of all these cytological indices is relative, i.e. they can be used only for comparing the actual value of the index with that of a previous test in the same patient. The interindividual variability as regards the sensitivity of the vaginal mucosa to ovarian hormones is considerable and moreover the index characterizes only one parameter of the cellular character in the vaginal smear, while it is biased by a personal error of approximately $\pm 10\%$ and cannot be considered specific for a certain ovarian steroid.

As far as the evaluation of the oestrogenic activity of the product is concerned, it must be always taken into account that the minumum effective dose and period of administration of the oestrogenic product are markedly lower than the histological response of the endometrium and that the effect on the vaginal mucosa regresses substantially more slowly than that on the endometrium (therefore during oestrogenic stimulation of the vaginal mucosa we can already detect an atrophic endometrium) (55).

## VAGINAL CYTOLOGY AND OVULATION

Usually we differentiate only between late proliferation and the early secretory phase. If the ovulation period is manifested at all characteristically in the vaginal

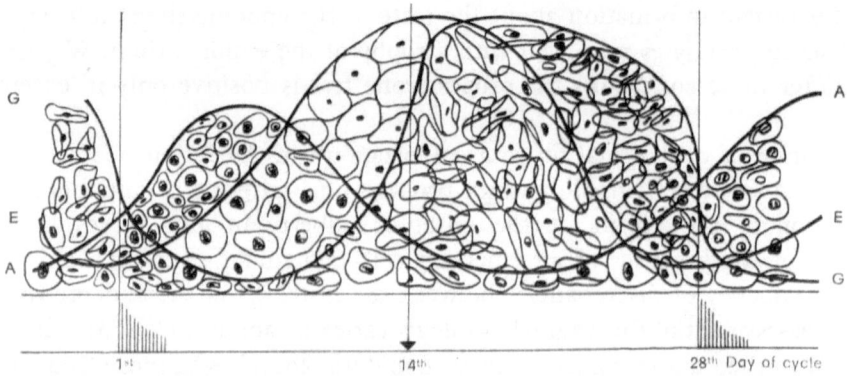

*Fig. 33.* Cellular types in vaginal smear during menstrual cycle; E — predominantly oestrogenic picture, G — predominantly gestagenic picture, A — predominantly androgenic picture; under physiological normal conditions these "pure" pictures are not encountered in smears, the resulting cytological picture is characterized by their overlapping (288).

smear, then a predominance of fully developed and isolated surface cells together with a maximum value of the karyopyknotic and eosinophil index is described (Fig. 33).

## VAGINAL CYTOLOGY AND SECRETORY TRANSFORMATION OF THE ENDOMETRIUM

To obtain evidence of implemented ovulation, i.e. secretory transformation of the endometrium, in vaginal cytology as a rule the necessity of comparing repeated smears, at least late proliferation and late secretion, is emphasized. Vaginal cytology in the luteal phase of the menstrual cycle cannot replace the histology of the endometrium. In the differential diagnosis of functional sterility the dating of endometrial biopsy is essential. The vaginal mucosa is a less suitable target tissue for evaluation of gestagens than the endometrium.

# FUNCTIONAL BIOPSY OF THE ENDOMETRIUM

The endometrium reacts very sensitively to sex hormones. It responds by cyclic changes which in the proliferative phase are influenced by oestrogens, and in the secretory phase mainly by progesterone on the basis of oestrogen action. Histology is thus a very good test which provides information on the action of these steroids in chronological sequence. Biopsy of the endometrium, sometimes also described as microabrasion, is a rapid, safe and inexpensive examination method by means of which we obtain information in particular on the action of progesterone, and also whether ovulation has taken place. We obtain, however, also information on the action of oestrogens and finally on many functional disorders of the cycle and pathological conditions which are reflected in the histology of the endometrium.

## COMPARISON OF ENDOMETRIAL BIOPSY AND CURETTAGE

A number of authors compared the results of microabrasion with the results of curettage. Up to the fifties when abrasions developed on a clinical basis the majority preferred curettage. Advocates of microabrasion, on the other hand, found both methods equally effective (386) in non-malignant as well as in malignant cases (accuracy 88–96%). In a review of 13 papers a 75–96% accuracy of biopsy checked against surgical specimens was reported (3). Microabrasion, however, does not replace curettage when there is suspicion of a malignant process of the endometrium

219

and in case of some pathological changes which affect only part of the uterine cavity; it is, however, of equal value for diagnosing the phase of the cycle. More recent comparisons based on dating of the endometrium from 272 curettages revealed a chronological coincidence from the first day of the last menstruation with an accuracy of $\pm 1$ day in 59%, and in 144 biopsies agreement was recorded in 51%. The values did not differ significantly (466). The **advantages and disadvantages of biopsy** can be summarized as follows: an *advantage* is (1) the small loss of time for patient and doctor during the out-patient examination, (2) rapid diagnosis, (3) economy, (4) a smaller risk of infection, dissemination of carcinoma, haemorrhage, (5) equal accuracy in the diagnosis of the phase of the cycle and its disorders as in curettage. *Disadvantages* are: (1) it does not detect polyps quite reliably, (2) it may miss a small focus of carcinoma, (3) severe haemorrhage is stopped more effectively by curettage. Even nowadays microabrasion is occasionally refuted for fear of missing endometrial carcinoma. Our attitude towards microabrasion is very favourable. We use it for the diagnosis of disorders of the cycle in women up to the age of 38 years. Only when there is suspicion of a malignant process or polyp or in case of very profuse haemorrhage we use curettage. For diagnosis in women older than 38 years we use curettage only. In tens of thousands of microabrasions thus indicated practically not a single case of carcinoma was missed.

## COLLECTION OF SPECIMENS AND EVALUATION OF ENDOMETRIUM

Material for histology is obtained by means of special metal curettes such as Novak's curette with a toothed opening at the end of the bent tube, Randall's or Meig's curette with a hook at the end. Most common is Novak's curette with or without aspiration. Flexible polyethylene cannulae with aspiration (Smith cannulae) can be also used which are a transition to the method described as aspiration cytology of the endometrium (brush technique) where by means of a mandrin with transverse grooves material is obtained for the dynamic investigation of cyclic changes or by rinsing cellular material for the diagnosis of ovulation which has taken place (Gravler jet washer). Collection of specimens by rinsing on the first day of menstruation ensured practically the same percentage of suitable specimens for histological diagnosis as collection by means of Novak's curette (95.5% as compared with 97.4%).

Specimens may be collected on any day of the cycle, however, preferably 2–3 days before menstruation in a regular cycle, and in infertility sometimes also on the 21st day of the cycle. In unforeseeable irregular cycles we perform the collection during the first few hours of menstrual bleeding. Timing to the onset of the cycle, so as to avoid interference with possible pregnancy, is not suitable in our opinion, as a detailed diagnosis from the menstrual decidua is difficult and inaccurate. The risk of damage is minimal as microabrasion performed during conceiving cycles practically never causes damage to the foetus development of which proceeds normally.

Data reported in the literature show that in 21 cases of microabrasion performed during conceiving cycles only two women aborted whereby in one case a patient with habitual abortion was involved and microabrasion was not necessarily the cause.

## RELATIONSHIP OF ENDOMETRIAL BIOPSY TO OTHER CRITERIA

The diagnostic value of endometrial biopsy was compared with other criteria of hormonal action. Comparison with the **basal temperature** has already been mentioned previously and showed the advantages of biopsy. Comparison with **vaginal cytology** also revealed the advantages of biopsy. Vaginal cytology gave 16–18% of incorrect results, as compared with biopsy. Dating of the endometrium correlated with the day of the cycle calculated from the **peak of LH** with a standard deviation of 1.2 days, the peak of plasma oestradiol preceded by one day (275). In another paper statistical analysis revealed that there is no difference between the appearance of the dated endometrium $E_{14}$ according to Noyes et al. (372), the appearance of the dated **corpus luteum** $C_1$ according to Corner (92), the LH peak in plasma and the oestradiol peak in plasma (313). This confirms the high diagnostic value of dating of the endometrium.

The secretory phase in biopsy of the endometrium correlated with **progesterone values** >2 ng/ml plasma 15 times from a total of 17 cases. In another publication the secretory endometrium corresponded with the secretory progesterone level 16 times from a total of 18 cases and only twice was it lower. The proliferative endometrium corresponded with the proliferative phase in 19 out of a total of 20 cases. The correlation of both values in infertile women agreed much less and thus e.g. from a total of 59 paired results only 34 (57 %) agreed within three days when dating was applied. In other instances in infertile women a secretory progesterone level of >3 ng/ml plasma was recorded in 90% of the cycles and a secretory endometrium in 81% (473). This is natural as in infertile women inadequate response of the endometrium was much more frequent.

# CLINICAL IMPORTANCE OF ENDOMETRIAL BIOPSY

The clinical value of endometrial biopsy is considerable. We are either satisfied with a simple description of the proliferative or secretory phase or we demand a more detailed characterization of the pathological condition by means of *dating of the endometrium* based on the ideal 28-day cycle (372). The authors described pictures of the endometrium in the course of the cycle as $E_1$–$E_{28}$. They assumed that ovulation occurred at the lowest point of the basal temperature, i.e. on the 14th day and specified this picture as $E_{14}$ or $E_1$ of the secretory phase. $E_{14}$ corresponds to the first picture of corpus luteum dating according to Corner (92). The authors reported that the dating error was $\pm 1$ day. When the subjective factor of two independent authors was evaluated, then in 80% of the endometria the deviation was $\pm 2$ days. The objection that the local specimen obtained does not represent the entire mucosa of the uterine cavity is refuted by comparison of four independently collected specimens. From a total of 82 and later 100 patients with ovulation, uniformity was recorded in 64 (with a standard deviation of $\pm 1$ day), a difference of more than 3 days was found in 18, with a standard deviation of 1–5 days, and six patients showed a greater variability (371). According to some authors dating of the phase with an accuracy of one certain day is not real, as they found during repeated dating 2-day variations in 15% and 3-day variations in 5%. Therefore sometimes a more simplified classification into sub-phases proves useful: menstruation (1st–4th day), early proliferation (5th–8th day), developed proliferation (9th–11th day), advanced proliferation (12th–14th day), early secretion (16th–18th day), developed secretion (19th–22nd day), advanced secretion (23rd–24th day), secretion in regression (25th–28th day).

Biopsy of the endometrium ensures diagnosis in pathological conditions. (1) It confirms the diagnosis of an anovulatory cycle when the basal temperatures remain for several months monophasic. (2) Biopsy is essential for the diagnosis of the majority of disorders of ovarian activity manifested by a menstrual disorder, sterility or infertility. In disorders with excessive bleeding it is a fundamental question from what type of endometrium the bleeding occurs. By biopsy we assess the diagnosis of dysfunctional haemorrhage and irregular shedding of the endometrium. In women with inadequate haemorrhage or an impaired rate of bleeding biopsy provides information on the action of oestrogens and progesterone. In sterile and infertile women dating of the endometrium must be done to detect retardation or inadequate secretory transformation which may have their cause in the endometrium or in insufficiency of the corpus luteum. Biopsy also reveals subtle disorders of the secretory transformation in the glands or stroma. (3) The diagnosis of inflammation of the endometrium and in particular of a tuberculous inflammation is very important. Tuberculous endometritis is diagnosed in biopsy material when regular biopsies are made in disorders of the cycle or in sterility much more frequently than from clinical symptoms. (4) For the diagnosis of adenocarcinoma of the endometrium curettage is more suitable (see p. 219). (5) Sometimes biopsy of the endometrium is used to study the effects of oestrogens and in particular new gestagens after their therapeutic administration.

The information which can be derived from endometrial biopsy when investigating hormonal influences is greater than that of other criteria on the genital periphery (basal temperature, vaginal cytology, cervical mucus). It is therefore a reliable test for the diagnosis of a normal endometrium, for the analysis of menstrual disorders and for the follow up of hormonal treatment.

## LAPAROSCOPY AND CULDOSCOPY

Both endoscopic methods (the first via the transabdominal and the second via the transvaginal route) render visualization of the ovaries, and in laparoscopy also ovarian biopsy, possible (for technical details we refer to special monographs). It is beyond doubt that direct visualization of the ovaries provides more accurate information on their macroscopic appearance than pneumopelvigraphy (and the possibility of photographic documentation provides an apt supplement). It is also beyond doubt that the risk of endoscopic methods and the stress inflicted upon the patient is greater.

Indications for visualization of the ovaries are primary amenorrhoea, secondary menstrual dysfunction with hirsutism and secondary amenorrhoea or oligomenorrhoea in sterility not responding to clomiphene. We can supplement the list by the syndrome of premature menopause. Unless the gonads are streak-like and dysgenetic or entirely lacking, which is extremely rare, the following suggested **classification of ovaries with regard to their macroscopic appearance** can be applied (500):

I. active ovary (normal, rugose white ovary with visible growing follicle or corpus luteum),

II. atrophic ovary (shrivelled yellowish ovary resembling ovary after menopause),

III. polycystic ovary (enlarged, smooth, pearl-white ovary often with thickened capsule),

IV. resting ovary (normal-sized, smooth, whitish without thickened capsule and without visible growing follicle or corpus luteum).

Some authors confine the indication for laparoscopic ovarian biopsy only to cases of primary amenorrhoea, while others supplement it by cases which need for therapeutic prognosis of menstrual dysfunction and sterility a confirmation or exclusion of the presence of the follicular apparatus, but they draw attention to the fact that in particular in severely hypoplastic ovaries further diminution of the tissue by biopsy may be an issue. The recommended **classification of ovarian laparoscopic biopsy** differentiates between a) normal, b) reduced and c) absent follicular apparatus. A more detailed classification evaluates moreover stimulation of follicles and ovarian stroma (130):

a) normal ovary (more than 10 follicles in the visual field of the biopsy specimen, maturation at least up to formation of antrum, vital stroma without fibrosis);

b) normal ovary — slight fibrosis of the stroma (otherwise the same as a));

c) reduced stock of follicles — normal stimulation (less than six follicles in visual field of bioptic specimen, otherwise the same as a));

d) reduced stock of follicles — slight fibrosis of stroma (less than six follicles, otherwise the same as b));

e) absence of follicles — normal stimulation (in the whole biopsy specimen not more than 1 to 2 follicles can be found; the stroma is vital; the atretic follicles still bear signs of stimulation, i.e. appearance of ovary in the postmenopausal period);

f) absence of follicles — slight fibrosis of the stroma (stroma and scars manifest fibrous transformation, otherwise the same as e)).

The most serious objection against laparoscopic biopsy of the ovaries for this indication is that the specimen is not representative for the entire ovary. A case-history was reported where according to laparoscopic biopsy of the ovary the absence of the follicular apparatus was diagnosed, where, however, the reaction to the gonadotropin stimulation test was positive and after treatment with HMG the woman became pregnant. Even the authors of the above mentioned classification of the laparoscopic biopsy of the ovary (500) recorded in a case with apparent absence of the follicular apparatus a regular menstrual cycle during a subsequent follow-up. The reduction of the follicular apparatus described does not rule out even later eumenorrhoea or pregnancy. We prefer therefore the gonadotropin stimulation test which, as compared with simple morphological description, frequently of a non-representative specimen, confirms or excludes the sensitivity of the ovary to exogenous gonadotropins (see p. 213). Only in cases with a negative reaction we consider biopsy justified; we also indicate it in premature ovarian failure (see p. 293).

We refute laparoscopic biopsy of the corpus luteum in functional sterility, but we may obtain reliable information of its function by dating of endometrial biopsy, by assessing the level of circulating progesterone and by means of the gonadotropin stimulation test (see p. 215).

# GENETIC EXAMINATION (SEX CHROMATIN AND KARYOTYPE)

The rapid development of human cytogenetics which renders it possible to assess the karyotype has pushed the assessment of sex chromatin (chromatin test) to the background and it is now used only as a screening test.

## SEX CHROMATIN TEST

The essence of sex chromatin was discussed on p. 1. Most frequently smears of the oral mucosa are used [for details we refer to special monographs (208)]. As positive we evaluate a finding of more than 10% nuclei with sex chromatin or five or more typical nuclei in one smear. The test is negative, if in one smear no nucleus with a Barr body is found; doubtful cases call for repeated examination. In healthy men in rare instances 1% and in exceptional cases 2% positive nuclei are found.

Less frequently used is evaluation of cell nuclei in skin biopsy or so-called drumsticks (Davidson's sign) in nuclei of segmented neutrophils in peripheral blood smears. Better than skin biopsy is the use of epidermal cells of the outer hair sheath obtained by pulling out a single hair.

In polysomia of gonosome X excessive sex chromosomes X undergo heteropyknosis and thus the number of Barr bodies in the nucleus increases. It is a rule that the intermitotic cell contains as many Barr bodies as are heterochromosomes X in the gonosome complement minus one. The necessity of further detailed chromosome analysis of all abnormal findings is obvious.

The informative value of the chromatin test is substantially increased by the possibility of detecting gonosome Y in the cellular nuclei of the oral smear (or skin biopsy) by fluorescent staining. In normal men the "male sex chromatin" is found in 20–50% of nuclei as a fluorescent spot.

## ASSESSMENT OF KARYOTYPE

When examining chromosomes it is necessary to process mitotic cells of the examined tissue in a suitable way after cultivation *in vitro* lasting several hours (bone marrow cells), days (lymphocytes of peripheral blood) or weeks (e.g. fibroblasts). For details we refer to special monographs (208).

Indications for assessment of the karyotype in phenotypic women are:

A. primary amenorrhoea,

B. premature ovarian failure (so-called premature menopause or syndrome of premature climacteric),

C. menstrual dysfunction in subjects with very small (less than 152.5 cm) or very tall stature and in somatic malformations and abnormalities,

D. intersexual malformation of the genitalia.

When evaluating the karyotype it is essential to realize that for the classification of the case the clinical aspect is decisive. The sexual phenotype depends above all on the cellular line predominating in the gonad in the germ cells, while the karyotype is usually assessed from lymphocytes from the blood. Therefore we may encounter a discrepancy between the karyotype and the clinical picture (e.g. menstruation in cases with 46,XO or mosaic). Fundamentally, it is almost impossible to rule out the possibility of mosaic. If the latter is revealed, then it is almost impossible to assess its extent and distribution. It varies not only in different tissues but also in the same tissue. By destruction of less vital cells it may also change during the life time of the affected person.

# FUNCTIONAL TESTS OF THE HYPOTHALAMO-HYPOPHYSEAL SYSTEM

Many tests were proposed for the diagnostic differentiation of the site of disorder in endocrine disorders of central origin and for a pathogenetic classification. For the assessment of trophic functions of the pituitary the assessment of trophic hormones in plasma is used nowadays and also functional tests which investigate their change after a specific stimulus.

The integrity of gonadotropic function is tested by the clomiphene test, LH-RH test and the oestrogen provocation test.

## CLOMIPHENE TEST

In the clomiphene test we administer 100 mg clomiphene citrate for at least 5 days and investigate the response of LH and FSH in serum and sometimes also total oestrogens and pregnanediol in urine. A rise of all these values indicates a normal response and in disorders it provides evidence of their hypothalamic origin. A low or negative response suggests an inadequate pituitary reserve. The test is sometimes supplemented by administration of dexamethasone and investigation of the androgen response.

## LH-RH TEST

The LH-RH test is used to assess the gonadotropic reserve of the adenohypophysis. It can thus be decided whether the disorder is in the hypothalamus or higher or whether it is due to inadequate function of the adenohypophysis. Usually 100 µg are administered (sometimes 10–15 µg) of synthetic LH-RH by the i.v.

*Fig. 34.* LH-RH test in normal cycle (in follicular phase, n = 10, mean values ± ± SE) (216a).

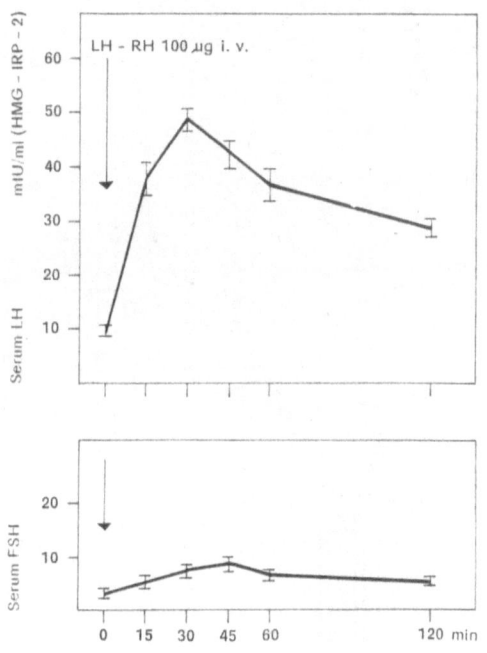

route and LH and FSH in plasma is assessed before administration and then at 15-minute intervals for one hour and again after two hours. The maximum rise of LH occurs after 30 min, and in FSH after 45 min (Fig. 34) (450, 517). In hypophyseal disorders (Sheehan's syndrome, condition after hypophysectomy) the responses are negative or only very low. Groups with hypergonadotropic hypogonadism have a significantly higher response than groups of women with hypogonadotropic hypogonadism which means an increased functional reserve of the adenohypophysis.

The response of the adenohypophysis, however, changes during the menstrual cycle and against a different steroid background, i.e. due to the modulating action of oestrogens; furthermore it depends on the basal level of LH and FSH (345). Therefore some work doubted the clinical value of the test (53) and modified it either by reducing the LH-RH doses to 25 µg or LH-RH was administered in an i.v. infusion (71), in particular when it was found that there are two pools of gonado-

tropin release. Finally a *double stimulating test* was suggested involving the administration of 2 × 25 μg LH-RH i.v. after a 2-hour interval (435), although the self-
priming effect of LH-RH is known. We cannot expect from the test that it will
characterize different clinical units, as was originally assumed, but it will differen-

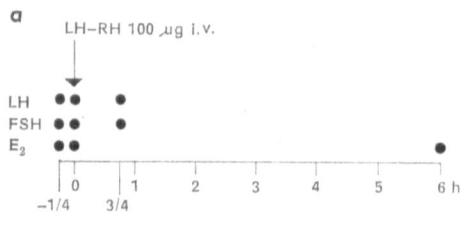

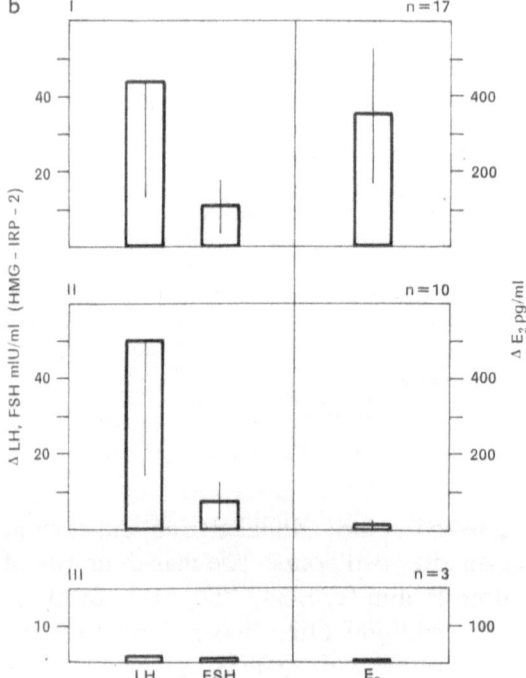

*Fig. 35.* Six-hour LH-RH test
with double response: a) schema
of test, b) results (I — hypothalamic disorders, II — ovarian disorders, III — hypophyseal disorders,
⊿ — difference between basal and
maximal level, n = 30, mean values ± SD) (220).

tiate readily the origin of a disorder in the hypothalamus or a disorder due to the
impaired sensitivity of the adenohypophysis, when we respect factors which
influence the dynamics of the gonadotropic response.

The *LH-RH test with a double response*, where we assess after administration of
100 μg LH-RH i.v., LH and FSH after 45 min and oestradiol in plasma after
6 hours enables us to differentiate at the same time the disorder of the cycle into
hypothalamic, hypophyseal and ovarian ones (Fig. 35) because it assesses also the
sensitivity of the ovary (220).

228

It has been clearly demonstrated that the stimulated release of gonadotropins causes a significant rise of plasma oestradiol only when the receptivity of the ovary is normal. A *quantitative graduation of the sensitivity of the ovary* is achieved by increasing the stimulating dose of LH-RH, i.e. by the use of a superactive analogue and the oestradiol response is assessed after 8–9 hours.

## OESTROGEN PROVOCATION TEST

The oestrogen provocation test is based on the positive feedback of oestrogens which also experimentally imitates gonadotropin release as in the follicular phase of the normal cycle. The oestrogen provocation test evaluates the functional capacity of the hypothalamo-hypophyseal axis for gonadotropin release and may predict whether clomiphene treatment will provoke ovulation or not. For the test 1 mg oestradiol benzoate is administered by the i.m. route and the significance of the rise of plasma LH is evaluated during the interval between 48 and 72 hours (468).

Similar experience was also accumulated with the modified oestrogen test where 6.6 mg oestradiol benzoate are administered and the rise of LH and FSH in plasma is followed up for four days. The criterion of positivity is >200 ng/ml LH for three days and >250 ng/ml FSH. By a negative test a disorder in the mechanism of the positive feedback can be diagnosed (532).

Nowadays it is possible to evaluate by means of *combined functional stimulation tests* all partial functions of the adenohypophysis simultaneously. One of these tests is a combination of insulin hypoglycaemia and the LH-RH test which renders it possible by assessing STH, LH and ACTH (and cortisol resp.) to evaluate the somatotropic, gonadotropic and adrenocorticotropic function. Another integrated direct test of the adenohypophysis is the administration of an arginine infusion (0.5 g/kg 5% arginine chloride) for 30 min, during the subsequent 90 min LH-RH (150 μg) are administered and TRH (500 μg) by the i.v. route. Before stimulation, during and after stimulation serum levels of LH, FSH, STH, PRL and TSH are assessed at 15-minute intervals for a period of 6 hours. Together with the assessment of cortisol it is then possible to evaluate accurately all trophic functions of the adenohypophysis (418).

## LABORATORY EXAMINATION OF THYROID FUNCTION

**Thyroxin T₄** — At present the most suitable isolated test of thyroid function is according to some authors the assessment of serum thyroxin (T₄) by means of a bond to a protein macromolecule (CPB) or by the radioimmunological method (RIA). Both methods assess the total (free and bound) T₄; therefore false low or high values may be assessed when the binding proteins of the blood are altered. Their binding capacity rises e.g. during pregnancy, during oestrogen treatment, under the influence of steroid contraceptives etc. and declines e.g. under the influence of androgens, corticoids etc. In these instances it is necessary to assess free $T_4$ which may be normal, if in the euthyroid patient the level of binding proteins and total $T_4$ is elevated, or conversely if the level of binding proteins and total $T_4$ is reduced.

Stimulation by means of TSH renders it possible to differentiate more readily between primary and secondary hypothyroidism. $T_4$ is estimated 24 hours after i.m. administration of 10 IU of TSH; in primary hypothyroidism the reduced concentration of serum $T_4$ rises only slightly, in secondary hypothyroidism it increases many times.

**PBI** — Classical test assessing the amount of iodine precipitated with serum proteins which theoretically is the criterion of serum $T_4$ concentration, is because of its inadequate specificity replaced by the above mentioned assessment of $T_4$.

**TSH** — Radioimmunological assessment of the concentration of circulating TSH is suited in particular for the diagnosis of marginal and slight primary hypothyroidism where the values of serum $T_4$ are as a rule still within the range of normal variation. It is used also for differentiation of primary (thyroid) and secondary (hypophyseal or hypothalamic) hypothyroidism; in the former case the TSH level in peripheral blood is raised, and in the latter it is reduced.

**BM** — Assessment of the basal metabolism where the normal range of variation varies between $\pm 15\%$ is a method of low sensitivity as far as thyroid function is concerned. It does not lose its importance for detection of cases of peripheral hypometabolism (see p. 189).

For details of examination of thyroid function we refer to special literature (67, 455). For orientation of the gynaecologist there is a review of methods in Table 15. In particular the diagnosis of borderline or slight hypothyroidism is difficult and should not be based on a single abnormal laboratory test; clinical symptomatology is the criterion (67).

*Table 15* Values of $T_4$, PBI and TSH in thyroid dysfunction

|  | $T_4$ | PBI | TSH |
|---|---|---|---|
| Euthyroidism with normal level of binding proteins | normal | normal | normal |
| Euthyroidism with raised level of binding proteins | raised | raised | normal |
| Euthyroidism with reduced level of binding proteins | reduced | reduced | normal |
| Primary hypothyroidism | reduced | reduced | raised |
| Secondary hypothyroidism | reduced | reduced | reduced |
| Hyperthyroidism | raised | raised | reduced |

# LABORATORY EXAMINATION OF ANDROGENIC FUNCTION OF ADRENALS AND OVARIES

We are presenting only a list of several of the most important examinations in clinical practice:

a) urinary 17-oxosteroids,
b) total and free plasma testosterone,
c) TEBG.

The serum concentration of testosterone and oestradiol binding globulin (TEBG) is assessed using the method of competitive bond by precipitation with ammonium sulphate or equilibration dialysis; both variants give practically the same results. Laboratory values of normal subjects are essential. In the follicular phase of the menstrual cycle of healthy women the following are quoted as the mean value ($\pm$ SE): 30 $\pm$ 2 mIU per ml with a range of 18–42 mIU/ml.

The binding capacity of TEBG is also expressed as the so-called dihydrotestosterone precipitation index (DHT-PI). The laboratory values of normal subjects are again essential. For healthy women mean values $\pm$ SE of 1.22 $\pm$ 0.28 are quoted.

We have refuted the suppression-stimulation test of androgenic adrenal and ovarian function (with administration of dexamethasone in the 1st and the simultaneous administration of dexamethasone and hCG in the 2nd phase) after testing, as well as the test of sequential suppression (administration of dexamethasone in the 1st and dexamethasone with a combination of oestrogen and gestagen in the 2nd phase). The logical premise of these two tests is too simphfied. Suppression by dexamethasone is not specific for the adrenals but also acts on ovarian steroidogenesis. Moreover, there are also reports on the effects of hCG and oestrogens on adrenal steroidogenesis. The information provided by the two tests does not correspond to their laboriousness and cost.

## ASSESSMENT OF GONADOTROPINS

The assessment of gonadotropin levels in urine and plasma is one of the basic tests in disorders of the cycle in primary and secondary hypooestrogenic amenorrhoea. A review of methods for their estimation and values recorded in normal cycles has been presented elsewhere (see p. 53). Nowadays the biological assessment of total gonadotropic activity (TGA) in urine and the radioimmunological estimation of LH and FSH in plasma resp. and estimation of prolactin in serum are indispensable.

The **biological assessment** of the LH and FSH (methods described by Parlow and Steelmann-Pohley resp.) and the immunological estimation of LH is little used nowadays because it is laborious and expensive. TGA in urine gives a preliminary idea of the total gonadotropin level in which FSH and LH participate by unknown ratios. Comparison of biological activities of TGA and of LH and FSH separately in urine reveals mid-cycle peaks which coincide. The levels of their tonic excretion in the follicular and luteal phase are also comparable. Because of the wide variation of values in 24 hours the average of two or three values is always assessed.

**Radioimmunological assessment** of LH and FSH is possible in urine and plasma. These are as much as 200 times more sensitive than biological methods and the plasma values are given in mIU/ml or in ng of standard. At present they are being introduced in some departments, because when the necessary equipment is available, they are very rapid and make it possible to obtain results in large series. They characterize the actual levels of both gonadotropins very accurately. The basic tonic secretion in the cycle is for FSH on average 4–17 mIU/ml, for LH 6–25 mIU/ml (448), the cyclic preovulatory secretion of FSH is double to treble the amount, and of LH five to ten times as much. A considerable individual variation must be considered as well as discrepancies due to lack of integration of radioimmunological methods as far as antibodies, technique and standards are concerned.

WHO therefore adopted a programme for the standardization and quality control of RIA of hormones in reproductive physiology (195) and comparative standards are being elaborated for biological and immunological methods of urinary and hypophyseal gonadotropins (see p. 57). On principle comparisons should be made with a standard of the same or similar origin. Despite these differences the character of curves obtained by biological methods is similar to curves obtained by radioimmunological methods, as was revealed by some comparisons which nevertheless record such differences as a great increase of FSH at the onset of the cycle and a minimum FSH at the time of the preovulatory peak of LH when biological methods are used. The correlation between routine immunological and biological (TGA) estimations was significant and about 70% of the results among low and medium values were in agreement. As to high values (after the menopause) for FSH, agreement was recorded in 80%, but for LH only in 18% (70); LH assessed by immunological methods was as a rule lower.

The clinical importance lies, in particular, in the **diagnosis of disorders of the cycle.** For classification of disorders of the cycle cases must be divided into normogonadotropic, hypogonadotropic and hypergonadotropic ones. For this purpose it is sufficient to assess TGA in urine. In disorders of the cycle which have a biphasic BBT, cyclic or irregular bleeding, assessment of TGA is useless. There it will be better in future to assess more subtle deviations of LH and FSH by means of radioimmunological methods.

Another important clinical aspect is the investigation of gonadotropins after **treatment with gonadotropic hormones** or other ovulation-inducing substances. We test the response to the administered substance and prevent manifestations of hypersensitivity, however, other indirect criteria can be also used.

Finally the assessment of the LH peak enables us to determine **the time of ovulation** accurately (see p. 243). This assumes, however, the possibility of rapid estimation of LH by means of commercially prepared immunological kits, or by means of radioimmunological methods on the solid phase in the case of LH (487).

*Prolactin (human)* is estimated nowadays by homologous RIA using double-antibody techniques. The normal serum level varies between 5–20 ng/ml. Depending on the method, a level above 20–25 ng/ml is classified as hyperprolactinaemia. The clinical importance of the assessment of prolactin levels is currently increasing and in differential diagnostic procedures it holds an important place. This is so because it was found that in addition to rare syndromes associated with galactorrhoea and adenoma of the pituitary, so-called idiopathic hyperprolactinaemia is the basis of a high percentage of disorders of the menstrual cycle with impaired ovulation such as: the galactorrhoea-amenorrhoea syndrome, anovulatory cycle, luteal insufficiency. All types of hyperprolactinaemia are readily treated by agonists of dopamine from the series of ergot analogues.

# ASSESSMENT OF STEROIDS

Clinical practice in gynaecological endocrinology commonly uses the assessment of pregnanediol in urine and of progesterone in plasma, total oestrogens in urine and oestradiol in plasma, 17-oxosteroids in urine and testosterone in plasma. Methods of estimation and their values in the course of the cycle are given in more detail elsewhere in this work (see p. 89, 100 and 109), as well as correlations with indirect clinical tests (see p. 206, 208, 218 and 221).

## GESTAGENS

For quantitative assessment of **pregnanediol** in urine there exist two widely used methods — adsorption chromatography and, more recently, gas chromatography. Both methods can be easily combined with the assessment of pregnanetriol in urine. The estimation of pregnanediol is of clinical importance in particularly in disorders of corpus luteum function associated with infertility, for evidence of ovulation and finally in the follow-up of treatment with gestagens or other ovulation-inducing substances. In luteal insufficiency it can differentiate this condition from mere retardation of the secretory phase of the endometrium and characterize from the height and persistence of the level the corpus luteum function. The daily amount during the secretory phase varies between 3 and 8 mg/24 hours. Levels of 1.25 to 2.0 mg/24 hours are taken as a rule as the range signalizing ovulation. The estimation must be done every day, and values lower by more than 2 SD or SE from the mean are usually classified as reduced.

In disorders of the adrenals **pregnanetriol** in urine is the most sensitive indicator of impaired biosynthesis of cortisol, e.g. in adrenogenital syndrome. For verification of therapy it is more suitable than 17-oxosteroids or 17-hydroxycorticoids.

Only recently has the importance of quantitative assessment of **progesterone** in plasma increased. It has the same indications as pregnanediol. Methods of saturation analysis rendered it possible to elaborate very sensitive protein-binding methods and radioimmunological methods which can be used with very small amounts of plasma. During the secretory phase plasma progesterone reaches maximum values 5–8 days after ovulation, i.e. 8–15 ng/ml. It is maintained that a level above 5.2 ng/ml on the 4th to 10th day after ovulation with a 95% confidence limit suggests the presence of the corpus luteum (313). Similar data are reported also by other authors. In other publications the reported value is 1.8 ng/ml (13), 3 ng/ml (230) and 5 ng/ml in the mid-luteal phase (2). For the diagnosis of a defect of the luteal phase according to some authors one plasma progesterone value suffices, according to others the decline on the 6th day of the luteal phase, as the level is not only lower but declines sooner than in a normal cycle. As a rule, however, more values are needed. Recently doubts were expressed that it is possible to express by means of one value the quality of the luteal phase and a combination of three values is recommended between the 11th to 4th day before menstruation, whereby the total value should not exceed $3 \times 5$ ng, i.e. 15 ng/ml (2). For the diagnosis of ovulation one value in the mid-luteal phase suffices. It seems that modern methods of progesterone assessment in plasma will gradually replace pregnanediol estimations in urine which are more tedious and less accurate.


## OESTROGENS

The clinical value of oestrogen assessment is less than that of progesterone. Nowadays **total oestrogens in urine** are still assessed. The borderline between a normal and reduced level is about 10 µg/24 hours, the highest normal level during the preovulatory peak is 30 to 100 µg/24 hours. In practice there are three indications for the estimation of urinary oestrogens. A rare indication is suspicion of oestrogen-active tumours (granulosa-cell tumour, thecoma, feminizing mesenchymoma in young girls or in women after the menopause). The second indication is the diagnosis of hypooestrogenic conditions where indirect tests cannot be used. The most serious indication is the follow-up of gonadotropin treatment. By means of a semi-automatic method the total oestrogen value can be obtained in three and a half hours and hyperstimulation syndromes can be prevented. When the values exceed 200 µg/24 hours, treatment must be discontinued.

Recently very sensitive protein-binding methods and radioimmunological methods assessing **plasma oestradiol** are used. Antisera are highly specific and in RIA individual steroids need not be separated which considerably shortens the procedure. Normal values are, according to our own experience, during the follicular phase on average 68 pg/ml with a lower range of 30 pg/ml. According to various RIA methods the normal average values are 50–100 pg/ml. The preovulatory peak on the day preceding ovulation is on average $175 \pm 16$ pg/ml, and according to other authors 100–400 pg/ml. The levels during the secretory phase are between 100–250 pg/ml. The indication for the assessment of oestrogens and oestradiol are restricted for several reasons: normal and pathological values overlap due to the wide range of variations in 20%. In practice we possess sufficiently suitable, rapid and simple indirect tests of oestrogenic activity. A positive progesterone test informs us rapidly and simultaneously about the presence of oestrogens and also whether the endometrium is satisfactory from the functional aspect and that there is no mechanical obstruction.

# ANDROGENS

In practice it is frequently necessary to analyze hyperandrogenic conditions. Many clinical tests were proposed but they were soon subjected to criticism (17-oxosteroids, fractions of 17-oxosteroids, functional tests such as e.g. Jayle's test for the differentiation of ovarian and adrenal androgens, etc.). Although we know that only a small proportion of **17-oxosteroids** in urine originates from testosterone, their estimation may be recommended as a screening test in hyperandrogenism, as they are usually elevated in these conditions, while in polycystic ovaries they are usually at the upper normal range which is 15 mg/24 hours. More recently **testosterone** was estimated in plasma, the normal range of values being 300–600 pg/ml. From an analysis of the testosterone metabolism it may be concluded (see p. 106) that the level of this hormone in plasma does not give an accurate idea of its production. Only about 70% cases of hirsutism have raised testosterone plasma levels. Better results are obtained by the simultaneous assessment of **free and bound testosterone and the binding capacity** (TEBG) or estimation in ovarian venous and adrenal blood. So far, however, we are lacking sufficient experience and practical data.

# X-RAY EXAMINATION

In disorders of the menstrual cycle some X-ray examinations may contribute towards the diagnosis.

The latter include: vaginography, hysterography, hysterosalpingography, pneumopelvigraphy, X-ray examination of the sella turcica, retroperitoneal insufflation and the assessment of ossification age. We consider them special examinations which are indicated only in some patients to assess the diagnosis.

**Vaginography** is a simple method for the visualization of the relations of the efferent urinary pathways and the vagina in developmental anomalies. It is indicated in case of a common urogenital duct to visualize the urogenital sinus and in anomalies of the vagina in primary amenorrhoea to visualize the length and terminal portion of the vaginal recess when visual access is lacking.

**Hysterography** has proved useful as a diagnostic method in all menorrhagias, in particular in the secondary type, and to differentiate anatomical from endocrine causes of disorders. It revealed the presence of submucous myomas or polyps which frequently were not detected by sound or curettage. Moreover hysterography detects anomalies in the shape of the uterus.

**Hysterosalpingography** is not a special endocrinological method but we use it when the disorder of the cycle is associated with sterility and infertility. It provides objective evidence of hypoplasia of the uterus and its changes after therapy resp., it detects abnormalities of the uterus and cervix, in amenorrhoea and hypo-menorrhoea it reveals secondary synechiae obliterating the uterine cavity. We assess polyposis of the endometrium and a suspect specific process of the endometrium and tubes resp. An occlusion of the oviducts must always be ruled out before treatment of an anovulatory cycle by ovulation-inducing substances. The hysterosalpingographic diagnosis is discussed in the chapter on sterility (see p. 333).

**Pneumopelvigraphy** makes use of the contrast of the gaseous filling and the mass of the uterus and ovaries and enables visualization of the shape, size and syntopy of the organs of the pelvis. In addition to general gynaecological diagnosis it is very useful in disorders of the cycle. In the first phase we make a transparietal puncture of the mesogastrium and pneumoperitoneum by insufflation with 600 to 1,000 ml $CO_2$, in the second phase we take a picture in the genupectoral position. In view of the irradiation load an apparatus must be used with an amplifier and possibly a television screen. The main indication is primary amenorrhoea where we can demonstrate changes in the size of the ovaries from normal via hypoplastic ovaries to aplasia of the ovaries and confirm dysgenesis of the gonads. We can also demonstrate aplasia and gross malformations of the uterus. In secondary, and rarely also in primary amenorrhoea, bilateral enlargement of the ovaries provides evidence of the syndrome of polycystic ovaries. It was also possible to provide evidence of ovarian tumours which could not be reliably detected by palpation. The finding of calcifications in the space of the inner genitals in primary amenorrhoea suggests a specific process contracted and usually terminated in the postnatal period. Pneumopelvigraphy can also be combined with hysterosalpingography — so-called **gynaecography.** When comparing pneumopelvigraphy with culdoscopy, the latter provides in addition to information about the shape, information on another characteristic, i.e. colour, and is thus of greater diagnostic value.

**X-ray of the sella turcica** must be made in all primary and secondary cases of hypohormonal amenorrhoea or when a hypophyseal process is suspected. We can thus detect tumours of the pituitary or the parasellar spaces, or an adenoma of the anterior lobe in acromegaly. In combination with a pneumoencephalogram we can diagnose the "empty sella syndrome". The appearance of the sella must be known in galactorrhoea and hyperprolactinaemia. A reduced size of the sella is typical of a primarily hypophyseal origin in an ovarian disorder and helps to differentiate it from a primarily ovarian pathogenesis with a normal sella. The standard lateral X-ray projection is usually supplemented by another three projections and tomography resp.

**Retroperitoneal insufflation** is indicated when an adrenal disorder is suspected and we thus facilitate the diagnosis of adrenogenital syndrome. We perform it by means of filling the perirenal spaces with $CO_2$ and take an X-ray picture of the adrenals.

**Ossification age.** In developmental disorders it is often important to know the developmental retardation. For this purpose X-rays of the ossification nuclei of the long bones are made. By comparison with tables of normal ossification times we can evaluate the examined patient because the time during normal growth when the ossification nuclei of the epiphyses of some bones develop is constant. A marked retardation of bone development is found e.g. in hypothyroidism and in nanism.

## ANTHROPOMETRIC EXAMINATION

Anthropometric measurements are used for the objectivization of skeletal proportions. The proportions of the skeleton together with the maturation of the facial features, bone, dental, mental and sexual development serve to evaluate the growth and development of the individual.

The basic anthropometric data are: height, the span of the hands (the distance between the finger tips with outspread arms), the upper and lower portion of height (measured from the symphysis to the top or base) and their ratio, the circumference of the head, chest and abdomen. By comparison with tables of normal values for different ages deviations in the development are assessed (Engelbach's tables).

Some anthropometric measurements were used to prepare so-called morphograms. Typical pathological curves develop in Turner's syndrome, eunuchoidism, nanism, etc. A certain quantification of impaired development is involved.

## OVULATION TESTS

Assessment of the ovulation time in women is of immense practical importance for the diagnosis of a normal ovulation cycle and for fertility control in the positive (best time of conception) and negative sense (contraception).

Therefore for years data on the physiological incidence of ovulation in relation to the cycle was in the foreground of interest, as well as the most suitable and most accurate clinical signs of the ovulation time. Based on laparotomies and direct observation of the ovaries it was established that ovulation occurs $14 \pm 2$ days before the next menstruation. When the relationship between the day of ovulation and the length of the cycle was confirmed, it was possible to assess the time of ovulation statistically in women pregnant after a single intercourse; on average it was found to be the 12.8 day from the beginning of menstruation in a cycle with an average length of 28.7 days. For marginal lengths of the cycle, 23 and 34 days, the day of ovulation is on the 10.7th and 14.8th day according to the equation: $y = 2.2 - 0.37x$, where $SE = 1.1$ and $r = 0.63$ (350).

Due to the variability of the follicular phase of the cycle the variability of the ovulation time, counting from the onset of the cycle, is between the 10th and 15th day whereby about two thirds of cycles have ovulation between the 12th and 14th day. This is consistent with data obtained by dating of fertilized ova, where ovulation appears to be on the 11th–17th day of the cycle or $14 \pm 2$ days from the onset of the subsequent cycle.

Clinical ovulation tests based on almost all factors which displayed marked cyclic variations during the ovarian cycle (see p. 71–129) were proposed. Reviews will be found in several publications (140, 164). Ovulation tests can be evaluated from several aspects: accuracy, early response, and simple procedure in practice. It must be added, however, that so far there is no completely reliable test which can be carried out rapidly and easily under clinical conditions.

## DIRECT CRITERIA OF OVULATION

(1) Observations during laparotomy, culdoscopy and laparoscopy helped to assess the day of ovulation; these data are, however, rare and therefore cannot be used in practice.

(2) Pregnancy after a single intercourse or after insemination can determine ovulation *ex post*. The assessment is, however, not accurate although the fertilization period of the ovum is short, usually only 12 hours. Sperm cells are able to fertlize not only for 48–72 hours as is usually maintained, but they may preserve their motility for as much as seven days.

(3) The removal of non-fertilized ova during operation from the oviducts may also be evidence of ovulation. It is, however, difficult to assess accurately the age of non-fertilized ova. Collection of fertilized ova provides accurate information on the date of ovulation with a variation of about half a day. For practice this evaluation is, however, not suitable and is rather an exception.

(4) Histological dating of the corpus luteum can *ex post* determine the day of ovulation (92) but there are also some objections. First of all this implies comparison with a standard 28-day cycle, secondly the criteria were elaborated from material obtained in monkeys or from evaluation of the condition of the endometrium (140).

(5) The difference in size of the ovaries during ovulation assessed by an electromagnetic technique provided evidence that ovulation had taken place. In women the ovary is largest during the luteal phase. In practice this test was not introduced on a larger scale.

(6) Intermenstrual or ovulation pain, an associated manifestation of ovulation, has been recorded for a very long time. Some reported its occurrence before the rise of basal temperature and after the peak of cervical mucus, while others reported that it persisted for several days before the rise. By comparison with new criteria, e.g. the peak of LH, it was revealed that intermenstrual pain

238

occurred before the peak of LH (334), on the day of its peak and after the peak of LH. If we add to this the inconstant incidence of this phenomenon, it may be said that its value as an ovulation test is dubious.

(7) Assessment of plasma proteins in cervical mucus estimated electrophoretically was also proposed as a direct ovulation test. This sudden rise was supposed to be due to the follicular fluid taken up by the oviducts after rupture of the follicle. Other authors, however, could not demonstrate this fluid by its antigenic properties.

To sum up it must be said that so far there is no suitable direct ovulation test.


## INDIRECT CRITERIA OF OVULATION

In clinical practice indirect criteria are most frequently used, based on the action of oestrogens and progesterone on peripheral tissues during the cycle. Some of these tests precede ovulation and are thus of value for the investigated cycle, others provide an answer only after ovulation and give retrospective information. The follow up must extend over several days.


## CERVICAL MUCUS

Cervical mucus has many properties which change periodically during the menstrual cycle (see p. 124), and this has led to the elaboration of various ovulation tests among which the viscosity test and fern test are best. Because the changes take place under the influence of oestrogens and in conjunction with their preovulatory peak, these are early tests which are positive before ovulation or on the day of ovulation.

a) "**Spinnbarkeit**" test was introduced 30 years ago. It is a short period of reduced viscosity of cervical mucus when from a drop of mucus on a slide or tampon forceps a filament on average 14 cm long (10–25 cm) can be drawn, as compared to days of high viscosity when it is only 0–5 cm. The period of decreased viscosity lasts 3–6 days. The peak of "Spinnbarkeit" is usually correlated with the basal temperature. The day of maximum "Spinnbarkeit" precedes according to the majority of authors the rise of basal temperature by 1–2 days, sometimes by as much as four days. The maximum "Spinnbarkeit" is on average one day before the peak of LH (339) or during the interval —2 to +1 day in relation to the peak of LH (42). From the data thus ensues that the maximum "Spinnbarkeit" is 0–2 days before ovulation. In practice this test is the most suitable one.

b) **Fern test.** This test is based on the formation of crystals in the shape of tree- or fern-like formations in a drop of cervical mucus after drying. Crystals of NaCl are formed which during ovulation account for 97% of all chlorides in mucus; the positivity of crystals is due to oestrogens. Experimentally it was, however, shown that for maximum crystallization in addition to oestrogens progesterone is also needed. The presence of crystallization is quantified subjectively from 0 to $+++$, it is sooner positive than "Spinnbarkeit" and persists longer. The day of maximum crystallization coincides with the day of maximum "Spinnbarkeit". If we compare the peak of crystallization with the peak of LH, both maxima are recorded on the same day. Some work evaluated this test favourably, other authors are critical to this test because crystallization persisted for some days, while "Spinnbarkeit" declined already.

c) **Half-open external cervical orifice.** This serves in practice as a preliminary sign of the ovulation time. The external orifice is flabby and with the transparent mucus creates the impression of the pupil of a fish eye.

d) The **amount of cervical mucus** is greatest during ovulation time. The amount of mucus and its transparency, absence of leucocytes and half-open external orifice are sometimes expressed quantitatively e.g. as Rauscher's index (419). Based on a correlation with the basal temperature and biopsy of the endometrium the attainment of 9 and a half points is considered the preovulation time which lasts 2–3 days. Other types of cervical score include moreover "Spinnbarkeit" and crystallization (228).

e) An increased **amount of sodium chloride** in cervical mucus during ovulation could be proved only in dried mucus. In fresh mucus the NaCl content is roughly isotonic ($0.93 \pm 0.12\%$) and does not display cyclic variation. On the other hand, in dry mucus it has a sharp maximum at the time of ovulation (40–70%), as compared with the other phases of the cycle (2–20%). For the so-called *spot test* (test of McSweeney and Sbarra) filter paper impregnated with a mixture of silver nitrate and potassium chromate is used; with sodium chloride a white or yelllow colouration of silver chromate is obtained. The mucus on the filter paper begins to alter the brown colour on the paper to white four days before ovulation and the maximum white colouration is found at the time of ovulation. The advantage of the test is the simple procedure and that the woman can carry it out herself. In practice, however, the results are rather variable (202).

f) The **burning phenomenon** is another simple ovulation test based on the change of colouration after rapid drying of a smear of mucus over a flame. The colour change from milky white to dark brown is recorded on a scale from 0–3. During ovulation the colour is white and the course of changes is the mirror image of crystallization (60).

g) The **ovulation method** is a simple test where the woman herself learns to recognize the clinical symptoms of changes of cervical mucus, i.e. so-called dry days, the onset of the mucus symptom and the peak symptom of transparent mucus. The correlation between the ovulation time, assessed as the first day after the peak of LH pregnanediol and oestrogens revealed that the peak symptom preceded ovulation on average by 0.9 days ($+3$ to $-2$ days). For the first time the mucus symptom was found on average 6.2 days (3–10) before ovulation (42). This natural ovulation test is made by the woman herself and she controls accordingly conception or abstinence without any examination. However, so far we have little practical experience with this test and critical comments on the test are increasing.

h) **Glucose test.** This test detects either glucose or glucosamine by a colour reaction and is described also as Test-Tape indicator. It is made with test papers for sugar in urine, and the colour change signalizes the increased glucose concentration in cervical mucus at the time of ovulation. The favourable results of the original authors were countered by the negative experience of others. The test is no longer used.

i) Assessment of **enzymes in cervical mucus** revealed typical cyclic changes during the menstrual cycle and it is therefore recommended as an ovulation test. Alkaline phosphatase declines significantly closely before the peak of LH and begins to rise after ovulation. Similarly a significant preovulation decline is found in esterase, while the decline of aminopeptidase is not significant.

## RISE OF BASAL BODY TEMPERATURE

The rise of basal temperature gives retrospectively the approximate time of ovulation (see p. 203). Because the woman records it herself, it is used commonly to regulate pregnancy.

## KARYOPYKNOTIC OR EOSINOPHIL INDEX

The karyopyknotic or eosinophil index reaches its peak in conjunction with the peak of oestrogens 1–3 days before ovulation or at the time of ovulation, while the oestrogenic type of smear during the luteal phase disappears quickly. In correlation with other signs of ovulation, it corresponds to the cervical score. In view of the longer persisting peak it is used in practice for the diagnosis of ovulation less frequently than the basal temperature and "Spinnbarkeit". As compared with urinary oestrogens, the cytological peak appears 1–3 days after the oestrogen peak somewhat later than the peak of cervical mucus. In relation to the peak of LH secretion the peak of the karyopyknotic index is delayed by 0.6 days with a variation range of 4 days before the LH peak to 3 days after it (333).

# BIOPSY OF THE ENDOMETRIUM

Biopsy of the endometrium also provides retrospective evidence of ovulation. The first changes which can be evaluated as an ovulation test occur according to older work only 24–36 hours after ovulation, while more recent correlations with LH provide evidence that the basal glycogen vacuoles in the glandular cells are already present on the first, and latest on the second day after the LH peak. Even before vacuoles at the basal pole of the glandular cells, after staining, nitroformazan granules can be observed. Chronologically they correspond to the onset of LH release. Biopsy is suited for the retrospective diagnosis of ovulation but not for regulating conception.

# HAEMATOLOGICAL PARAMETERS

Cyclic changes of various parameters in the peripheral blood stream were observed a long time ago in conjunction with the ovarian cycle (haemorrhagic diathesis, capillary permeability, coagulation tests, and number of blood elements). Only some were recommended as ovulation tests: changes of eosinophil cells, thrombocytes, basophil cells and alkaline phosphatase in leucocytes.

a) The number of **eosinophil cells** has a postovulation minimum which occurs $1.57 \pm 0.91$ days before the rise of the basal temperature. Some authors report positive results, while more recent data indicate an insignificant difference (331), as is the case for the total number of leucocytes, monocytes or neutrophil cells.

b) The number of **platelets** during ovulation rises steeply and remains at an elevated level throughout the secretory phase. It was recommended generally as an ovulation test or evidence of the secretory phase. Comparison with the basal temperature revealed that the rise of thrombocytes occurs earlier, there being a marked difference between the pre- and postovulatory period (196). Recently a rise of thrombocytes two days after ovulation was recorded (331). Negative results were also published.

c) The number of **basophil cells** declines briskly on the day of ovulation and reaches the average value of $27.5 \pm 12$/cub.mm. These relations were detected only recently. A significant decline of the absolute and relative number of basophil cells, as compared with the otherwise only slightly varying level, is recommended as a suitable ovulation test. So far the cause of this phenomenon remains obscure.

d) **Alkaline phosphatase in neutrophil leucocytes** reaches its maximum in the mid-cycle during the rise of the basal temperature. This maximum is consistent with ovulation within a range of 3–5 days. Oestrogens are the cause of the rise of this enzyme, while progesterone inhibits it. Alkaline phosphatase may be assessed also in saliva.

## ASCORBIC ACID RETENTION

Ascorbic acid retention during ovulation and the sudden decline of its urinary excretion after excess doses (200 mg per day) was recommended as Pillay's ovulation test and was confirmed by other authors. More recently 500 mg ascorbic acid per day are administered and the maximum decline precedes the rise of basal temperature by two or three days, occurring as a rule on the 13th to 14th day (383). Comparison with the curve of LH secretion shows agreement; the increased ascorbic acid excretion after a previous decline seems to be metabolically associated with the LH peak. The use of this method as an ovulation test in practice is limited, as it is necessary to make repeated laboratory estimations.

## ELECTROPOTENTIALS

The original experiments of authors who recorded electropotentials by a vaginal and suprapubic electrode at the time of ovulation were renewed in the sixties. At ovulation time flat electropositive curves with a range of 10–20 mV were recorded. Devices that measure electropotential differences in finger-to-finger contact were introduced on a clinical scale. Recent results have found this method unreliable for detection of ovulation.

## HORMONE LEVELS

Assessment of hormones in urine has become the basis of a number of ovulation tests. Practically none of them has proved useful. Most widely recommended were tests based on **pregnanediol** estimation in urine (see p. 233). A great variation of pregnanediol values and their overlapping, raised values during luteinization without ovulation, and the relatively difficult assessment were the reason why none of these tests was introduced. Similarly assessment of **oestrogens** in urine for diagnosis did not prove useful. The same applies to Farris test which assessed LH during the preovulation period by hyperaemia of the ovaries after injection of urine in infantile rats.

Accurate, rapid and therefore perspective methods of assessment of hormones in peripheral blood are ovulation tests which record the peak of plasma LH and the plasma progesterone level.

**LH** release into the blood stream is of decisive importance in the mechanism of ovulation. Therefore this peak is frequently considered the zero day in relation to ovulation and other laboratory methods are referred to it. Actual ovulation occurs within 36 hours after the LH peak, and according to other authors 12–24 hours after the peak. It is thus correct to speak of a preovulatory release of LH; while as regards ovulation, this is day —1. The urinary oestrogen peak is —2 to +1 day from the LH peak, while the plasma oestradiol peak is —3 to 0 days. The first progesterone rise is within —2 to 0 days from the LH peak. So far LH estimation is little used for the diagnosis of ovulation because immunological methods although rapid are expensive. By using RIA modifications on a solid phase the results can be obtained within 5–7 hours. Even more rapid for LH estimation is the radioreceptor method which gives results within 4 hours (453). Thus the clinician obtains an accurate and rapid ovulation test.

Plasma **progesterone** is nowadays a reliable index not only of ovulation but more of luteal function. Its correlation with other parameters in the secretory phase was mentioned before (13).

## PHOSPHATE IN SALIVA

Cyclic changes of some constituents of saliva in conjunction with the normal cycle of women have been previously detected. As ovulation test it was suggested to estimate the glucose, sialic acid, alkaline phosphatase, and peroxidase concentration. A simple test seems to be the estimation of phosphate concentration in saliva. In 16 of 18 normal cycles a one-day but very striking increase of phosphates was observed in correlation with the rise of the basal temperature. Further confirmation by practical experience is needed.

# DIFFERENTIAL DIAGNOSIS OF MENSTRUAL DYSFUNCTION IN PRACTICE

The pathogenetic classification of disorders of the menstrual cycle (for details as regards difficulties of their aetiology see p. 197) begins at the level of out-patient practice. Further steps call for some laboratory and clinical examinations which can be performed only in collaboration with in-patient departments which have laboratory facilities.

Schematically, a simple and rational strategy for investigation of menstrual dysfunctions is presented in the form of stepwise flow charts (decision trees with decision and chance nodes) (Figs. 36–38). It also shows which examinations are considered basic at the particular stage of decision, how far we can get in ambulatory practice and when it is essential to refer the patient to an in-patient department. The schematic presentation naturally involves a certain amount of simplification; but nevertheless we assume that it may serve as a guide and starting point for selecting the procedures [e.g. on Fig. 37 secondary amenorrhoea with hirsutism which needs a special examination (see p. 230 and 275) is not mentioned].

A quite special approach is needed in primary amenorrhoea. It is essential for these women to be examined in a specialized department, and for the differential diagnosis pretentious laboratory and clinical methods are essential. For intersexual malformations we refer to special literature (239, 382). As far as phenotypic females are concerned, the starting point for the differential diagnosis may be any basic clinical or laboratory examination given on p. 174. As an example we are quoting the modified flow sheet for diagnostic approach (540).

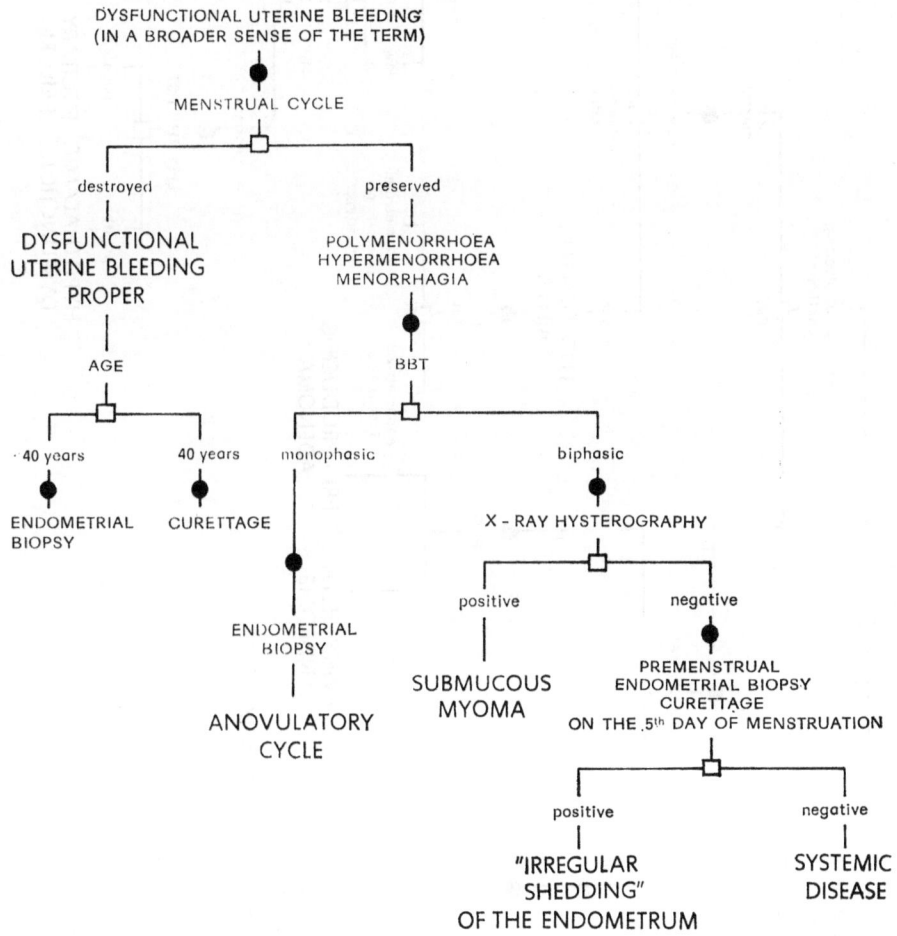

*Fig. 36.* A stepwise flow chart for the diagnostic approach to dysfunctional uterine bleeding (● — decision nodes, ☐ — chance nodes).

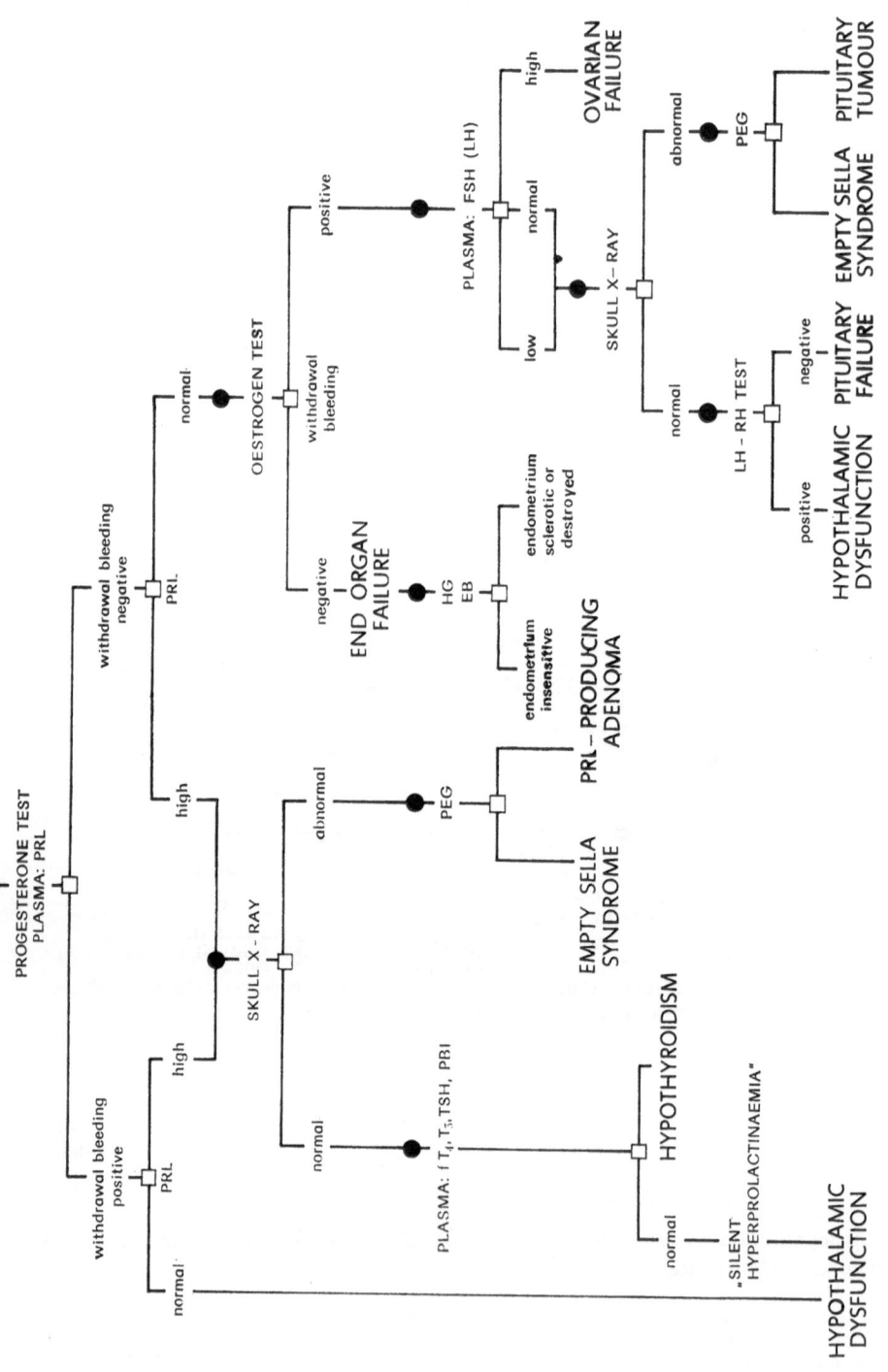

*Fig. 37.* A stepwise flow chart for the diagnostic approach to secondary amenorrhoea according to the positivity or negativity of the progesterone withdrawal-bleeding test and plasma PRL level (PEG – pneumoencephalography, HG – hysterography, EB – endometrial biopsy).

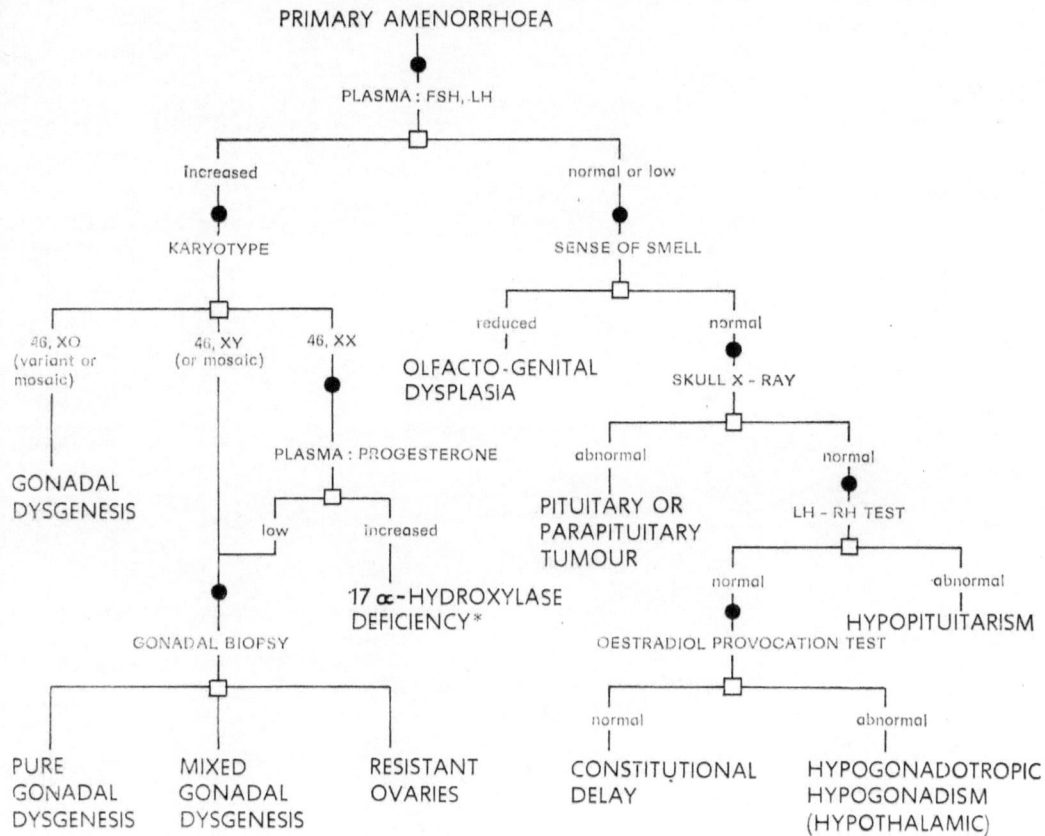

Fig. 38. Flow sheet for investigation of primary amenorrhoea (modified after 540) (* the presence of hypertension suggests a congenital deficiency of 17α-hydroxylation of progesterone with cortisol, oestradiol and testosterone biosynthesis alteration).

# Clinical Aspects of Disorders
# of the Menstrual Cycle

## PSYCHOGENIC DISORDERS

The pathogenesis of psychogenic menstrual dysfunction and sterility and their aetiology was discussed in detail in previous paragraphs (see p. 177 and 201).

## SECONDARY AMENORRHOEA

A recent epidemiological investigation of secondary amenorrhoea (157) revealed a surprisingly high incidence of psychogenic factors in the affected women. The incidence of stressful life events with frustration, depression, the sensation of loss and isolation was statistically significantly higher (in about one third of amenorrhoic women) than in a control sample of the population. Secondary amenorrhoea was also found more frequently in unmarried women and in women with an intellectual occupation. On the other hand, there was no significant difference in the incidence of secondary amenorrhoea in women with psychoneurosis and women without this disease. Gonadotropic patterns in psychogenic amenorrhoea with a negative progesterone test are very different. Plasma LH and FSH concentrations may be normal, lowered and even elevated (185, 396). However, cases with normal urinary TGA and normal total oestrogen excretion have also been reported. Moreover, alterations in PRL secretion are known in women with psychogenic disturbances (see p. 178).

### "SCHRECKAMENORRHOE"

After acute and very brief psychic trauma (so-called psychic or mental shock) an expected menstruation may be missed; cases of sudden arrest of menstruation which has already started are also known. We assume that the initial parahypophyseal nervous mechanism participates followed by a transhypophyseal disorder in the control of ovarian function.

# "NOTSTANDSAMENORRHOE"

This term covers cases of secondary amenorrhoea with a mass incidence occurring under difficult conditions during the last world war in women in concentration and internment camps, prisoners and refugees.

In the Terezín concentration camp (29) 54% of the women developed amenorrhoea; 60% during the first month after imprisonment, and during the second month another 25%, i.e. it was not yet associated with the gradually developing malnutrition, protein and vitamin deficiency. Conversely, menstruation was spontaneously restored in 94% of the affected women within one to one and a half years of imprisonment, as a rule during the second half of the first year. Menarche, with rare exceptions of retardation, did not occur at all in young girls in concentration camps. Half the women in the internment camp in Hong Kong also developed temporary amenorrhoea lasting several months. Later, in conjunction with drastic protein restriction a second wave of the disorder developed.

Initial amenorrhoea is, no doubt, psychogenic and affects subjects with a less resistent higher nervous activity. Spontaneous restoration of the menstrual cycle suggests that the psychic stress has been overcome, and higher nervous activity has been normalized.

In amenorrhoic women of the Terezín concentration camp it did not prove possible to induce uterine bleeding even with large oestrogen doses; therefore the existence of a parahypophyseal, neurodystrophic disorder of the receptivity of the endometrium cannot be excluded in addition to the possible alteration of specific receptor protein synthesis in the target tissues due to malnutrition. In about one half of 5% of the women where amenorrhoea persisted for one and a half years climacteric phenomena in addition to uterine atrophy were present. Since more detailed examinations were not done, the possible development of a primarily psychogenic ovarian lesion (premature ovarian failure) as one of the manifestations of corticovisceral pathology cannot be verified.

In a certain number of women after the amenorrhoic interval a period of menorrhagia and metrorrhagia followed. This type of disorder occurred instead of the initial amenorrhoea only in a small number of imprisoned women.


## PSEUDOCYESIS (PSEUDOPREGNANCY)

Pseudocyesis is the syndrome of phantom or false pregnancy (for review see 351). The woman is amenorrhoic; the abdomen is enlarged — however, without effacement of the umbilicus; the breasts are also enlarged and tense, they secrete colostrum or milk. The uterine cervix is congested and softened, the uterus is as a rule also enlarged, sometimes very markedly; the woman reports that she perceives foetal movements. The body weight is increased. Morning sickness is frequent (even a case of EPH toxaemia was described, the symptoms disappearing when the diagnosis of pseudopregnancy was made). In some instances an increased urinary gonadotropin excretion was described, so that the pregnancy test (biological and immunological) therefore can be falsely positive. In other instances, however, a decline of circulating gonadotropins was observed. An increase in plasma PRL level seems to be common. The contemporary literature still lacks representative results of systematic examinations of circulating gonadotropin and steroid levels. Reports published hitherto are incomplete and the conclusions are not unequivocal.

To rule out pregnancy the following are important: an inverted umbilicus on the enlarged abdomen, the absence of foetal parts of the X-ray and diminution of the abdomen under anaesthesia (the enlargement of the abdomen is due to a special position of the abdominal musculature and hyperlordosis of the lumbar spine).

As to the aetiology depression from an unfulfilled intensive desire for pregnancy or conversely fear of unwanted pregnancy play a part. The pathogenesis is corticovisceral (see p. 177). Persistence of the corpus luteum is assumed (in several instances restoration of the menstrual cycle was observed after its exstirpation). In other instances, however, laparoscopic examination did not reveal the presence of a corpus luteum and the endometrium was, consistent with the reduced secretion of hypophyseal gonadotropins, in a state of inactive proliferation.

Women with an unrecognized syndrome of pseudopregnancy are frequently subjected to attempts of legal abortion and laparotomy because of suspected extrauterine pregnancy; they may, however, also be admitted to the labour ward with an apparent onset of labour and pseudocyesis is diagnosed only there, in extreme cases after laparotomy performed for indication of Casearean section because of assumed danger to the foetus (for review see 62). The syndrome of phantom pregnancy may occur repeatedly in the same woman.

Therapy is beyond the possibilities of gynaecology. Unequivocal elimination of pregnancy is a potently acting factor in the liquidation of the syndrome itself. However, treatment is impossible without psychotherapy supplemented by psychopharmacotherapy. Cooperation with a psychiatrist is essential.


## ANOREXIA NERVOSA

The syndrome the incidence of which is extremely rare (0.0002–0.0006%) is typical as to its onset, usually before the age of 25 years. Anorexia with a weight loss of at least 25% of the body weight is characterized by a distorted attitude to food intake, which resists arguments and threats, denial of the pathological condition (without alarm caused by the weight loss), and sometimes with the development of an ideal of attractiveness identical with extreme thinness. Vomiting is frequent (sometimes provoked by the patient) and conversely there are periods of bulaemia. The condition is frequently associated with hypotension, bradycardia, hypothermia and constipation.

Secondary amenorrhoea is the rule, and in younger women also primary amenorrhoea (only rarely, in about 10%, it is absent). Its relationship with anorexia and loss of weight is variable. In about half the patients it starts with anorexia; it may, however, already have developed before the first manifestations of anorexia or just after their onset, roughly equally often. As far as the onset of weight loss is concerned, sometimes it precedes, only rarely it follows and most frequently (in 80%) it coincides with it, i.e. it occurs before a significant loss of body weight. Amenorrhoea persists in as many as half the patients even after the body weight has reached normal levels, even when the levels of circulating FSH and LH are normal. Some consider this as evidence of a primary functional lesion of the hypothalamus. The question has, however, not yet been resolved unequivocally.

Gonadotropin secretion, in particular LH, is practically always reduced. The pattern of LH secretion usually corresponds to the pattern typical for prepubertal or pubertal premenarcheal girls (see p. 18). Thus in mental anorexia with primary amenorrhoea arrest of development and, in cases with secondary amenorrhoea, regression — in both instances reversible — of the pattern of LH secretion is involved. This "immature" pattern of LH release becomes normal when normal body weight is restored (58). The above fact provides evidence in favour of the "critical" body weight (see p. 17). Even in women after the menopause an extreme weight loss leads to a decline of circulating LH levels and to a regression of the secretory pattern to the pubertal type (58).

The reduced gonadotropin concentration in the peripheral blood stream does not respond to clomiphene stimulation; after realimentation the typical response is restored. The reactivity of the hypothalamus is thus closely associated with the metabolic condition of the organism. The result of the LH-RH test, when the weight loss is smaller than 25%, is usually normal. If the adenohypophysis does not react to the LH-RH test, as is usually the case when the body weight drops to less than 46 kg or when the weight loss is greater than 25%, the condition improves after realimentation. Therefore the idea is plausible that initial amenorrhoea in anorexia nervosa is of hypothalamic origin. However, developed malnutrition may aggrevate the disorder and lead to a hypophyseal defect of gonadotropin secretion. In this connection it is an interesting observation that during the postwar period in amenorrhoic women with weight losses restitution of the menstrual cycle occurred after amino acid substitution during treatment with protein lysates.

In the diagnosis all possible organic causes must be ruled out (in particular tuberculosis, malignant tumours and hypophyseal cachexia) and primary psychiatric causes (in particular schizophrenia and severe psychoneuroses).

This syndrome is classified also among corticovisceral pathological conditions. Premorbid neurotic complaints in as many as 3/4 of the patients suggest an increased vulnerability of the higher nervous activity. The provoking psychogenic trauma was identified in almost 1/2 of the patients (most frequently family conflicts, conflicts in the erotic and sexual sphere, at school, at work; in about 10% the extreme "diet" was started after a traumatizing comment on fatness).

Recently, a classification of anorexia nervosa according to 4 different chromatographic patterns of urinary peptides has been demonstrated (514): (1) similar to normal women, (2) similar to patients with schizophrenia, (3) to patients with a hysteriform type of neurosis, and (4) a primary "hypothalamic" type of anorexia nervosa. Only in the latter group were fractions influencing appetite in mice found. An anorexigenic peptide was identified and verified by the synthesis of the tripeptide, pyroGlu-His-GlyOH. The structure of the second appetite stimulating peptide has not yet been determined.

Treatment comprises realimentation (incl. forced feeding by stomach tube or by the i.v. route) and psychiatric treatment, preferably during hospitalization.

The condition is serious and proves fatal in approximately 7% of cases. The cause of death is, as a rule, deterioration of the electrolyte balance or septicaemia with frequent leucopenia. The aim is restoration of normal body weight. If the menstrual cycle is not restored (or does not start) cyclic substitutional treatment with ovarian steroids must be administered.


## PSYCHOGENIC STERILITY

We have in mind particular patients with a regular menstrual cycle and anovulation (a so-called complete anovulatory cycle). That the ovulatory mechanism can be influenced by psychogenic factors is apparent from double blind tests where at least 25% of patients with deficient ovulation respond with ovulation to placebo administered instead of clomiphene (86a, 90b).

Psychogenic sterility in the narrower sense of the word implies that in a particular patient contemporary examination methods do not enable us to reveal any morphological or functional causes of infertility, the fertility of the husband being normal. Corticovisceral pathology is suggested by the following:

(1) Frequent conception (in 20–40% of cases) after simple exploratory examination of the patency of oviducts with a normal finding or after hormonal therapy when the menstrual cycle is normal.

(2) Conception after a change of partner who in a subsequent marriage also proves fertile.

(3) Frequently reported conception after adoption of a child. Although the gynaecologist may know such cases from his own practice, they seem to be only of importance as case-histories. In large groups this relationship was not proved.

In the aetiology probably the most frequent factor is fear of possible sterility, of failure to implement the basic biological function in marriage, in particular if wanted pregnancy does not occur in the expected short period. A similar role is played also by more complicated emotional conflicts. The pathogenesis is, no doubt, corticovisceral.

In cases with preserved ovulation uterotubal spasm is blamed which may simulate isthmic obstruction of the oviducts in KI or HSG (a spasmolytic effect is produced by instillation of a superficial anaesthetic several minutes before the examination or inhalation of amylnitrite in "obstruction").

The diagnosis of psychogenic sterility must not be based only on negative results of a gynaecological clinical examination. It is essential to have also a psychological examination of both partners focused on conflicts and tension in their relationship. A different approach to the diagnosis is obviously the reason why data on the incidence of psychogenic sterility differ greatly; from 0.2% to 24% of all cases.


## PSYCHOGENIC DYSFUNCTIONAL UTERINE BLEEDING

### "SCHRECKBLUTUNG"

This is uterine bleeding which occurs within a relatively short period following psychic trauma ("mental shock"), regardless of the phase of the menstrual cycle or even in atrophy of the endometrium in the menopause (497). A parahypophyseal mechanism of the development via the autonomic (vasomotor) innervation of the endometrium is probable (see p. 152).

### PSYCHOGENIC ANOVULATORY DYSFUNCTIONAL UTERINE BLEEDING

This differs from other cases of anovulatory dysfunctional uterine bleeding only by its aetiopathogenesis. The provoking factor is usually chronic emotional disorder. There is no agreement whether sexual factors are of greater importance than factors from the non-sexual sphere — data reported in the literature are controversial.

# TREATMENT OF PSYCHOSOMATIC DISORDERS
# OF THE MENSTRUAL CYCLE

Treatment of psychogenic menstrual dysfunctions and sterility ought to be and could be causal. The mere verbalization of the conflict releases the emotional tension of the patient. A sympathetic attitude of the doctor and the development of a positive interpersonal relationship between him and the patient is the prerequisite. This should be followed by psychotherapy. The gynaecologist can provide rational explanatory psychotherapy and adjuvant psychopharmacological treatment, specially anxiolytic drugs (antiphobic drugs and tranquillizers). In case of failure and in serious cases (e.g. in the above mentioned case of pseudocyesis and in mental anorexia), cooperation with the clinical psychologist and psychiatrist is essential.

Symptomatic medicamentous treatment, a positive progesterone or oestrogen test in psychogenic amenorrhoea or arrest of anovulatory dysfunctional bleeding are, no doubt, of positive value and help to establish the patient's confidence in the doctor, sometimes enabling her to "retreat" from her disease without losing her face. There is no doubt, however, that successful symptomatic or pathogenetic medicamentous (hormonal) treatment masks the psychogenic cause of the impaired menstrual cycle or sterility, if the doctor does not consider corticovisceral pathology and possible relapses do not draw his attention to it. Advocates of the extreme view recommend in secondary amenorrhoea and anovulatory dysfunctional bleeding, as soon as organic causes are ruled out, consideration of the possibility of psychosomatic disease.

## EONISM

At the end of this chapter we are adding a short comment on so-called *eonism*, also called *psychic hermaphroditism*. It includes transvestitism and transsexualism.

**Transvestitism** is episodic fetishist wearing of clothes of the opposite sex which relieves the patient's psychic tension and facilitates the accomplishment of orgasm. In women it is found only in exceptional cases.

**Transsexualism**, on the other hand, is complete reversal of the gender identity (for review see 274). It is a psychosexual identification with the opposite sex, despite the existing gonosomal, gonadic, genital, somatic and hypothalamic sexual determination. In the affected woman (the incidence of this disorder in women is reported to be 0.001–0.004%) we do not detect any anatomical and functional abnormalities except that in the phenotypic female there is male identity. The extreme are subjects who before they developed the disease became pregnant and delivered a child. Careful psychiatric and sexological examination and long-term follow up are essential. Attempts to treat these patients with gonadal steroids are doomed to failure. It is remarkable that in approximately half the patients there are detectable changes in the area of the temporal lobe. Some reports indicate a certain relationship between dysfunction of the temporal lobe and disorders in the sexual sphere.

The only therapeutic effects achieved so far were obtained with antiepileptics or temporal lobectomy. Cases are also known of return to the original gender identity and suicide committed after performed surgical correction.

# HYPOTHALAMIC DISORDERS

## LUTEAL INSUFFICIENCY

Luteal insufficiency is a manifestation of abnormal ovarian function characterized by inadequate progesterone production. This condition is often described as a defect of the luteal phase, as an inadequate luteal phase, short luteal phase or retardation of the progestational phase of the endometrium. It becomes a pathological entity only when assessed repeatedly (at least three times). Only then it can be the cause of sterility and in particular infertility. Until recently, in a common group, primary disorders of the corpus luteum, as well as primary disorders of the receptivity of the endometrium, were included. As for the diagnosis mainly microabrasion of the endometrium was used. Only recently is it possible to diferentiate by assessment of progesterone or pregnanediol in combination with microabrasion, between central and peripheral origin of the disorder.

The first time an inadequate response of the endometrium was described as the cause of sterility some 40 years ago. It participates in primary sterility by 11–17% of cases, and in habitual abortions, however, much more, the estimate varying between 35 and 38%.

A short luteal phase may be a contributing factor to adolescent sterility, as has been shown in the monkey (147). An inadequate luteal phase was detected also in other pathological entities such as benign breast diseases and premenstrual syndrome.

The impact of inadequate progesterone production on disorders of reproductive physiology, i.e. sterility and infertility, depends on the degree of progesterone deficiency and its action on the (1) endometrium, (2) tubes, (3) myometrium. On the endometrium there is not sufficient secretory transformation nor an adequate glycogen supply for the nidation of the fertilized ovum. The effect of oestrogen on motility, not inhibited by progesterone, leads to an impaired tubal transport of the ovum. A low progesterone level does not sufficiently inhibit the motility of the myometrium which is necessary for the localization of implantation. While the majority of authors emphasize the importance of luteal insufficiency in disorders of reproduction and achieve by its treatment therapeutic results (245), others apparently achieve pregnancy high rates: 56–60% without treatment (388), and according to some, treatment does not influence the already achieved high pregnancy rate (352). The chronological incidence and degree of retardation of the progestational phase remain uncertain factors. The criterion of the shift of this phase is sometimes two, three or four days or more and it is assessed sometimes twice or three times before the establishment of the diagnosis. The spontaneous evolution of the retarded progestational phase must also be taken into consideration (388).

## PATHOGENESIS AND AETIOLOGY

In the pathogenesis of the disease according to investigations assessing the levels of circulating plasma hormones, the following play a part: (1) inadequate progesterone production, (2) oestrogen deficiency, (3) the inability of the endometrium to respond to a hormonal stimulus, (4) excessive or low prolactin secretion. The impaired steroidogenesis is due to a disorder of the central impulse. According to some authors evidence of this is provided by an inadequate cyclic release of LH, while according to other workers reduced FSH is more likely to be responsible for the inadequate development of the corpus luteum. Sometimes a disproportion of FSH to LH is given as the cause.

Although aetiological factors are not known, they obviously are similar as in the anovulatory cycle. They include psychogenic or neurogenic factors, metabolic disorders, nutritional and iatrogenic factors. Different drugs (tranquillizers and antihistaminic drugs) may interfere with the neurotransmission in the hypothalamus. Aetiological factors may act temporarily and the luteal insufficiency is only episodic, in other instances they may act permanently.

An example of metabolic influences are luteal insufficiencies in oligomenorrhoic obese women with reduced FSH and progesterone (474).

A model of the central action on the development of inadequate function of the corpus luteum are patients with induced ovulation. After clomiphene administration, in addition to induction of normal function, we find a considerable discrepancy between induction of ovulation and pregnancy, an increased percentage of impaired pregnancies, lower progestesterone production and an inadequate secretory phase on the endometrium.

Normal function of the corpus luteum requires a certain prolactin level. An excessive rise of serum prolactin ( >20 ng/ml) causes an alteration of the positive feedback mechanism of oestrogens on gonadotropins, as was demonstrated in women where sulpiride-induced artificial hyperprolactinaemia caused injection of conjugated oestrogens not to produce a response in the positive feedback on LH and FSH (297).

Conversely a reduced serum prolactin level (3 ng/ml) also leads to inadequate progesterone synthesis without changes in the tonic secretion of LH and FSH and with unaltered or only slightly reduced oestradiol plasma levels, as was demonstrated in work where large doses of bromocryptine were administered to women with a normal cycle (459), or when, in hyperprolactinaemias, oversuppression was caused by bromocryptine.

Experiments *in vitro* also suggest, however, an alternative idea about the direct action of increased or reduced amounts of prolactin on progesterone formation in the cultivated granulosa of the human ovary (see p. 69).


DIAGNOSIS

Insufficiency of the luteal phase is diagnosed in practice in particular by the following methods:

(1) **Microabrasion of the endometrium** on the 25th–26th day of the cycle and by dating in order to assess the difference of at least two days retardation in the secretion, as compared with criteria of the normal cycle. The sometimes recommended 21st day (time of implantation) or the first day of menstruation are less suitable. The above procedure is described sometimes as the histochronological definition of the luteal phase. However, in addition to the chronological shift, the histological picture may also display signs of dissociation between the development of glandules and decidualization of the stroma.

(2) It is of fundamental importance to confirm the diagnosis by assessment of the urinary **pregnanediol** or plasma **progesterone** level. We thus differentiate a primary disorder of receptivity of the endometrium while the corpus luteum function is normal. So far only one study differentiated, by parallel investigations of different criteria, the so-called retardation of the luteal phase into primary and secondary caused by luteal insufficiency (155).

The borderline of luteal insufficiency regarding urinary pregnanediol depends on the methods used, 1.25–2.5 mg/24 hours, and for plasma progesterone usually less than 10 ng/ml assessed in the mid-luteal phase. Sometimes the sum of three values assessed between the 11th–4th day before menstruation which is 15 ng/ml or more is considered an index of satisfactory function. The length of the luteal phase in insufficiency is shorter than 10 days. A short luteal phase is characterized by means of hormonal parameters as a general form of luteal insufficiency with infertility. In addition to a length of < 10 days and reduced progesterone, the preovulatory peak of oestradiol and FSH peak are also reduced.

(3) **Basal temperature** does not suffice for the quantitative evaluation of the corpus luteum. It can be used only as a subsidiary criterion or for screening but it must be always supplemented by microabrasion of the dated endometrium and the progesterone level. The basal temperature reveals a short luteal phase; from a low biphasic curve conclusions can be drawn less readily. Correlation with

other parameters reveals that luteal insufficiency may also be present when there is a normal biphasic basal temperature, and conversely.

(4) **Vaginal cytology** or signs of cervical mucus cannot be used either for the quantitative evaluation of progesterone production.

(5) Values of circulating plasma **oestradiol** were assessed only infrequently. In a short luteal phase, the preovulatory oestradiol peak is reduced and the decline also persists during the luteal phase, while in the type of inadequate luteal phase the same authors found normal oestradiol plasma levels (474). Furthermore unexpectedly low total urinary oestrogen levels were found in the follicular phase.

(6) Assessment of LH and FSH **gonadotropins** in plasma gives interesting, although so far not unequivocal, results. A number of research workers revealed a relationship between the LH level and the length of the luteal phase, i.e.lower LH levels in the short luteal phase, either once or repeatedly. This would sugget a causal relationship with reduced plasma progesterone. Other authors found, however, normal LH levels in defects of the luteal phase. Conversely another group of authors uses as a basis findings of a reduced FSH and reduced oestradiol respectively during the period of follicular growth, and they consider this fact a causal factor (499).

In about 50% of short luteal phases, a raised serum prolactin level is found (20 ng/ml) along with a relatively reduced serum FSH level and reduced oestradiol plasma level during the luteal phase (349).

TREATMENT

Treatment should be focused in particular on aetiological factors which are, however, not sufficiently clear. Usually we are restricted to pathogenetic treatment, i.e. substitutional hormonal therapy. In oestrogen deficiency we recommend small doses of oestrogens (0.05 mg mestranol per day) administered continously or intermittently for three weeks from the 5th day of the cycle. In progesterone deficiency, for a period of 10 days from the 17th to the 26 th day of the cycle, oestroprogestational oral substitution can be administered (0.15 mg mestranol and 10 mg norethisterone), or on the 17th day substitution by injection (10 mg oestradiol valerate + 125 mg 17α-hydroxyprogesterone caproate), or finally it is possible to induce three-month therapeutic pseudopregnancy (0.15 mg mestranol + 10 mg acetoxyprogesterone or norethisterone acetate daily). Less frequently we use stimulatory treatment with choriongonadotropin, 2,500 IU per day or on alternate days. On an ever increasing scale drugs stimulating ovulation are used (clomiphene citrate, cyclofenil, bromocryptine).

The aim of oestroprogestational treatment is to retard menstruation in cycles with a short luteal phase and to increase circulating progesterone in infertile women.

Evidence of positive results is an increase of the number of completed pregnancies (245). Sometimes, however, doubts are expressed as regards these results (388). Only in rare instances was the effect of this therapy investigated objectively, i.e. how it influences circulating progesterone. Progesterone protracted the luteal phase by three days, but did not raise the level of circulating progesterone (246). In other instances the effect was rather luteolytic and a rapid decline of circulating progesterone occurred (250). Choriongonadotropin protracted the luteal phase and raised the progesterone level by its luteotropic action (246).

Clomiphene citrate and cyclofenil have proved successful in the treatment of infertility caused by luteal insufficiency. The response in the steroid spectrum to clomiphene citrate is not always the same. In rare instances it is reported after 100 mg/day of clomiphene citrate that oestradiol as well as progesterone levels are higher than in healthy women.

Bromocryptine or other analogues with a dopaminergic effect are indicated in all cases of luteal insufficiency where raised serum prolactin is detected. The results (normalization of the cycle and pregnancy) are equally satisfactory as in anovulatory cycles and amenorrhoea with hyperprolactinaemia. A satisfactory effect also was observed in a group of women with so-called dysprolactinaemia, i.e. with normal serum prolactin but with galactorrhoea. In euprolactinaemia with impaired ovulation views on the results of bromocryptine treatment are not uniform (for review see 111).

## ANOVULATORY CYCLE

An anovulatory cycle is characterized by periodic bleeding resembling menstruation without previous ovulation and corpus luteum formation, persisting for at least 6 months. It belongs to the group of anovulation in the wider sense which comprises also amenorrhoea, anovulatory oligomenorrhoea, dysfunctional bleeding and the syndrome of polycystic ovaries.

The anovulatory cycle in women was first described and defined as pseudo-menstruation 40 years ago; soon after that its pathological picture was revealed and explained. However, at the beginning of the century it already had been found that monkeys can menstruate without a corpus luteum, and later it was confirmed that anovulatory bleeding occurs in monkeys as a rule in summer, during puberty, during lactation and after an illness. In women anovulatory cycles cumulate after menarche (physiological sterility of women), after childbirth and in the premenopause. These are periods of the onset and termination of the physiological activity of the ovaries. In women during maturity, occasionally or temporarily anovulatory cycles might occur, in particular during mental and physical stress and in neurotic conditions. The percentage incidence of anovulatory cycles thus depends on age and the reports of different authors vary. Older data report 5–30%, more recent ones report between the ages of 20–40 years anovulatory cycles in 3–10% (116), another group reports 13.3%. Only a minor part of anovulatory cycles occurs after regular 28-day intervals. More frequently the interval is shorter (anovulatory polymenorrhoea) or protracted (anovulatory oligomenorrhoea). Sometimes regular anovulatory cycles are described as aluteal.

## PATHOGENESIS AND AETIOLOGY

From the pathogenetic aspect, anovulatory cycles were partly elucidated on the basis of histological findings on the endometrium and in the ovary (210, 457).

The former simplified idea explained anovulatory cycles by the persistence of a mature follicle which does not ovulate and persists for a short period. Long-term persistence is then the basis of dysfunctional haemorrhage. The mechanism is probably not so uniform, since on the basis of steroid assessment, some authors differentiate between three types of anovulatory cycles and assume two (63) or three different mechanisms (200). One group can be described as the short-term persistence of the follicle with bleeding which occurs immediately after the drop of the raised oestrogen level, i.e. withdrawal bleeding. The second group has as its basis the regression of mature follicles, with normal oestrogen levels where only the corpus luteum is lacking and breakthrough bleeding occuring with the formation of haemorrhagic infarctions of the endometrium (210). The third group is formed by non-maturing follicles with low oestrogen levels.

The proper causes of anovulatory cycles are not known. It may be said, however, that it is a disorder of the central regulatory mechanism in the hypothalamus where the positive oestrogen feedback is not implemented and LH is not released in sufficient amounts for ovulation. By modelling the menstrual cycle, it is possible to imitate spontaneous anovulations by short interference of some factors or marginal phenomena which influence secretion or clearance of hormones, while the remaining mechanism is normal. Thus no clearly defined pathological factor conditions an anovulatory cycle (52). The position is probably different in permanently anovulatory cycles where a decisive part may be played by factors of psychic and physical stress which interfere with central control or factors associated with the development or termination of ovarian function which explain anovulatory cycles after menarche and before the menopause. The following conditions thus may be the cause of anovulatory cycles and defects of the luteal phase: (1) central defects (direct mechanism of interference with LH secretion), cerebral damage, psychogenic factors, drugs, or hereditary defects, (2) disorders of the intermediary metabolism, metabolic diseases, chronic diseases, nutritional disorders, (3) ovarian defects leading frequently to premature menopause, defective luteinization of the granulosa-luteal cells, (4) raised or reduced prolactin secretion.

DIAGNOSIS

For the diagnosis of anovulatory cycles we presently use as a rule the **basal temperature curve** which should be monophasic for at least 6 months. To confirm the preliminary diagnosis we perform always premenstrual microabrasion, as a certain small percentage of monophasic curves is found even when the action of progesterone is developed (see p. 203). In the diagnosis of anovulatory cycles we find continuous transitions to related pathogenetic entities such as dysfunctional bleeding or a defect in the luteal phase. In some instances anovulatory cycles develop into acyclic bleeding either alternately or permanently. In other instances the defect of the luteal phase changes into an anovulatory cycle and sometimes both lead to amenorrhoea. This suggests a close pathogenetic origin, and sometimes the classification can be only arbitrary. Conversely, post-partum amenorrhoea changes into a normal ovulatory cycle preceded by an anovulatory cycle. According to the basal temperature from a total of 105 controlled cycles after childbirth (the 2nd–4th cycle were involved) 14% of cycles were anovulatory, 34% had a reduced hyperthermal phase, suggesting a defect of the luteal phase and only 52% were typical biphasic cycles (116).

**Histological examination of the endometrium** reveals in the majority of patients with anovulatory cycles a mucosa in the proliferative stage, but there are also transitions from the atrophic stage to hyperplasia in conjunction with a wide variation of oestrogen values. Contrary to the normal proliferative edometrium, in the proliferative endometrium of anovulatory cycles in the 4th week before pseudomenstruation no alkaline phosphatase activity is detected. After the decline of oestrogens, focal haemorrhagic necroses or new haematomas into the stroma without dislocation of the stromal cells and without release of fibres develop. During the short persistence of the follicle among the proliferated glands, cystically enlarged glands also appear, and sometimes a small amount of glycogen in the glandular epithelium as a manifestation of circumscribed abortive luteinization (95).

By means of old inaccurate methods in anovulatory cycles high and low levels of urinary **oestrogens** were assessed. Moreover, groups with constant total oestrogens of 15–30 µg/24 hours with persistence of the follicle and fluctuating oestrogens of 10–45 µg/24 hours with one maximum and early regression of the follicle without rupture were differentiated (63). In other instances three types of oestrogen curves were differentiated: raised curves with one peak, normal curves with two peaks and low ones to which speculatively different types of follicles were allocated — all this being based on a very small number of cases (200).

Urinary **pregnanediol** in the second half of the anovulatory cycle never exceeded 2 mg/24 hours which provides evidence of the absence of corpus luteum. Plasma **progesterone** in the second half on the cycle had values of 0.6 to 1.1 ng/ml which did not differ from those recorded during the first half (0.5–0.8 ng/ml). Depending on the methods used, higher values also were reported, but these values never exceeded 3 ng/ml which is considered the borderline between ovulatory and anovulatory cycles.

**Gonadotropins** have a normal, sometimes reduced tonic secretion. The periodic mid-cycle peak of LH and FSH is, however, lacking. In the urine in the first half a reduced FSH level is repeatedly found.

## TREATMENT

Two types of treatment must be differentiated: induction of ovulation and oestroprogestational substitution. Induction of ovulation is indicated in sterile women who want a child. Drugs of the diphenylalkene series are used (clomiphene citrate, cyclofenil) or from the series of retrosteroids or menopausal gonadotropins, or bromocryptine, because induction by means of steroids is not quite suitable, and induction by means of LH-RH has not been sufficiently elaborated (see p. 330). In women with anovulatory cycles who do not want a child and in irregular cycles where there is imminent bleeding due to the protracted persistence of the follicle, we indicate substitutional treatment with gestagens or oestrogens and gestagens (see p. 315).

## DYSFUNCTIONAL UTERINE BLEEDING

Dysfunctional bleeding is defined as irregular prolonged uterine bleeding which is not associated with a specific tissue defect, neoplasm or pregnancy and which is due to impaired ovarian function based on persistence of the follicle. This is dysfunctional bleeding in the narrower sense of the word. The broader term also comprises other types of dysfunctional bleeding, e.g. due to persistence of the corpus luteum and irregular shedding of the endometrium. It does not include irregular organic heamorrhage in carcinoma of the cervix or uterine body, polyps, myoma, endometritis, disorders of early pregnancy or choriocarcinoma. Many authors use, however, much vaguer definitions, and thus the term dysfunctional bleeding becomes very heterogeneous particularly as some differentiate between functional and dysfunctional bleeding, while others identify it with glandular hyperplasia (for review see 10, 527).

Dysfunctional bleeding occurs in all periods of a woman's life, most frequently, however, at the onset and at the end of generative function of the ovary or after pregnancy. At the onset of sexual maturity it is described as **juvenile bleeding.** During the premenopause, when it is most frequent, we speak of **climacteric bleeding.**

Dysfunctional bleeding is one of the most common gynaecological diseases and is the main cause of work incapacity of women from gynaecological indications. From this ensues the great social impact of its diagnosis and treatment.

## PATHOGENESIS AND AETIOLOGY

It is generally accepted that dysfunctional haemorrhage is a disorder of hypothalamic origin where the positive feedback of oestrogens is lacking. Thus there is not a sufficient cyclic release of LH for ovulation and a corpus luteum is not formed. So far there are few **investigations of plasma FSH and LH.** The findings in three types of dysfunctional bleeding differ (7). In juvenile bleeding the FSH values are lower, LH slightly raised and correspond to anovulatory cycles caused by a central defect (immature hypothalamus). In the premenopausal group there is a markedly raised FSH level, a slightly elevated LH level without a mid-cycle peak; anovulation seems to be due to inadequate ovarian activity. A group of women of mature age comprises cases of the two above types. Other workers also report the disappearance of the LH peak (154, 521); the values of tonic gonadotropin secretion differ only little from normal.

A **non-ruptured follicle** has different fates: either it persists only for a short time and undergoes atresia, as is the case in anovulatory cycles, or there is prolonged persistence and small cysts are formed, as is the case in dysfunctional bleeding. If this occurs repeatedly, a large number of thin-walled small cysts are formed in the ovary, sometimes incorrectly described as microcystic degeneration. The persisting follicles produce varying amounts of oestrogens which cause a permanent proliferative stage or glandular hyperplasia of the endometrium. Thus an anovulatory cycle and dysfunctional bleeding have a similar pathogenesis. The reason why one or the other type of disorder develops has not been fully elucidated so far. Older authors who provided evidence of a relation between dysfunctional bleeding, glandular hyperplasia and persistence of one or a major number of follicles simultaneously (457), assumed that it depends on the period of persistence of the follicle: longer persistence leads to hyperoestrinism, this in turn to hyperplasia and the decline of oestrogens to bleeding. Today we know that persistence of the follicle is not always associated with glandular hyperplasia and dysfunctional haemorrhage does not depend only on the absolute oestrogen level.

The **mechanism by which bleeding occurs** in this pathological entity is of two types. It is either withdrawal bleeding (Entzugsblutung), which occurs during the decline of oestrogen levels which are as a rule elevated, or breakthrough bleeding (Durchbruchblutung) with a constant oestrogen level (433). However, even the drop of the oestrogen level does not always bring about bleeding. It occurs only if the oestrogen level declines below 50% of the original level. In breakthrough bleeding a relative deficiency of hormone is involved in relation to the target tissue, although the level is equal and any haemorrhage of this type can be arrested by increasing the hormone level.

Experiments concerned with the effect of steroids in climacteric women elucidated sufficiently the principles according to which uterine bleeding is induced or arrested. These principles can be applied in the interpretation of dysfunctional bleeding as well in the therapy of bleeding by means of steroids (see p. 317). From this it ensues that bleeding may occur in any type of endometrium — from atrophic to glandular cystic hyperplasia. Hyperplasia and dysfunctional bleeding respectively depend on the following: (1) the time factor, i.e. sufficient duration of the suprathreshold oestrogen level (at least 19 days), (2) suprathreshold stimulus, i.e. a certain but not always equal oestrogen level as it depends on receptivity and reactivity of the endometrium resp., (3) absence or deficiency of progesterone which leads to an uninhibited effect of oestrogens. Bleeding caused by dysfunction differs from menstrual bleeding by the fact that ischaemia and necroses in the spiral arteries develop in a focal manner and gradually. Thus the desquamation of the mucosa and bleeding are more protracted. The glandular cells in the necrotic tissue are of a proliferative character, leucocytes are only few in number, and a thrombo-infarsation process is in the foreground.

**Oestrogen levels** assessed by older methods were either raised (25–40 µg/24 hours) or normal. Dynamic investigation of the course of amenorrhoic or haemorrhagic phases originally also revealed normal values independent of the phase. More recent dynamic investigations, using better methods, revealed two types of oestrogen excretion (68). In one type urinary oestrogens were permanently roughly on the same level which was raised (40–50 µg/24 hours) during bleeding as well as during the amenorrhoic interval; this type corresponded to breakthrough bleeding. In the second type the level varied. High values were attained during the interval (30–90 µg/24 hours); during the decline bleeding occurred and occasionally also during the rise. These findings were confirmed also by other authors (521). The oestradiol and oestriol plasma levels in dysfunctional bleeding were within the normal range. Dynamic investigations of plasma oestradiol revealed variations in juvenile bleeding from 60–90 pg/ml without LH peaks (154), which corresponds to a normal concentration. In other instances the levels were slightly elevated (50 to 200 pg/ml) (7). Further long-term investigations of oestrogens in relation to the onset of bleeding will be needed.

The **cause of dysfunctional bleeding** which is primarily in the hypothalamus is obscure so far. It is also obscure why with the same pathogenesis once an anovulatory cycle occurs and in another instance dysfunctional bleeding. It seems that in the former case rhythmic impulses from the hypothalamus were preserved, while this did not occur in the latter case. The relatively constant interval of spontaneous bleeding (13.3 days) after a single dose of gestagen from the proliferative oestrogen-pretreated endometrium in women with prolonged amenorrhoea is of interest. This type of bleeding which differs from the two types described above suggests that the hypothalamus acts as a promotor of rhythmic impulses for bleeding (455).

Among **additional** or **aetiological factors** which participate in the development of dysfunctional bleeding, are nervous factors and stimuli from the second signal system. In young women, new social situations, conflicts, dramatic events, complicated emotional situations may play a part. Evidence of this is e.g. the striking increase of bleeding and glandular hyperplasia during the Second World War. After psychic trauma dysfunctional bleeding has been observed also by other authors.

Other potential causes include vascular factors and sympathicotonic influences. In the aetiology of obscure bleeding an impaired vascular permeability is found due to interference of the vegetative system. It is assumed that as much as 20% of obscure haemorrhages develop as a result of vegetative dystonia and a so-called haemorrhagic factor of a neurovegetative nature is assumed.


## CLINICAL PICTURE

The clinical picture develops in the first phase as short-term hyperhormonal amenorrhoea persisting for 6–8 weeks. Contrary to hypohormonal amenorrhoea, the clinical picture displays signs of an adequate amount of endogenous oestrogens. After this first phase more or less intense irregular acyclic bleeding from the uterus occurs which is markedly protracted. Sometimes these two phases precede an anovulatory, but otherwise regular cycle, or a disorder of the cycle manifested by oligomenorrhoea or polymenorrhoea. Less frequently irregular bleeding develops without transition from a normal cycle. Terms like so-called metropathia haemorrhagica in Schröder's concept (457), or the clinical syndrome of hyperoestrinism defined by Dreyfus, a French author, are only defined units on the same pathogenetic basis. Dreyfus' hyperfolliculinia, defined as mastopathy, hyperaemia of the mucous membranes and neuropsychic manifestations revealed only a slight correlation with hyperoestrinic manifestations in endometrial biopsy (5%), vaginal cytology (15%) and oestrogen levels (10%). Prolonged blood losses lead frequently to anaemia and without treatment to severe conditions. Sometimes after a prolonged period irregular intervals occur when bleeding stops. However, it did not prove possible to assess a regular rhythm of intervals or the length and intensity of bleeding. The uterus is frequently slightly enlarged, the cervix relaxed, the cervical mucus bears signs of oestrogenic action. The basal temperature is monophasic, under the influence of oestrogens frequently on a low level.

The **histological picture of the endometrium** in dysfunctional bleeding has, similar to anovulatory cycles, a varying character. We encounter proliferation of different forms, from simple ones to hyperplasia. The degree of proliferation, however, does not depend on the onset of dysfunctional bleeding; after prolonged bleeding hyperplasia is not always found. The association of peristent follicles with glandular hyperplasia was shown a long time ago, similar to the relationship of hyperoestrinism and glandular hyperplasia in experiments. The incidence of glandular hyperplasia in dysfunctional bleeding varies between 23–68%. The forms of hyperplasia also vary. We differentiate between homologous hyperplasia with concomitant proliferation of the glands and stroma, which is most frequent, and heterologous hyperplasia which is either interstitial (with a predominance of proliferation of the stroma) or glandular (with predominant proliferation of the glands). Special forms are adenomatous, limited, polypous hyperplasia and hyperplasia of the basal layer (for review see 95). In a small number of cases, also in case of persistence of the follicle and glandular hyperplasia, slight signs of secretory transformation are found on the endometrium (3–6%), similar to the end of the normal proliferative phase, which perhaps are due to transient luteinization in the persisting follicle (210).

## DIAGNOSIS

The diagnosis of dysfunctional bleeding is based on microabrasion of the endometrium or curettage and monophasic basal temperature, which provides evidence of anovulation, while the gynaecological finding is normal. In the differential diagnosis we must rule out all organic disorders causing irregular uterine bleeding. As to the order of importance and frequency these are: carcinoma of the uterine cervix and body, pathology of early pregnancy, cervical polyps, submucous myoma, inflammatory bleeding, ovarian tumour, syndrome of polycystic ovaries, impaired blood clotting, a cyst of the corpus luteum, and an irregular secretory phase. Histological examination is essential in our opinion; up to the age of 38 we use microabrasions, in older women always complete curettage. It is known that haemorrhage from a carcinoma also responds to hormonal treatment by arrest and without microscopic examination the carcinoma could be missed for a long time. An exception can be made only in juvenile bleeding where we do not hurry with microabrasions and curettage in virginal patients and when the case-history is typical we use hormonal treatment. Arrest of bleeding within 72 hours after oestrogen-progestational treatment is a test indicating that probably dysfunctional haemorrhage was involved.

# TREATMENT

In treatment of dysfunctional bleeding several procedures are used: (1) operation (curettage, in rare instances hysterectomy), (2) hormonal treatment, (3) non--hormonal treatment. The age of the patient is decisive, as well as the risk of the treatment and other findings (coagulopathies, relapses, failures). We differentiate between two phases of treatment: arrest of bleeding and prevention of relapses; these are supplemented nowadays by induction of ovulation in women suffering from sterility.

**Surgical treatment** is an exception nowadays. We restrict it to women above 38 years of age, as was explained in detail in the section dealing with diagnosis. After curettage prevention of relapses is attempted by hormonal treatment, and if this fails, we repeat curettage. In younger women, and in particular in juvenile patients, curettage is used only when hormonal treatment failed. Failures are, however, rare and they indicate practically always a different origin of haemorrhage. Therefore another surgical operation — hysterectomy — on account of dysfunctional bleeding was never necessary, unless there was concomitant myomatosis or pathological ovarian findings in older women.

Nowadays the best treatment is **hormonal treatment,** in particular with norsteroids or with a combination of oestrogens and progesterone. Norethisterone acetate in doses of 15 mg per day per os for 10 days leads within 1–3 days to haemostasis. Termination of ten-day-treatment is followed within 2–3 days by withdrawal bleeding (pseudomenstruation); the first day of bleeding is the onset of artificial cycles which we induce for 3–6 months by repeating 10-day-treatment with 15 mg norethisterone acetate per day, always starting on the 17th day. Later the doses can be reduced either to 10 mg per day or we administer 15 mg only for five days from the 21st or 22nd day of the artificial cycle. The advantage of this treatment is that it is simple and the same preparation is used for haemostasis and for prevention of relapses. Haemostasis can be achieved also by administration of oestrogens. For the prevention of relapses gestagens only can be used or oestroprogestational contraceptive mixtures (see p. 317).

**Non-hormonal treatment** includes general roborating treatment, physical therapy, psychotherapy, and interference with blood clotting. The haemostatic action of toluidine blue and protamine sulphate proved useful. Nowadays we use mainly antifibrinolytic preparations such as ε-aminocaproic acid, $3 \times 2$–4 g per day, or p-aminobenzoic acid, 1–2 g/day, whereby the dosage of both substances is gradually reduced. Another antifibrinolytic preparation is the specific protease inhibitor from the pancreas, administered by the sublingual route, 1 tablet after three hours. Haemostasis as a result of enhanced capillary resistence is produced by ethamsylate cyclonamine 1.5 g/day ($3 \times 2$ tablets). Anticoagulants and haemostatic preparations are, however, important mainly as adjuvant treatment or in patients with menorrhagia or where hormonal treatment is contraindicated. Actinotherapy in dysfunctional bleeding is used in case of great surgical risk instead of hysterectomy.

## STEIN-LEVENTHAL SYNDROME
## (POLYCYSTIC OVARY SYNDROME)

In the symptomatology of Stein-Leventhal syndrome (492) three complexes of symptoms dominate: (1) chronic anovulation, (2) manifestations of hyperandrogenism and (3) enhanced anabolism. The incidence of individual clinical symptoms is demonstrated in Table 16. With the exception of enlarged polycystic ovaries

*Table 16* Symptoms of Stein-Levanthal syndrome in a group of 1,079 cases published in 187 papers (172)

| Symptom | Incidence (%) mean | Incidence (%) range |
|---|---|---|
| Sterility | 74 | 35–94 |
| Hirsutism | 69 | 17–83 |
| Amenorrhoea | 51 | 15–77 |
| Obesity | 41 | 16–49 |
| Dysfunctional uterine bleeding | 29 | 6–55 |
| Dysmenorrhoea | 23 | |
| Corpus luteum present in ovarian wedge resection | 22 | 0–71 |
| Virilization | 21 | 0–28 |
| Biphasic BBT | 15 | 12–40 |

(PCO), none of the symptoms is obligatory. Objective evidence of bilateral enlargement of the ovaries is the basic prerequisite of Stein-Leventhal syndrome. The finding of PCO alone, however, is not sufficient for the diagnosis, if the clinical symptoms are absent. PCO are a substantially more frequent finding than the Stein-Leventhal syndrome proper, the latter affecting only a fraction of patients with PCO. The incidence of PCO in sterile women is reported to be 0.6% to 4.3%. In a series of 740 autopsies of women including children and old women, necropsy disclosed as much as 3.5% of these cases. In a group of more than 12,000 gynaecological laparotomies the incidence of PCO was 1.4% (for review see 171).

## PATHOLOGICAL ANATOMY OF POLYCYSTIC OVARIES AND THEIR SUBSEQUENT DEVELOPMENT

Polycystic ovaries are markedly enlarged, greyish white, and have a smooth surface. The tunica albuginea is in typical cases thickened (so-called peripheral sclerosis of the ovary). The ovaries contain, in particular beneath the capsula, a large number of follicular cysts of varying size. The cysts are as a rule lined by a thin layer of granulosa; the thickening of the theca interna is typical, sometimes with cellular luteinization. This appearance was described as hyperthecosis. [Since at present the term **hyperthecosis** or **thecomatosis** (see p. 275) is used to describe the condition when the ovarian stroma contains isolated cell aggregates and nests which morphologically cannot be differentiated from luteinized thecal cells without any connection with follicles, we call the thickening of the theca interna *follicular hyperthecosis* and the above described thecomatosis *stromal hyperthecosis*.] Some conceive thickening of the theca as hypertrophy, others as hyperplasia, as suggested by numerous mitotic figures; some speak only of a condensated theca.

Peripheral sclerosis of the ovary does not correspond to the severity of the clinical picture. It is also found in ovaries without subcapsular cystic follicles and without follicular hyperthecosis.

Similarly, follicular hyperthecosis is described not only in PCO but also in some other abnormalities (e.g. retroflexion of the uterus, oophoritis, endometriosis of the ovary) and even during pregnancy. It is thus not specific for Stein-Leventhal syndrome.

The finding of a corpus luteum in PCO is rather an exception (see Table 16), but similarly as an anamnestic pregnancy even a corpus luteum does not rule out Stein-Leventhal syndrome.

Thus the statement from forty years ago still holds (492) that "the pathologist is unable to demonstrate the anatomical structure or typical change in the ovary which would enable him to describe the clinical picture" and "that the only consistent pathological finding is the presence of follicular cysts lined with thecal cells".

In addition to common static descriptions of ovarian morphology in PCO, which is extremely variable and is the source of never ending controversies, the dynamic aspect, taking into account the further development of this ovarian pathology, is unique.

One system of classification (491) differentiates between two principal stages: the 1st *thecal-granulosal synergistic phase* (early, intermediate and late) with PCO and proliferative hyperplastic endometrium, and finally with glandular cystic hyperplasia with gradual development of menstrual dysfunction from menorrhagia and irregular cycle to dysfunctional bleeding; and the 2nd *thecal dominant phase* (early, intermediate and late), where in the ovaries the first islets of thecal cells appear in the stroma, their number increasing until they eventually take up the entire stroma. In the endometrium the mitotic activity declines gradually and finally atrophy develops; oligomenorrhoea changes into amenorrhoea. Thus, for the last period of the thecal dominant phase, the syndrome of stromal hyper-thecosis (see p. 275) is typical and is the further developmental stage of "Stein--Leventhal" PCO.

The other systematic classification (20) foresees the developing imbalance between secretion of LH and FSH with gradual relative or absolute predominance of LH. It differentiates between the 1st, *early imbalance phase* with polycystic changes of the ovary, the 2nd *intermediate imbalance phase* with cirrhotic cystic changes or diffuse cirrhosis of the ovary and finally a 3rd *late imbalance phase* with cirrhotic or cystic atrophy of the ovary. The original PCO (the 1st phase) wrinkles, cortical tissue is destroyed, the cysts diminish, similar to follicles which are able to develop up to the stage of generalized collagen infiltration, and fibrosis of the stroma is complete. Oestrogen formation is markedly reduced. The ovaries are reduced in size and are hard (the 2nd phase). The substance of the ovary diminishes gradually, the ovary atrophies and reaches a size amounting to one half or one third of the normal size, the surface becomes again smoother, and follicles do not mature (the 3rd phase). Oestrogen production declines further, and hypooestrogenic amenorrhoea develops.

## ABNORMAL STEROID BIOSYNTHESIS IN THE POLYCYSTIC OVARY

**Androgens in the polycystic ovary syndrome.** The glandular source of hyper-androgenism in Stein-Leventhal syndrome is variable. Pretentious clinical studies with concurrent retrograde venous ovarian and adrenal catheterization in hirsute women revealed that the following can be sources of androgen hypersecretion: (1) ovaries, (2) adrenals, (3) ovaries and adrenals and (4) peripheral conversion of relatively non-androgenic precursors into testosterone. Although hitherto assembled results of the ovarian and adrenal vein catheterization experiments have been and still are controversial, it seems that the combined ovarian and adrenal source of testosterone and androstenedione hypersecretion is equally frequent as the isolated ovarian one.

The site of abnormal steroid biosynthesis in the polycystic ovary is the thickened theca of the cystic follicles. The concentrations of testosterone and androstenedione in polycystic ovarian tissue are actually higher than in the normal ovarian cortex. Studies with the incubation of tissue from polycystic ovaries *in vitro* reveal the existence of three types of abnormalities regarding ovarian steroid biosynthesis:

(1) *Deficiency of the system of aromatizing enzymes* which convert androstenedione into oestrogens results in excessive androstenedione formation, with oestrogen production lagging behind. The decline of oestrogen formation may be compensated by peripheral conversion of androstenedione or enhanced gonadotropic stimulation at the price of an even greater increase of androstenedione production. The administration of progesterone in these instances enhances the 17-oxosteroid excretion.

*Table 17*  Conditions altering the metabolic clearance of testosterone and its plasmatic bond in women (according to 248)

|  | Metabolic clearance | Plasmatic bond |
|---|---|---|
| Hirsutism and virilization | raised | reduced |
| Testosterone administration | raised | reduced |
| Dexamethasone administration | raised | reduced |
| Gestagen administration | raised | reduced |
| Obesity |  | reduced |
| Hypothyroidism | raised | reduced |
| Pregnancy |  | raised |
| Oestrogen administration | reduced | raised |
| Hyperthyroidism | reduced | raised |
| Ageing | reduced |  |

(2) *Deficiency of the 3β-hydroxysteroid dehydrogenase* converts pregnenolone into progesterone, 17α-hydroxypregnenolone into 17α-hydroxyprogesterone and finally dehydroepiandrosterone into androstenedione. The result is an excessive formation of dehydroepiandrosterone which cannot be converted directly into oestrogens; their production lags behind. In urine the excretion of pregnanetriol, a metabolite of 17α-hydroxypregnenolone, rises.

Androstenedione and dehydroepiandrosterone are weak androgens, they can be, however, converted into testosterone in the ovary as well as in the periphery.

(3) *Abnormal testosterone biosynthesis* directly from progesterone without 17α--hydroxyprogesterone and androstenedione as intermediary products via testosterone acetate, similarly as in the testes.

In all instances only partial defects are involved, not complete blocks, and thus oestrogen production proceeds. The most frequent disorder seems to be excessive androstenedione formation, the main precursor for peripheral conversion (in the liver, adipose tissue and skin) into testosterone. Evidence of the ovarian source of hyperandrogenism is the marked decline of the androstenedione and testosterone plasma level after a wedge-resection of the ovaries.

In contrast, a recent study has been unable to demonstrate any deficiencies in the steroidogenic potential of the PCO *in vitro*. Isolated granulosa, theca and medullary tissue of normal and polycystic ovaries had a similar capacity to secrete $C_{19}$ and $C_{21}$ steroids. It seems probable, therefore, that the chronic anovulation and elevated androgen production in patients with PCO are not caused by an obvious inherent abnormality in the *de novo* steroidogenic potential of these ovaries (537b).

**Plasma testosterone** levels are often within normal limits (see p. 110), although occasionally subjects have levels beyond the normal range. However, it has also been demonstrated that the concentration of **TEGB** in plasma of hirsute patients is reduced, as compared with normal women. Thus the **free, unbound, testosterone** levels are much more consistently abnormal. Testosterone production rates and metabolic clearance rates are also raised (Table 17). Many more patients have **plasma androstenedione** levels above the normal range. Since androstenedione is not bound to the TEBG and since the androstenedione metabolic clearance rate is reported to be normal in hirsute patients, the plasma levels of androstenedione presumably reflect elevated androstenedione production more accurately than testosterone levels reflect testosterone production.

**Urinary 17-oxosteroids** are only to a small extent products of testosterone metabolism. Therefore, not even a five- to tenfold increase of testosterone production is necessarily manifested by an increase of 17-oxosteroid excretion.

A manifestation of the participation of the adrenals in hyperandrogenism, in addition to the ovaries, is hyperresponsiveness of androstenedione secretion to exogenous ACTH in some women with polycystic ovaries in addition to a LH-dependent ovarian source. However, only few of these women have elevated plasma levels of 11-deoxycortisol or 17-hydroxyprogesterone, thus meeting the diagnostic requirements for congenital adrenal hyperplasia. The adrenal abnormality involves only the androgen-secreting mechanism. Simultaneously the raised level of pregnenolone, 17$\alpha$-hydroxypregnenolone (or its urinary metabolite pregnanetriol) and dehydroepiandrosterone suggests a deficiency of the 3$\beta$-hydroxysteroid dehydrogenase system. It is not known whether the adrenal abnormality is primary or secondary due to some other hormonal dysfunction. Dexamethasone suppression resulting in attenuated suppression of plasma androstenedione and testosterone levels in peripheral blood does not provide evidence of their adrenal origin. Glandular vein catheterization experiments reveal a decline of plasma androstenedione and testosterone concentrations following dexamethasone administration even in hirsute women whose androgen hyperproduction was of ovarian origin (138, 263). Recently, a glucocorticoid receptor protein in rat ovaries has been demonstrated (310).

**Oestrogens in polycystic ovary syndrome.** The levels of circulating oestradiol were found to be equivalent to those observed during the early follicular phase while the oestrone levels corresponded to levels found in the preovulation period in healthy women. The ratio of plasma oestradiol to oestrone is thus reversed, as compared with the condition in normal ovulating females. More than half the concentration of circulating eostrone is the product of peripheral androstenedione conversion. The source of low basal oestradiol plasma levels can be the ovary or peripheral conversion of oestrone or testosterone.

**Abnormal gonadotropic secretion in the polycystic ovary syndrome.** Contemporary radioimmunological methods provide evidence in most patients of erratic or inappropriately elevated LH secretion and relatively constant and low secretion of FSH; they confirm thus the defect of cyclic release of pituitary gonadotropins. This pattern of gonadotropin secretion is most probably the result of a functional derangement of the hypothalamo-pituitary system due to inappropriate steroid feedback in the polycystic ovary syndrome. Clinical experiments provide evidence of the existence of an intact mechanism of an inhibitory (negative) and in most patients also stimulatory (positive) feedback of oestrogens. Ovulation after administration of the antioestrogen clomiphene provides evidence that the stimulatory oestrogen feedback on LH release is intact (for review see 248). The elevated plasma LH levels appear to be related to an increased pituitary responsiveness to LH-RH, due to the chronically inappropriate plasma oestrogen levels found in these patients (421).

In addition to cases of the polycystic ovary syndrome with a raised plasma level of LH ("typical" PCO), there are patients with a normal or low level ("atypical" PCO); the FSH levels in the two groups do not differ nor does the concentration of circulating free testosterone. (Plasma androstenedione and plasma TEBG binding capacity appears to be greater in the high-LH group than in the normal LH group.) A correlation between ovary size and LH secretion was not confirmed by all authors (i.e. macroscopically markedly enlarged ovaries with translucent follicular cysts and raised plasma LH levels, small to slightly enlarged ovaries without evident cysts without a raised LH level). In "atypical" PCO there is, however, a more frequent tendency towards stromal hyperthecosis and slightly raised 24-hour urinary 17-oxosteroid values.

"Atypical" PCO is sometimes considered a later developmental stage of PCO (168), and in other instances as secondary PCO of probable adrenal origin. A possible mild adrenal block syndrome is suggested by the relatively frequent elevation of urinary pregnanetriol with the ACTH stimulation test in these patients. Treatment of anovulation with clomiphene is not very successful in these patients. Adrenal suppression alone is recommended or as a background for clomiphene administration (37, 417).

Recent investigations reveal mild hyperprolactinaemia in as much as 20% of women with the polycystic ovary syndrome. Inhibition of PRL secretion by bromocryptine (see p. 282) leads to restitution of the ovulatory cycle and even to a drop in plasma levels of adrenal androgens, similar to exogenous corticosteroids.

A quite unexpected aspect is the finding that PRL probably can modulate adrenal cortical biosynthesis of steroids.

## DIFFERENTIAL DIAGNOSIS OF STEIN-LEVENTHAL SYNDROME

Stein-Leventhal syndrome is suspected in the presence in particular of the three most frequent symptoms: anovulatory sterility, hirsutism and menstrual dysfunction. For the clinical diagnosis of Stein-Leventhal syndrome, objectively proved bilateral, symmetrical enlargement of the ovaries (by pneumopelvigraphy, laparoscopy or culdoscopy) is decisive. The finding of polycystic ovaries with a typical microscopic appearance confirms the clinical diagnosis.

Assessment of 17-oxosteroids, 17-hydroxycorticosteroids and possibly testosterone in urine is useful only for orientation. Normal values do not rule out the diagnosis; markedly raised values suggest instead adrenal dysfunction, so-called borderline adrenogenital syndrome, or "mild" adrenal hyperplasia. When the values are markedly raised and there is concomitant virilization, we must consider the possibility of acquired adrenogenital syndrome due to hyperplasia or the presence of an adenoma with androgenic activity or a malignoma of the adrenal cortex, or more rarely, androgen-producing tumours of the ovary.

Most reliable for confirmation of androgen hypersecretion is in our opinion evidence of raised plasma levels of free testosterone and a decline of the binding capacity of TEBG. We refute clinical tests with dexamethasone and hCG for the identification of the source of hyperandrogenism. Dexamethasone does not produce a selective suppression of adrenal androgen secretion (138, 263). Although views are not uniform in this respect, it is probable that hCG is not a selective stimulator of ovarian steroidogenesis and also acts at the same time on the adrenal cortex (138). Oestrogens used in another variant of tests for the evidence of gonadotropin--dependent hyperandrogenism also act on the adrenal cortex. The conclusive differentiation of the ovarian and adrenal form of hyperandrogenism may be provided only by blood analysis obtained by ovarian and adrenal vein catheterization; in clinical practice it is, however, justified only in malignant hirsutism and virilization if less pretentious examination methods are not sufficient for the differential diagnosis.

**Syndrome of hyperthecosis.** Marked hirsutism along with obvious signs of virilization (clitoromegaly), oligomenorrhoea or amenorrhoea and usually obesity and frequent failure of anovulation treatment with clomiphene, differentiate the syndrome of hyperthecosis, so-called thecomatosis, from the spectrum of polycystic ovary syndrome and Stein-Leventhal syndrome respectively. In the ovaries we find stromal hyperthecosis (described also as diffuse stromal luteinization) and a marked decline of primordial and developing follicles. By direct catheterization of venous blood, the ovaries were identified as the source of excessive hypersecretion of androstenedione and testosterone. The urinary excretion of 17-oxosteroids is usually slightly raised or

275

normal, and the cortisol production rate is normal. The amount of oestrogen produced per day exceeds the average oestrogen production rate of ovulatory women; the principal oestrogen is oestrone which is formed at extraglandular sites from plasma androstenedione. The endometrium frequently displays hyperplasia, increased oestrogen formation being associated with an increased risk of endometrial carcinoma. A raised plasma level of LH and decline of FSH are found.

Hyperthecosis (thecomatosis) is considered by some to be the extreme variant or developmental stage of the same disorder as Stein-Leventhal syndrome (see p. 271). Sometimes it runs in families, similarly as Stein-Leventhal syndrome.


## AETIOPATHOGENESIS OF STEIN-LEVENTHAL SYNDROME

The aetiopathogenesis of Stein-Leventhal syndrome is obscure. In about half the cases the anovulatory menstrual dysfunction and clinically definable hirsutism are already manifested at the onset of or shortly after menarche. An interesting hypothesis draws attention to the striking similarity of the polycystic ovary and the pubertal ovary and to some common clinical features of Stein-Leventhal syndrome and postmenarcheal adolescent sterility. The polycystic ovary is considered typical only for chronic anovulation during prolonged acyclic gonadotropin action (9a, 330). The question why pathological persistence of premenarcheal or adolescent anovulation respectively develops when the hypothalamo-pituitary system is able to respond under certain conditions (exogenous oestrogen, clomiphene, ovarian wedge resection) by release of ovulatory hormone (an adequate complex of both gonadotropins), and the ovary is able to respond by ovulation to an adequate gonadotropic stimulus, remains open.

The cause of the disorganized steroid biosynthesis may be an increased responsiveness of the polycystic ovaries to gonadotropins, apparent during administration of exogenous gonadotropins. This could be the manifestation of a certain hereditary potential for the development of polycystic ovaries and Stein-Leventhal syndrome. This is suggested by genetic studies of families and investigations of monozygotic twins with Stein-Leventhal syndrome. So far it is not clear whether the dominant inheritance of this potential (gene mutation?) is autosomal or linked to gonosome X. The alternative is an altered sensitivity of the ovary to gonadotropin acquired during the prenatal period of development of the ovary.

The existence of severe hirsutism with a preserved ovulatory ovarian cycle and fertility, as well as ovulation in Stein-Leventhal syndrome induced by the antioestrogen clomiphene, provides evidence against the decisive role of androgens, mediated by non-aromatizable testosterone metabolites, in the development of anovulation. The stimulatory (positive) feedback of oestrogens is preserved, while in men it is manifested only after orchidectomy. However, as demonstrated in subhuman primates, in orchidectomized males even continuous substitution with physiologic doses of testosterone or dihydrotestosterone fails to block the oestrogen-induced gonadotropin surge (495). The inhibiting principle proper appears to be a testicular water-soluble peptide. Ovarian hyperandrogenism seems to accompany chronic anovulation in cases of pathologically increased sensitivity of the ovary to gonadotropins, rather than cause anovulation. In chronic anovulation of hypothalamic origin, with persistent tonic secretion of pituitary gonadotropins without primary alteration of ovarian responsiveness, hypersecretion of androgens is lacking.

## TREATMENT OF STEIN-LEVENTHAL SYNDROME

*Treatment of anovulatory sterility* in Stein-Leventhal syndrome is initiated with clomiphene (see p. 324). If its action fails even when potentiated with subsequent administration of hCG or oestradiol and when "atypical" PCO is suspected, we try to suppress adrenal function, preferably with dexamethasone. Its inhibitory action on ACTH secretion is maximal [0.75 mg corresponds to 5 mg prednisone or 20 mg cortisol (hydrocortisone)], mineral corticoid action (sodium retention, potassium excretion) is negligible. The effect is checked on the 17-oxosteroid excretion and should be maintained at 10 mg/24 hours or less with a daily dose of prednisone ranging from 2.5 to 10 mg (or with a corresponding dose of dexamethasone). If suppression with dexamethasone or prednisone alone does not suffice to induce ovulation, we administer in addition again clomiphene. When treatment fails it is advisable to assess the PRL plasma concentration, in case of accidental hyperprolactinaemia bromocriptine should be administered, if necessary combined with clomiphene.

Failure of conservative treatment of anovulation is an indication for ovarian wedge resection, with a risk, however, of postoperative adhesions resulting in sterility. If necessary after operation, clomiphene is administered again.

For *treatment* of severe cases *of hirsutism*, the antiandrogenic gestagen cyproterone acetate is used along with ethinyl oestradiol or mestranol to inhibit possible ovulation in the sequential reverse pattern of administration for a period of 6 to 9 months. For the prevention of frequent relapses we proceed with the therapeutic administration of a one-phase steroid contraceptive, the optimal gestagenic component of which in that case is medroxyprogesterone acetate, the least suitable norethisterone. It is also possible to use continual administration of medroxyprogesterone acetate alone in amounts of 10–20 mg per day. This gestagen reduces markedly the plasma level of total and free testosterone and its production rate and enhances the metabolic clearance rate of testosterone. The initial mechanism is probably the inhibited secretion of pituitary LH; medroxyprogesterone acetate, however, also inhibits adrenal steroidogenesis (137). The oestrogenic component of steroid contraceptives acts favourably by inhibition of LH secretion and by increasing the binding capacity of TEGB (see Table 17). Plasma testosterone is checked every 2 to 3 months, and depending on the results, the administration may be temporarily discontinued.

In less severe cases of hirsutism, a daily dose of 30 mg of medroxyprogesterone acetate for 2 to 3 months is sufficient. Then the dose is reduced or discontinued, depending on the plasma testosterone level. In the mildest cases we administer therapeutically a one-phase steroid contraceptive.


## HYPOTHALAMIC AMENORRHOEA

From the pathogenetic classification of disorders of the menstrual cycle it is apparent that the majority of disorders is of hypothalamic origin but only in a minor number are the causes known.

Hypothalamic tumours, inflammations and degenerative processes are rare causes of primary or secondary amenorrhoea. The symptoms then depend on the woman's age, and the site and size of the lesion. In some instances hypogonadotropic hypogonadism as a consequence of a hypothalamic lesion is involved.

Functional hypothalamic defects without a detectable organic lesion are, however, the most frequent cause of hypothalamic amenorrhoea. This group comprises "idiopathic hypogonadotropic hypogonadal primary amenorrhoea" with a low LH and FSH concentration and a low oestradiol plasma level with normal developmental, nutritional and genetic parameters which can be differentiated by the sequential pituitary stimulation test (268). This group also includes "hypothalamic chronic anovulation" with secondary amenorrhoea and distinct psychological disturbances, with normal gonadotropins and oestrogens but an increased sensitivity and pituitary reserve regarding the FSH response (287). Among functional hypothalamic disorders we must also include the so-called "oversuppression syndrome" (post-pill amenorrhoea) (see p. 365) if it is an independent entity.

In the classification of secondary amenorrhoea by means of the progesterone test and the gonadotropin level, a group of disorders is described called "hypothalamo-hypophyseal dysfunctions" with a positive progesterone test, normal LH and FSH and oestradiol levels in plasma and a normal clinical and somatic finding (266). The conclusion could be drawn that the cause of the disorder may be at different levels of hypothalamic control.

The diagnosis of hypothalamic amenorrhoea still has shortcomings. It is not always possible to define the primary defect in the hypothalamus or in the anterior lobe of the pituitary and the conclusions reached after elimination of a hypophyseal lesion need not be correct. So far it is not possible to assess the LH-RH plasma level in clinical practice. And a single LH-RH stimulation test need not always differentiate reliably between a hypothalamic and hypophyseal disorder.

A reduced response may be the result of chronic lack of hypothalamic stimulation of the pituitary, and conversely, in hypophyseal tumours the response may be also normal. It seems that the sequential pituitary LH-RH stimulation tests will be able in future to make the diagnosis more reliable (289, 467).

Hypothalamic amenorrhoea is treated by oestrogen-progesterone substitution or by inducing ovulation with clomiphene in normoestrogenic women and by HMG/hCG in hypoestrogenic patients or after failure of clomiphene.

## OLFACTOGENITAL DYSPLASIA (KALMANN - DE MORCIER SYNDROME)

Olfactogenital dysplasia is characterized by a combination of primary amenorrhoea and sexual infantilism with anosmia. The incidence of this syndrome is extremely rare, the estimate being 1:50,000. The karyotype of the affected women is normal, 46,XX. An irregular autosomal pattern of inheritance is assumed; however, an X-linked probably dominant mechanism of transmission cannot be excluded. Reports of a higher incidence in children from marriages of related parents were not generally confirmed.

The primary cause of olfactogenital dysplasia is a developmental disorder of the CNS, absence of the olfactory bulbs and tracts and hypoplasia of the hypothalamus. The syndrome may be considered an attenuated form of holoprosencephaly; a number of facial stigmata have been noted in females with olfactogenital dysplasia.

The ovaries are small, not stimulated, resembling prepubertal ovaries. They contain primordial and primary follicles, growing follicles are usually lacking. The plasma level of FSH and LH is regularly reduced, and it displays a typical pulse-like secretion. The response to exogenous LH-RH usually suggests that the capacity of hypophyseal gonadotropin secretion is normal. In some instances a defect of hypothalamic control of pituitary PRL secretion was also observed. By adequate gonadotropic stimulation (HMG) ovulation can be induced; deliveries of healthy infants were recorded. Cyclic substitutional treatment with oestrogens and gestagens stimulates the development of secondary sex characteristics (for review see 247).

(An impaired sense of smell was observed also in some women with chromatin negative gonadal dysgenesis, more frequently in mosaicism than in the pure karyotype 45,X0. Developmental anomalies of the hypothalamus and limbic system are assumed.)

# AMENORRHOEA WITH GALACTORRHOEA

Galactorrhoea implies bilateral secretion of a milk-like fluid during periods other than pregnancy and the post-partum lactation period. (Under this heading we do not include the secretion of transparent, opalescent, purulent or sanguinolent fluid.) Milk-like fluid is secreted spontaneously in drops or it can be expressed on examination. Some authors also include under the term of galactorrhoea the secretion of serous fluid resembling colostrum. The excreted fluid differs from milk in that it contains approximately 20 times less lactose, three times less lipids and somewhat less protein.

The incidence of galactorrhoea is low. It is reported to amount to 0.5–1.0% in a group of gynaecological patients comprising several thousand women. Data on the incidence of amenorrhoea in women with galactorrhoea vary, some report that approximately one third of these women menstruate and some of them became pregnant. Conversely, galactorrhoea is described in 10–15% women with amenorrhoea. In women with anovulatory menstrual dysfunction, galactorrhoea is encountered about three times more frequently than in women with normal ovulatory cycles (there in about 1% of all cases).

In galactorrhoea combined with amenorrhoea, depending on the nature of onset of the disorder, its duration and on the X-ray finding on the sella turcica, three basic syndromes are differentiated (Table 18) (394).

*Table 18*  Syndromes of amenorrhoea with non-puerperal galactorrhoea (for review see 480a)

|  | Chiari-Frommel | Ahumada-Argonz-Del Castillo | Forbes-Albright |
|---|---|---|---|
| Onset of disorder | after delivery | spontaneous | after delivery or spontaneous |
| X-ray finding on sella turcica | normal | normal | enlarged |
| Persistence of disorder | usually transient | usually permanent | permanent |

According to its causes galactorrhoea can be divided into several groups (5):
(1) tumour-induced galactorrhoea;
(2) drug-induced galactorrhoea (it may be caused by phenothiazines and other major psychotropic drugs, anti-hypertensives and oral steroid oestrogen-containing contraceptive agents);
(3) idiopathic galactorrhoea with or without amenorrhoea (including post-partum patients);
(4) galactorrhoea due to primary hypothyroidism;
(5) miscellaneous uncommon causes (including local chest wall diseases and diseases of the CNS).

Differentiation of tumour-induced galactorrhoea from other patients with galactorrhoea is of utmost importance. It is maintained that in about 20% of women with galactorrhoea X-ray signs of an intrasellar expansive process are found; in women with galactorrhoea and amenorrhoea the incidence is even higher, sometimes as much as one third of all cases. In all cases of galactorrhoea therefore radiography of the sella turcica is an essential examination; a negative finding, however, does not rule out PRL-secreting pituitary microadenomas which may not visibly alter the architecture of the sella turcica. Visual field testing is obvious. Non-tumourous galactorrhoea is an indication for prolonged dispensarization; plasma PRL is examined roughly once a year, X-ray examination of the sella not less than once in three years. Local examinations must not be omitted either: mammography, ductography, thermography and cytology of the secretion from the mammary glands.

Demonstrable sellar enlargement indicates further special examinations to differentiate pituitary tumours from primary **empty sella syndrome,** i.e. non-tumourous enlargement of the sella resulting from herniation of the suprasellar cistern through a congenitally defective sella diaphragm into the subarachnoid space of the sella turcica leading to compression and flattening of the pituitary gland. Pneumoencephalography is the conclusive diagnostic test.

The most frequent mechanism of the development of galactorrhoea is hyperprolactinaemia (see p. 64), functional or tumour-induced. Unfortunately, there is no unequivocal relationship between hyperprolactinaemia, galactorrhoea and amenorrhoea. One third to three quarters of women with hyperprolactinaemia have also galactorrhoea; galactorrhoea is, however, also found in about 15% of normoprolactinaemic women with amenorrhoea. There are also cases of galactorrhoea in menstruating women; in the majority, the PRL plasma level is normal. In two thirds of these cases galactorrhoea persists after delivery despite the return of the menstrual cycle. Secretory adaptation of the mammary gland to relatively low levels of PRL stimulation is assumed. Hyperprolactinaemia is encountered in 15–30% women with functional amenorrhoea and it is not always associated with galactorrhoea. A raised PRL plasma level is also found in some women without galactorrhoea and with an ovulatory cycle with luteal insufficiency (see p. 256).

Tumour-induced hyperprolactinaemia is associated, as a rule, with high levels of circulating PRL and does not respond at all or very mildly to suppression of hypothalamic PIF by means of chlorpromazine and to direct stimulation of PRL release by the action of exogenous TRH. Only in exceptional instances is a 100% increment of plasma PRL obtained after TRH. Either the tumour cells are secreting already at maximum capacity or the receptor sites for TRH on tumour cells are altered.

The mechanism of the development of amenorrhoea is either central or peripheral. It is probably not the raised plasma level of PRL which inhibits the stimulatory (positive) feedback of oestrogens (therefore most of these women do not react to clomiphene by ovulation), but an alteration of the dopaminergic control system in the CNS. Also an interference of hyperprolactinaemia with ovarian gonadotropin-mediated steroid production is possible. The pituitary response to exogenous LH-RH in idiopathic hyperprolactinaemia is, as a rule, enhanced regarding LH secretion, while in cases with an enlarged sella it is lower than normal. The basal plasma level of FSH and LH usually corresponds to an early follicular stage of the cycle. The secretion of ovarian oestrogens in amenorrhoea with galactorrhoea usually does not suffice for the positivity of the progesterone withdrawal-bleeding test.

**Therapy** depends on the cause. Pituitary PRL-secreting tumours can be treated by resection or heavy particle irradiation. In hypothalamic dysfunction it is essential to interfere with pathogenetic mechanisms (discontinue hyperprolactinaemia-inducing drugs, treat hypothyroidism) and similar to idiopathic forms inhibit the secretion of PRL. An effective drug is brominated ergot alkaloid ergocryptine (2-Br-α-ergocryptine, brom-ergocryptine, bromocryptine, CB 154). It reduces the concentration of circulating PRL and normalizes the gonadotropin secretion. It has a dual effect; it stimulates synapses of dopaminergic tubero-infundibular neurons of the hypothalamus — dopamine itself is believed to be the most important PIF — and secondly, above all, being a dopamine agonist, it activates the inhibitory dopamine receptors on the PRL-secreting pituitary cells and hence inhibits PRL secretion. Bromocryptine is administered before meals. We start with a dose of 1.25 mg per day, after 2–3 days we increase it to 3.75 mg/day and then to 5.0 mg per day. This dose is administered for at least one month, and usually it is not necessary to increase it further (to 7.5 mg or more per day). First the galactorrhoea recedes; then menstruation develops and later also ovulation. The effect of bromocryptine does not persist. We use it therefore mainly for the treatment of anovulatory sterility. If the patient becomes pregnant, we terminate the administration of bromocryptine immediately after the first missed menstruation.

Surprisingly a considerable proportion of patients with normoprolactinaemic secondary amenorrhoea responded to bromocryptine treatment by menstruation and/or ovulation. These were women who became amenorrhoic after discontinuation of oestrogen-containing oral contraceptives, weight loss, or emotional distress. Since the plasma PRL levels decreased significantly in these normoprolactinaemic patients, PRL suppression at the physiological level cannot be ruled out as an explanation of favourable bromocryptine action, and we need not assume a peripheral or undefined central bromocryptine effect.

If with bromocryptine we achieve only menstruation without ovulation, it is an advantage to administer clomiphene while continuing with bromocryptine in the usual way.

Treatment with L-dopa, a precursor of dopamine which during prolonged administration raises the catecholamine level in the hypothalamus, is much less effective, probably because it is difficult to achieve sustained suppression of plasma PRL levels. Also the use of pyridoxine (vitamin $B_6$) — 200 mg three times a day — is not very successful. Pyridoxine is a coenzyme required for decarboxylation not only of dopa to dopamine but also of 5-hydroxytryptophan to serotonin. It may increase both dopaminergic and serotoninergic activities in the brain; the net effect on PRL release thus cannot be predicted.

# HYPOPHYSEAL DISORDERS

Hypophyseal disorders may have several pathogenetic backgrounds (inflammatory, traumatic, tumourous or degenerative) (see p. 180). As to the site of origin, they may be primary or secondary (acquired), and as to the extent of the affection the disorders are complete or partial.

## SHEEHAN'S SYNDROME

Synonyms of this pathogenetic unit are: Gliński's syndrome, and post-partum panhypopituitarism. It is a special (and most frequent) form of secondary hypopituitarism which develops as a consequence of necrosis of the anterior lobe of the pituitary after severe post-partum haemorrhage or shock.

Its reported incidence is $0.1^0/_{00}$ of the population (for review see 226, 472) or 4 cases in 35 post-partum shocks. It is also known that the severity and duration of shock is more important for the development of the syndrome than the blood loss. According to post-mortem findings, it is a true ischaemic infarction caused by thrombosis of the portal vessels, 90% of which are final vessels. Only affection of 97–99% of the tissue of the anterior lobe leads to elimination of all three tropic functions and to the development of the complete clinical picture. Experimental removal of 75–95% of the anterior lobe in dogs led only to loss of ovarian function and in some also to loss of thyroid function. Therefore, partial insufficiencies or insufficiencies restricted to a particular function are much more frequent. Fatal cases due to acute necrosis are very rare. Usually the syndrome develops in the course of months or years and sometimes due to the regenerating power of the anterior lobe, minor tissue damage may become compensated and after prolonged ovarian insufficiency normal activity develops. From this ensues a great variety of clinical symptoms and laboratory findings.

The main early **symptoms** are agalactia and amenorrhoea. Other symptoms which develop later are: adynamia, apathy, fatigue, sensation of cold, genital atrophy, loss of libido, loss of hair, pubic and axillary hair, depigmentation and atrophic skin (alabaster- or marble-like skin). The loss of body-weight is, however, slight and the cachexia described by Simmonds is an exception. When the symptom develops, the different functions are eliminated in a typical way: first the somato-tropic ones, then the gonadotropic functions, then the thyrotropic, and finally the adrenocorticotropic ones. The basic aldosterone secretion and minimal thyroid function remain preserved. Elimination of functions of the anterior lobe of the pituitary leads to severe psychic changes which may develop into psychoses. At the onset it is, as a rule, a reduced initiative, a loss of interest which may develop into complete indifference to oneself and the environment. The extinction of psychic functions may also be followed by acute hallucinoses and deliria.

The **laboratory findings** include reduced levels of hormones or values of indirect ovarian, thyroid and adrenocorticotropic functional tests. The gonado-tropin level is reduced and thus also the oestrogen level. The progesterone test is negative, the vaginal smears and endometrium are atrophic. The LH-RH test or sequential pituitary stimulation test suggest a reduced response as evidence of an inadequate reserve of the anterior lobe. Accumulation of $^{131}$I, PBI, and BM give low values. The serum cholesterol is high. The 17-hydroxycorticoid and 17-oxo-steroid values are low and the negative metopiron test indicates an inadequate reserve of the anterior lobe for ACTH function. The increased sensitivity to insulin was used formerly for diagnosis as the insulin test. Hypotension and anaemia are also found.

For the **differential diagnosis,** the case-record, typical clinical findings and laboratory findings with the X-ray of the sella are most important. The following should be considered in the differential diagnosis: anorexia nervosa, Chiari-Frommel syndrome and Forbes-Albright syndrome, as well as other forms of panhypopituitarism and isolated functional disorders.

**Treatment** involves substitution with hydrocortisone (10–20 mg/day) or prednisone (2.5–5 mg day) and thyroxin (0.1–0.3 mg/day) or dried thyroid (0.3 mg/day). During stress (infection, operation) the doses must be increased. In younger women oestrogen substitution (ethinyl oestradiol 0.05 mg/day) is useful. Libido can be stimulated by anabolics (fluoxymesterone 2.5 mg/day). In individual patients ovulation may be induced by gonadotropins HMG and hCG or even pregnancy, similar to hypophysectomized women.

## ISOLATED GONADOTROPIN DEFICIENCY

Formerly this has also been described as monosymptomatic hypogonadotropic hypogonadism or partial hypopituitarism. It must be differentiated from partial Sheehan's syndrome. It has an obscure pathogenesis, but today we know that it is at least partly of hypothalamic origin. In these women primary amenorrhoea is associated with the absence of puberty and with hypogonadism, a low LH level and a low FSH level. The LH-RH test presents, however, a double response of the anterior lobe of the pituitary. In some instances it is normal and thus a selective hypothalamic deficiency of trigger hormones is involved. In other instances the response in the LH-RH test is low or negative and thus a disorder of the gonadotrops of the anterior lobe of the pituitary is involved (54). The thyroid and adrenal function are normal. So far very rarely isolated FSH deficiency has been assessed: it was in a woman with eunuchoid appearance with primary amenorrhoea where the response of LH was normal in the LH-RH test, while the FSH response was lacking. It is assumed that in that case, a defect in the synthesis of the β-subunit of FSH, i.e. at the pituitary level, was involved, as revealed by further analysis (34). Isolated deficiencies are, however, known also in other hormones (myxoedema of pituitary origin, isolated ACTH deficiency).

## TUMOURS OF THE PITUITARY AND SURROUNDING TISSUE

Tumours are a rare cause of disorders of the menstrual cycle. Three quarters of pituitary disorders lack substantial secretion (chromophobe adenoma, craniopharyngeoma), one quarter is manifested by excessive secretion of the anterior lobe cells and cause hypersecretion syndromes (eosinophil adenoma, basophil adenoma).

The picture of clinical symptoms is very variable. It is formed by symptoms ensuing from pressure on the surrounding tissues and from hypopituitarism with extensive damage to the parenchyma of the anterior lobe and hyperfunctional manifestations in active tumours. The common and early symptom is amenorrhoea with impaired ovarian function: in chromophobe adenomas it is almost always present, in the remainder in 90%, in craniopharyngeomas in about 50%. From the pressure exerted by the tumour on the surrounding tissue later neurological symptoms develop (headache, sometimes neuralgia of the trigeminal nerve, paralysis of the oculomotor muscles) and visual disorders (bitemporal hemianopsia, central scotomas, double vision, changes on the fundus). In hormonally active pituitary tumours there are also other symptoms: in eosinophil adenoma, acromegaly, skin changes (pigmentation, cutis gyrata), hypertrichosis, changes of the bones, splanchnomegaly, muscular atrophy, sometimes galactorrhoea; in basophil adenoma, there are symptoms caused by overproduction of corticoids (hypercortisolism), i.e. the Cushing's disease. Progressing atrophy of the anterior lobe of the pituitary finally leads to manifestations of panhypopituitarism, similar to Sheehan's syndrome. Tumours are, as a rule, small and grow for a long time; if they propagate into the hypothalamus, further symptoms develop: diabetes insipidus, somnolence, and impaired thermoregulation. Intrasellar calcifications revealed on X-ray of the sella suggest the presence of a craniopharyngeoma.

Tumours are treated by operation or irradiation. Substitution of hormone deficiencies is similar to Sheehan's syndrome.

## OTHER TYPES OF PANHYPOPITUITARISM

A similar symptomatology to Sheehan's syndrome is displayed by hypopituitarism after skull injuries, or after surgical or irradiation hypophysectomy. Inborn *hypophyseal nanism* has its own problem to be studied in childhood. *Simmonds' cachexia* is a panhypopituitarism with no association with childbirth and its problems belong in the sphere of internal medicine.

# GONADAL DISORDERS

The pathogenesis, aetiology and classification of gonadal disorders in women have been discussed in detail. Now we would like to deal with the most important clinical symptomatology of developmental gonadal disorders in women, or rather individuals with a female phenotype with developed female external genitalia, regardless of their gonosomal sex. For cases which are beyond this definition we refer to special literature (382).

Intersexuality implies individuals with ambiguous external genitalia (199). In hermaphroditism and pseudohermaphroditism, on the other hand, the gonads are decisive. In **true hermaphroditism** one (unilateral hermaphroditism) or both (bilateral hermaphroditism) gonads are of the mixed type (ovotestis or testovarium), or there is an ovary on one side and testis on the other (lateral hermaphroditism).) In **pseudohermaphroditism** both gonads are of the same sex, female (pseudohermaphroditismus femininus) or male (pseudohermaphroditismus masculinus). This type of developmental disorder may be complete when the external and internal genital corresponds to the opposite sex than the gonad, or incomplete when only the internal or external genitalia belong to the opposite sex. (According to this classification testicular feminization is pseudohermaphroditismus masculinus externus.) We encounter also the term of ovarian or testicular intersex. A **testicular intersex** is an individual with ambiguous but predominantly female external genitalia, a female phenotype and testes. An **ovarian intersex,** on the other hand, has ovaries and masculinized external genitalia and frequently a virilized phenotype [e.g. prenatal (congenital) AGS].

If we understand by the term **hypogonadism** a deficiency of ovarian hormones, in particular oestrogens, then the majority of individuals thus defined whom we shall discuss in detail, are individuals with a gonosomal complement of the female type with *peripheral hypogonadism*, i.e. with a disorder directly in the ovary (contrary to *central hypogonadism* or *hypogonadotropism* where the disorder is in the hypothalamus and, in rare instances, in the pituitary). This defined group of developmental disorders is with some exceptions clinically manifested by amenorrhoea.


## GONADAL DYSGENESIS

Gonadal dysgenesis is a typical morphological finding where regardless of the gono-somal sex of the individual, so-called *streak gonads* are present at the site of the ovaries. Those are narrow fibrous strips formed by cellular fibrous stroma, which are lacking any germinative constituents of the gonads in adults; in deeper layers there are irregular canals of the rete and canals of mesonephric origin. In their vicinity are usually nodules of so-called extragonadal interstitial cells (Berger's sympathicotropic cells). This *dysgenetic gonad* may be present on both sides or rarely on one side in Turner's syndrome, on both sides in pure gonadal dysgenesis or Swyer's syndrome, or on one side, if on the other one is a testis as it is the case in mixed gonadal dysgenesis.

The chromosomal classification of cases of gonadal dysgenesis comprises:
A. normal karyotype
   a) consistent with phenotype (46,XX dysgenesis)
   b) not consistent with phenotype (46,XY dysgenesis)
B. abnormal karyotype
   a) pure (45,XO in about 90% of cases, and 46,XXi, 46,XX—, 46,XXfr, 46,XYi and 46,XY—)
   b) mosaic (in addition to lines 45,XO we find further gonosomal complements).
Of interest are cases of gonadal dysgenesis with pure karyotypes 46,XX, also confirmed by cultivation of tissue from both gonads. They are found in about 5%. In exceptional instances, they have been observed in Turner's syndrome. Intra-chromosomal changes, molecular alteration of specific segments of chromosome X with submicroscopic deletion or defect of the gene complement with unrevealed translocation are assumed. Intrachromosomal changes may result not only from abnormal meiosis but may also develop during the zygote period or in the early postzygotic period. As gonadal dysgenesis in 46,XX were also observed in siblings, the possibility of autosomal, recessive heredity of this disorder is also taken into consideration.

From chromosomal findings it is apparent that by means of the chromatin test we can differentiate between two basic groups in gonadal dysgenesis, sex chromatin negative and sex chromatin positive (each of them comprises non-mixoploid and mixoploid cases).

In the differentiation of cases with gonadal dysgenesis it is not the chromosomal classification which is decisive, but the clinical symptomatology which may differ substantially even in the same karyotype.


## TURNER'S SYNDROME

Turner's syndrome, in addition to gonadal dysgenesis, is characterized in particular by stunted growth and sexual infantilism and some facultative somatic extra-genital anomalies (in the order of frequency: short neck with low borderline of hair and barrel-shaped chest, flexion groove on palm and abnormalities of the nails, cubiti valgi, pterygium colli, numerous pigmented naevi, "piscine" mouth and "gothic" palate); more detailed clinical examination reveals anomalies of the kidneys and ureters and inborn vitia cordis (usually coarctation of the aorta). Each of the symptoms displays a broad spectrum and extragenital anomalies may be absent altogether.

Stunted growth and other extragenital stigmas in Turner's syndrome are the result of loss of genetic material from the short processus of the X-chromosome. For the differentiation of the ovary and its further development two gene loci are essential, one on the long and one on the short processus of gonosome X. The loss of either of them causes the development of dysgenetic gonads. Where loss of the long processus of one of the chromosomes occurs, streak gonads develop, however, growth is normal and extragenital abnormalities are lacking.

In about 10% of patients with Turner's syndrome instead of the dysgenetic gonad a rudimentary anovulatory ovary is present with rare primordial small growing and atretic follicles, the product of severe primary hypoplasia of the ovary. This is usually the case in mosaic 45,XO/46,XX or pure karyotype 46,XX or in anomalies of the second X-chromosome with pure complement or mosaic 45,XO. Sex chromatin is therefore always positive. This type of gonad is also described as *dysgenetic ovary* (see p. 182). We do not agree with the wider concept of this term which in the literature is sometimes considered a synonym of dysgenetic gonad (199).

The incidence of chromatin negative Turner's syndrome in the population is estimated to amount to 0.03%.

The hormonal situation in gonadal dysgenesis and Turner's syndrome depends on the condition of the gonads. Dysgenetic gonads and ovaries do not produce oestrogens. Low levels of circulating and excreted oestrogens are of extragonadal origin, similar to women after the menopause or after ovariectomy. Oestradiol levels are extremely low. Oestrone is probably formed by peripheral conversion of adrenal androstenedione; its concentration in the peripheral blood declines after suppression with dexamethasone. The inhibitory (negative) feedback of oestrogens is preserved, while the TGA excretion and level of circulating FSH and

LH are increased, both of them displaying rhythmical and frequent oscillations, similar to normal women. There is also a typical prepubertal and pubertal pattern of elevated gonadotropin secretion during sleep which during the period corresponding to the attainment of sexual maturity disappears, similar to normal women. It seems that for the onset, normal course and termination of the programme of gonadotropin secretion normal ovarian function is not needed. Some sort of trigger role of adrenal steroids is assumed (57a, 90c). The gonadotropin concentration in the peripheral blood can be reduced by administration of oestrogen. The mechanism of stimulatory (positive) feedback is also developed and preserved.

Treatment of sexual infantilism and primary amenorrhoea is not started before the age of 14–15 years for fear of premature arrest of growth. The only treatment is cyclic substitution with oestrogenic and gestagenic preparations. Treatment of inadequate growth is limited to the dubious effect of anabolics or to the administration of minumum doses of oestrogens which promote growth and the general feminization of the individual. Only when — undesired — the first uterine bleeding occurs, typical cyclic substitution with full doses is started. Human hypophyseal GH fails in this respect. The target tissues do not respond to normal or raised levels of endogenous GH. More serious extragenital abnormalities call for the assistance of plastic surgery.


INCOMPLETE TURNER'S SYNDROME

Phenotypically it does not differ from true Turner's syndrome; however, menarche occurs spontaneously, and it usually is substantially retarded, and the menstrual cycle ceases after varying periods of time. The variability is considerable; one to several menstruations have been recorded as well as menstrual cycles persisting for several years.

As to the chromosome pattern, most frequently the mosaic 46,XX or 46,XX/ /47,XXX with karyotype 45,XO is found, and sometimes also a pure gonosomal complement 46,XX. The degree of development of the ovary depends mainly on the cellular line in the gonad (see p. 1–2).

Spontaneous menstruation rules out bilateral presence of dysgenetic gonads. Hypoplastic ovaries are present which by biopsy are often difficult to differentiate from rudimentary anovulatory ovaries (dysgenetic ovaries) in complete Turner's syndrome. Evidence of the extreme morphological variability of ovaries is provided by described cases with karyotype 45,XO and the phenotype of Turner's syndrome where the patient became pregnant (18, 357). Ovulating women have been described with Turner's phenotype and with 45,XO ovarian karyotype (260). A higher level of circulating ovarian oestrogens in these women is manifested by an advanced stage of development of secondary sex characteristics.

In some cases of incomplete Turner's syndrome unilateral gonadal dysgenesis is involved. A typical streak ovary may be found or a hypoplastic ovary. The oestrogen production influences the degree of development of secondary sex characteristics.

## ULLRICH'S SYNDROME (NOONAN'S SYNDROME, TURNEROID SYNDROME)

The syndrome is a phenocopy of Turner's syndrome and up to puberty it cannot be differentiated from chromatin positive Turner's syndrome. At that time the secondary sex characteristics begin to develop and after menarche, as a rule, a regular menstrual cycle follows.

The ovaries may be quite normal, as corresponds to karyotype 46,XX which is always present in this syndrome. The women are fertile, the disorder may be subject to autosomal dominant heredity, as often it has a familial incidence in several generations.

Submicroscopic structural chromosomal changes, i.e. point (gene) mutations, are assumed (for review see 208).

## PURE GONADAL DYSGENESIS

In pure gonadal dysgenesis, contrary to Turner's syndrome, inadequate growth and extragenital stigmas are absent. Secondary sex characteristics do not develop. Primary amenorrhoea is associated with an eunuchoid habitus, while the phenotype is a normal female one. The efferent genital pathways are of a female character, similar to the external genitalia. At the site of the ovaries are streak-like dysgenetic gonads.

About half the cases are chromatin negative, the remainder chromatin positive. The karyotype is usually normal, 46,XY (*Swyer's syndrome*) or 46,XX; mosaics are also encountered, however. A pure monosomia of the X-chromosome was never found (208).

Pure gonadal dysgenesis belongs among syndromes of early castration. In cases with chromosome Y in the gonosomal complement, early destruction of the foetal testis is assumed before testicular androgens and factor X could play a part in the masculine differentiation of the internal and external genitalia. Mutual exchange of genetic material is also possible between chromosome Y and X in the prophase of the first meiotic division of primary spermatocytes when the Y gonosome loses the genes which determine the differentiation of the testis. The sperm which carries it leads to the development of a zygote with the gonosomal complement

46,XY. However, the Y chromosome is inactive. Submicroscopic selective deletion of the critical locus with a regulatory gene on the Y chromosome is also considered.

In cases with karyotype 46,XX the mechanisms of the development of a dysgenetic gonad have been mentioned before (see p. 181).

Treatment is substitutional; cyclic administration of ovarian steroids should be started in time to suppress excessive eunuchoid growth. The purpose is to induce menstruation, while the uterus is developed and capable of this response.


## HORMONALLY ACTIVE OVARIAN TUMOURS

From the clinical aspect we differentiate between two basic hormonally active ovarian tumours, feminizing tumours and masculinizing tumours. We shall neglect the hitherto controversial and frequently confusing problem of histogenesis (for review see 346) and classify all ovarian tumours into three groups:
(1) ovarian tumours with primary (their own) hormonal activity
(2) ovarian tumours with secondary (induced in extratumourous tissue) hormonal activity
(3) hormonally active teratomas.


## OVARIAN TUMOURS WITH PRIMARY HORMONAL ACTIVITY

Ovarian tumours with their own hormonal activity include feminizing as well as masculinizing tumours. For pathological details we refer, similar to other groups of tumours of the ovary, to special literature. Regarding terminology, we adhere to Motlík's nomenclature (346).

**Feminizing ovarian tumours** are the most frequent hormonally active ovarian tumours and account for 0.5–10% of all solid ovarian tumours. They include:
granulosocellular tumour,
thecoma (thecocellular tumour) which is closely related to cortical stromal hyperplasia of the ovary, also called stromatosis or more frequently stromal hyperthecosis, thecomatosis (pseudothecoma) (see p. 275),
theco-granulosocellular tumour (gynoblastoma).

Granulosocellular tumour and gynoblastoma are potentially malignant (very approximate estimate — about one quarter of all cases), similar to arrhenoblastoma. Thecoma is, as a rule, benign. About one third of these tumours lack hormonal activity.

**Masculinizing ovarian tumours** include:
arrhenoblastoma,

gynandroblastoma, characterized as a combination of gynoblastoma and arrheno-blastoma,

interstitial-cell tumour (formed by hilar cells, Leydig cells of the ovary, Berger sympathicotropic cells, "adrenal-like tumour", and luteoma).

Androgens may also be produced, however, by feminizing hormonally active tumours of the ovary. Gynandroblastoma produces, as a rule, masculinizing as well as feminizing steroids with a predominance of one type. In some instances the character of steroidogenesis changes in the course of time.

## OVARIAN TUMOURS WITH SECONDARY HORMONAL ACTIVITY

Primary and secondary metastatizing tumours of the ovary which themselves are not hormonally active may induce steroidogenesis in the ovarian stroma which surrounds them (of oestrogens, androgens and in rare instances also gestagens). A mechanism resembling the effect of a growing follicle in the normal ovary is assumed. Abnormal hormonal activity associated with suspect growth of the ovary, therefore, does not always imply the presence of a tumour with steroidogenesis of its own, and does not rule out a secondary tumour (a metastasis of an extra-ovarian tumour).

## HORMONALLY ACTIVE TERATOMAS

Hormonally active teratomas are malignant embryomas, mixed tumours containing tissues with a low grade of differentiation, which as a rule do not reach the organoid stage. The epithelial component may contain tissue of a chorionepithelioma which produces hCG. Only in exceptional instances when in the fibrous portion (stroma?) of the tumour "interstitial" cells are present or a thecal reaction, do these tumours produce oestrogens or androgens. Malignant embryoma belongs among the most malignant tumours which soon develop metastases and accounts for about 2% of teratomas.

There are also some non-endocrine tumours, ovarian (e.g. dysgerminoma) and extraovarian (e.g. pulmonary carcinoma) which can produce gonadotropins. It is assumed that the hormonal activity is in this case the manifestation of functional dedifferentiation, the consequence of gene expression which occurs under physiological conditions only in highly specialized tissue of the endocrine gland.

## CLINICAL ASPECTS AND TREATMENT

In feminizing tumours the effect of continually produced oestrogens depends on the patient's age. It is manifested as isosexual pseudopubertas praecox (see p. 170) (in a fraction of these patients), dysfunctional uterine bleeding in reproductive age (in more than half the patients), or as "refeminization" in the postmenopausal period (in less than half the cases).

In masculinizing tumours the position is similar; heterosexual pseudopubertas praecox develops and later defeminization with secondary oligomenorrhoea, amenorrhoea and virilization. The reliable differentiation of a masculinizing ovarian tumour from an adrenal tumour (ovarian tumours have, as a rule, a markedly lower 17-oxosteroid excretion than adrenal tumours) is of extreme importance.

In hCG-producing tumours, the clinical picture depends on the stimulation of the contralateral ovary or both ovaries (in case of an extragonadal tumour).

Treatment involves the removal of the pathological source of steroids or hCG.


## PREMATURE OVARIAN FAILURE

We prefer this neutral term to the hitherto frequently used terms *"premature menopause"* or *"premature climacteric"*. The term climacteric is not pertinent in this condition. Premature ovarian failure, on the other hand, is a condition which corresponds to the menopause or postmenopause (in secondary amenorrhoea persisting for more than one year). Both the climacteric and menopause terms, moreover, suggest the incorrect idea of premature ageing. As will be apparent from what follows, premature ovarian failure need not always be irreversible.

There is no agreement on the chronological range of this syndrome. Some limit it to the age of 40 years, and others to 35 years. At present usually the range of 30 years is preferred. The purpose is to differentiate reliably premature ovarian failure from liminal cases of the physiological menopause; it is reported that in approximately 2.5 to $10\%$ of women it occurs before the age of 40 years. The incidence of premature failure of ovarian activity is estimated to account for $5\%$ of all cases of secondary amenorrhoea (for review see 491).

The criteria for the diagnosis are: (1) secondary amenorrhoea, (2) reduced production of ovarian oestrogens with a negative progesterone test (usually associated with atrophy of the endometrium found on bioptic examination), and (3) raised TGA levels in urine and elevated levels of circulating FSH and LH as a manifestation of hypersecretion of hypophyseal gonadotropins. Ovarian biopsy usually resembles the ovary during the postmenopausal period: normal stroma without primordial and atretic follicles or with a very small number of follicles.

In rare instances, however, numerous primordial and primary follicles are found with several growing follicles.

In roughly half the cases further symptoms of the postmenopausal period are lacking, such as circulatory, neuropsychic and general symptoms. In the remainder, where they are present, they are as a rule less marked than in women in the physiological menopause or after ovariectomy.

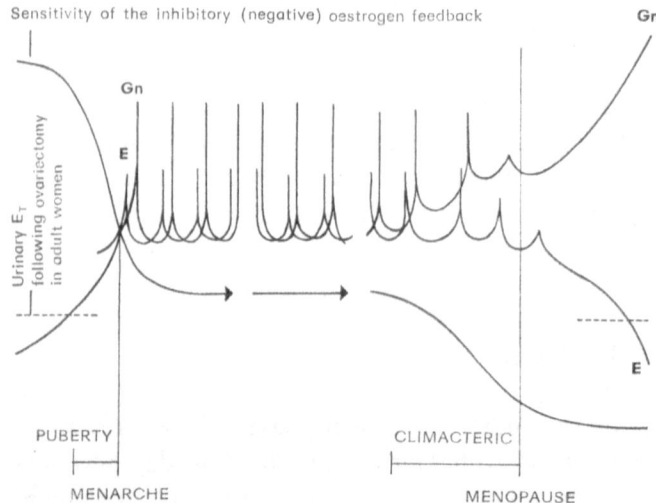

Sensitivity of the inhibitory (negative) oestrogen feedback

*Fig. 39.* Puberty and climacteric as a manifestation of "ageing" of the brain [assuming that the decline of sensitivity of oestrogen-sensitive areas in the inhibitory (negative) feedback of oestrogens proceeds during the climacteric (113)]. Gn — gonadotropins, E — oestrogens.

Long-term investigations have revealed that in about one quarter of the cases surprising periods of spontaneous restitution of ovarian function develop (from temporary positivity of the progesterone test to temporary oligomenorrhoea, in rare instances the patient became even pregnant). It is therefore probable that the aetiopathogenesis of premature ovarian failure is variable.

In 12.5% of patients subjected to cytogenetic examination, as reported, deviations of the karyotype were found, most frequently mosaics with a cellular line 45,XO. We consider them an extreme variant of incomplete dysgenesis. Frequently, however, the causes are different although even a normal gonosomal complement 46,XX does not rule out a developmental ovarian insufficiency (see p. 181 and 287). Autoimmune damage of the ovary is also considered (see p. 200). The mentioned cases of restitution of ovarian activity suggest a primary hypothalamic disorder of the inhibitory (negative) feedback of oestrogens. The decline of sensitivity of hypothalamic regulatory areas to oestrogens is also associated with the physiological onset of the climacteric and menopause (Fig. 39) (11); in the pathogenesis, not only toxiinfectious (see p. 199) but also psychogenic (see p. 177) factors might be involved.

For some cases in the group of premature ovarian failure which are still reversible, the term *"secondary amenorrhoea with increased secretion of hypophyseal gonadotropins"* which is prognostically neutral, is more pertinent, as the ovaries often respond to extreme doses of exogenous gonadotropins. This group may also include cases of resistant ovary syndrome (see p. 296). The only possible differentiation is by ovarian biopsy.

The prognosis is thus very serious, but remission cannot be ruled out. Long--term follow up is essential. Even biopsy of the ovary does not clarify the situation completely (see p. 223). The gonadotropin stimulation test may be of assistance (p. 213), preferably with the use of HMG.

Treatment is substitutional, cyclic administration of oestrogens and gestagens in amounts sufficient to induce menstruation.


## CASTRATION OF WOMEN

Castration of an adult female in reproductive age, i.e. bilateral ovariectomy, removes the most abundant source of oestrogens. The level of circulating oestrogens declines briskly (oestrone to a RIA level of about 40 pg/ml plasma, oestradiol to about 15 pg/ml), The excretion of total oestrogens in 95% of women is lower than 10 μg/24 hours, i.e. it reaches levels common in the postmenopause (6.4 μg//24 hours, with a range from 3.2–11.2 μg/24 hours). Their influence on the appropriate hypothalamic regulatory areas in the mechanism of the inhibitory (negative) feedback is thus eliminated and the disinhibited tonic secretion of hypophyseal gonadotropins rises markedly within one week after ovariectomy; it reaches the individual maximum about 3–6 weeks after castration. If ovariectomy was performed during the follicular phase of the menstrual cycle, the gonadotropin level in the peripheral blood rises more rapidly, than when the ovaries are removed in the luteal phase. At the end of the third week after operation, the mean level of circulating LH is 6–8 times, the FSH concentration 8–12 times higher: the change of the FSH LH ratio which after castration is higher than 1, is typical. Frequent investigations of circulating gonadotropins in monkeys reveal a significant rise of the LH concentration in peripheral blood already within two days after ovariectomy with the attainment of a plateau roughly after three weeks. Typical pulse-like release of gonadotropins with a mean frequency 1 pulse/hour (circhoral oscillation) is very rapidly inhibited by exogenous oestrogen and within several hours the plasma LH concentration decreases. It is assumed that the pulse-like gonadotropin release is superimposed on the continual secretion and the mean concentration of circulating hormone in a certain period of time corresponds to these two types of secretion. Mestranol (0.1 mg per day) in castrated women reduced the circulating FSH to initial levels rapidly (as a rule after 7 days), while the LH level declines only temporarily and rises even during administration.

The clinical consequences of castration depend on the woman's age. Intra-chromosomal changes of chromosome X in the gonosomal complement 46,XX or early destruction of the ovary and the development of a dysgenetic gonad cause peripheral hypogonadism, which is manifested as pure gonadal dysgenesis (see p. 290). Postnatal or prepubertal castration leads to sexual infantilism with eunuchoidism.

After castration of an adult woman in reproductive age, in particular when performed during the luteal phase of the cycle, frequently within several days endometrial bleeding occurs from the withdrawal of circulating oestrogens. Usually after five weeks postmenopausal neurovegetative symptoms develop, hot flushes and perspiration. They are twice as frequent than after the normal menopause and persist longer; according to reports in 20% of patients they persist for as long as four years and in about 10%, for as long as seven years after the operation. They are the most marked among other postmenopausal symptoms.

The residual level of circulating oestrogens after castration does not differ significantly from their level after the normal menopause, if we omit the period of the gradually regressing biosynthesis of ovarian oestrogens which follows immediately after the menopause.

## RESISTANT OVARY SYNDROME, INSENSITIVE OVARY SYNDROME (FOLLICULAR DYSGENESIS, SAVAGE SYNDROME)

The syndrome is characterized by a normal female phenotype with normal external genitalia, normal development of secondary sex characteristics and primary (in exceptional instances secondary) amenorrhoea.

Sex chromatin is of the female type, karyotype always 46,XX.

The ovaries are small, sometimes described as "fat" streak-like gonads. They contain numerous primordial follicles, but very few mature to the stage of cavitation and they do not develop further. Stromal cells are, in rare instances, hyperplastic and luteinized. However usually, these signs of stimulation are lacking.

These ovaries do not produce oestrogens. Oestrogens sufficient for the development of secondary sex characteristics are probably the product of peripheral conversion of androstenedione, which is produced by the stromal cells of the ovary or adrenals. The excretion of total oestrogens is less than 10 $\mu$g/24 hours, the TGA excretion is raised, similar to the plasma FSH and LH levels.

The cause of hypogonadism is deficiency of the follicular apparatus of the ovary to endogenous and exogenous hypophyseal gonadotropins. The mentioned deficiency need not be absolute. However, hyporeactivity is obligatory. The administration of more than 8,000 IU HMG-IRP-2 has been described without a rise in the excretion of total oestrogens and only a minimal response after 11,000 IU

HMG-IRP-2; in other instances the administration of approximately a triple dose has been needed to stimulate the ovaries in hypogonadotropic females.

The existence of an autoimmune mechanism which blocks circulating gonadotropins has not been proved. Excessive metabolic inactivation of oestrogens has also been ruled out. A defect of gonadotropic receptor proteins in the ovary and a developmental disorder are assumed (therefore the term *"follicular" dysgenesis* was suggested).

The resistant ovary syndrome as the cause of secondary amenorrhoea arouses scepsis. A differential diagnostic criterion against early ovarian failure would be provided only by biopsy of the ovaries. Regardless of the limitations of this examination method (see p. 224), the syndrome of premature ovarian failure — although defined fairly well from the clinical aspect — is very heterogeneous (see p. 293).


## TESTICULAR FEMINIZATION*)

**The complete syndrome of testicular feminization** is characterized by a normal female phenotype with well developed breasts, however, frequently with nipples and areolas of the juvenile type; the external genitalia are also of the female type. Axillary and pubic hair is lacking or only indicated. The vagina is formed. As a rule it is short, for coitus usually sufficient but with a blind end. As to the inner female genitalia usually not more than a streak-like "rudimentary uterus" is present. There are bilateral testes; in two thirds of the cases they are in the inguinal canal, frequently combined with bilateral inguinal hernia, sometimes intraabdominal or labial. Sexual feeling and behaviour is typically female.

In the testes there is a well differentiated tunica albuginea. The seminiferous tubules are narrow without lumen, lined with immature Sertoli cells and they contain only rare spermatogonia. In adult age the interstitium contains hyperplastic and hypertrophic Leydig cells. Non-specific degenerative changes are frequent.

**The incomplete testicular feminization syndrome** differs only by malformation of the external genitalia, most frequently only by hypertrophy of the clitoris (in rare instances masculinization is more advanced). There is also sparse axillary and pubic hair. The seminiferous tubules of the testes usually have a lumen, and maturing Sertoli cells, spermatocytes and rarely sperm cells are also found.

Chromosome examination reveals in 98% of all cases a normal male karyotype 46,XY (sex chromatin is of the male type); in the remainder in addition to the

---

*) Testicular feminization is discussed here only for practical purposes as an end organ failure due to inborn insensitivity to androgens.

Y chromosome polysomias of the X gonosome are found, in a pure karyotype or in mosaics (sex chromatin is of the female type).

The familial incidence of the disorder is striking; about half the male offspring are affected. Carriers are women who usually lack axillary hair and have sparse pubic hair and frequently delayed menarche or secondary amenorrhoea. More probable than autosomal dominant heredity limited to males is recessive heredity associated with chromosome X with one locus on gonosome X (376). Testicular feminization is about ten times less frequent than chromatin negative Turner's syndrome. The incidence in the population is estimated to amount to 0.002 to 0.005%.

The cause of testicular feminization is complete (or incomplete) insensitivity of target tissues to testicular testosterone with a typical disorder of the differentiation of internal and external genitalia of the foetus with a male gonosomal and gonadal sex.

The endocrine function of the testes is preserved also in adult age. The levels of circulating testosterone and oestradiol correspond to values found in normal males. The testosterone secretion and excretion are sometimes higher. The total oestrogen excretion is the same or higher than in normal women. The LH secretion rises with age, in adult age it is higher than in normal males, while the concentration of plasma FSH usually does not exceed values found in normal males. The gonadotropin and steroid secretion and excretion are continual and lack a cyclic character.

The biological ineffectiveness of testicular testosterone is due, in particular, to a genetically conditioned loss of sensitivity of target tissues to endogenous and exogenous androgens. Regarding the mechanism of insensitivity to androgens in humans, testicular feminization is heterogenous: the 1st type has a defective cytoplasmic androgen binding, the 2nd type has an altered chromosomal binding of the cytoplasmic receptor–androgen complex and further steps respectively. So far it is not clear whether in these instances a different allelle on the appropriate locus of the X-chromosome is involved or a mutation of another locus.

Female hypothalamic sex in testicular feminization is suggested when there is tonic secretion of hypophyseal gonadotropins with acyclic secretion of gonadal steroids and female sexual feeling and behaviour. The feedback inhibition of gonadotropins is, contrary to normal males, only partial, therefore in testicular feminization in adult age the level of circulating gonadotropins, in particular LH, is higher than in males. Orchidectomy leads to a further significant increase. It can be reduced by the administration of oestrogen or testosterone, but not with DHT or other non-aromatizable androgen (e.g. fluoxymesterone). It is thus obvious that the inhibitory feedback between the testis and hypothalamus is not mediated by DHT, but by oestrogen, which is formed from the testicular testosterone by local aromatization not only in normal men but also in subjects with testicular feminization. Heterotypic transplantation of the human ovary in two orchidecto-mized subjects with testicular feminization led to cyclic LH secretion and cyclic pregnanediol excretion (44). This observation provides evidence that testicular androgen, similar to normal males, did not impair the female pattern of hypotha-lamic control of secretion of hypophyseal gonadotropins in testicular feminization. It seems that the position is similar to pseudomasculinization of these regulatory mechanisms in normal males (see p. 9).

A frequently discussed question regarding the treatment of testicular feminiza-tion is whether the testes should be removed. We agree with the view that the only indication for orchidectomy in the complete syndrome is a suspected malig-nant tumour. Hormonal treatment is not necessary. Only in subjects where castration was performed (some recommend it after completed development of the breasts), is it essential to substitute oestrogens to prevent deficiency phenomena and later osteoporosis. In principle we do not inform the patients of the diagnosis. We inform them only of an inborn defect of the uterus and of irreparable sterility. In the incomplete syndrome with partial sensitivity of the target tissues to testi-cular testosterone there is the danger of virilization during puberty. We recommend therefore prepubertal gonadectomy when from the shape of the infantile genitalia the suspicion could already be confirmed. Even when signs of virilization develop during puberty, castration is necessary (for review see 353).

# UTERINE AND VAGINAL DISORDERS

## TRAUMATIC AMENORRHOEA (ASHERMAN'S SYNDROME)

The disease is also sometimes described as intrauterine synechia, atresia cavi uteri, Fritsch's syndrome, isthmic stenosis etc. It is a partial or complete oblitera-tion of the uterine cavity associated with reduced menstrual bleeding or ameno-rrhoea and with infertility or sterility.

Common factors in the aetiology of this syndrome are intrauterine trauma and a certain degree of endometrial inflammation. Therefore, intrauterine synechiae develop in particular after curettage during the puerperium or after abortions, if performed 1–4 weeks after a terminated pregnancy. On histological examination very frequently manifestations of acute or subacute endo-metritis are encountered. It seems that during involution and in the presence of infection the pregnant uterus responds very readily to curettage by the develop-ment of adhesions. Conversely diagnostic curettage, operations involving the endometrium (enucleation of a myoma, Caesarean section) only rarely promote the development of adhesions. It is usually assumed that the injury affects the basal endometrium. Granulation tissue is formed which combines with the opposite wall to form a firm ciccatrical bridge of varying extent and the latter reduces the uterine cavity or obliterates it completely. A frequent associated phenomenon is adenomyosis and the clinical symptom of pain (in 25%).

The main clinical symptoms are: (1) sterility and infertility, (2) disorders of late pregnancy, and (3) irregularities of the menstrual cycle. They depend on the extent of damage. An irregular cavity is an unsuitable medium for the implantation of the blastocyst and frequently renders implantation impossible. In other instances the pregnancy is threatened at an early stage by abortion, "missed abortion", ectopic nidation of the ovum and later by premature delivery. A frequent consequence is a placenta previa and placenta accreta. Secondary amenorrhoea develops in synechiae of the lower segment, or in case of extensive obliterations, in other instances, hypomenorrhoea is frequent, and sometimes menorrhagia or dysmenorrhoea. Ovarian function remains intact.

The diagnosis is based on the case-history (development after intrauterine injury), on a negative progesterone test in amenorrhoea, and on hysterosalpingography and exploration by sound.

For therapy various procedures were used. Nowadays we consider most suitable dilatation and destruction of adhesions by a catheter or curettage respectively. An intrauterine device is inserted into the uterine cavity for two months to prevent the formation of new adhesions. Broad-spectrum antibiotics before and after operation prove useful. Oestro-progestagen substitution for one month promotes the growth of the endometrium. Instead of an IUD some authors insert a child Foley catheter for a period of 10–14 days. In more serious cases the dilatation must be repeated several times, in rare instances implantation of the endometrium is possible. The therapeutic results are very satisfactory and complete recovery of the cavity is achieved in 90–100% of all patients; according to data of various authors 20–40% of the women become again pregnant.

## IMPAIRED RECEPTIVITY OF THE ENDOMETRIUM

It has been known for a long time that the target tissue of the action of steroid hormones, e.g. the endometrium, does not always respond to the same dose in the same manner. This disorder of receptivity was already previously described as "metrose de receptivité" and according to data reported by Moricard was present in about 10% of patients with secondary amenorrhoea. Factors which influence it include above all the central nervous system, tissue metabolism and the functional condition of cells. The receptivity has been studied little so far; only intensive investigation which gave some insight into the mechanism of hormone action at a subcellular level provides a basis for its objective evaluation in clinical pathology.

# IRREGULAR SHEDDING OF THE ENDOMETRIUM

Irregular shedding is clinically accompanied by menorrhagia caused by irregular or prolonged desquamation of the endometrium. We include it among uterine disorders although the true cause is not completely clear so far and is probably in the central regulation.

So far the endocrine basis has not been elucidated. Contrary to a normal cycle, the basal temperature is still elevated during bleeding. Urinary pregnanediol persisted during menstruation; the urinary levels of oestrogens and 17-oxosteroids were normal. Investigations of the corpus luteum revealed normal findings. It seems thus that the basis of this menorrhagia is a slowly declining functional activity of the corpus luteum (and thus not insufficiency) and haemorrhage ensuing from it, and not from a decline of progesterone.

Irregular shedding of the endometrium accounts for 10–17% of all functional menorrhagias. The maximum incidence is at the age of 30–40 years in women with an otherwise satisfactory fertility. A pathological condition frequently associated with it is concomitant hyperplasia of the endometrium, and, according to some authors, in many instances where prolonged shedding is assumed, hyperplasia of the basal layer of the endometrium is actually involved.

The main symptom is excessive protracted bleeding. In half the patients it persists for 8–10 days, in one quarter for 11–15 days. In the majority it is profuse and painless and often leads to the development of anaemia. The diagnosis is confirmed by taking a specimen by microabrasion on the first day of menstruation and then on the fifth day of menstruation we perform curettage. To eliminate submucosal myomas as the cause of menorrhagia, HSG is performed.

The specimen collected during the first 48 hours has the same histological appearance as tissue during normal menstruation. For this condition, a specimen of the fifth day of bleeding is typical. Most of the surface epithelium has disappeared, the endometrium displays a mixture of late secretory, necrotic, fragmented and involuting endometrium at a time when regeneration should have long since started.

Treatment is empirical. In less than half the patients the condition improved or has been cured by curettage. Major doses of progesterone are used 2–3 days before menstruation, so-called hormonal curettage. In other instances before and throughout menstruation oestrogens are recommended. Therapeutic failures call for castration (by X-ray or surgical operation).

## TUBERCULOUS ENDOMETRITIS

While non-specific chronic endometritis only rarely leads to disorders of the cycle, tuberculous infection of the endometrium which is an associated manifestation of genital tuberculosis is often accompanied by primary or secondary amenorrhoea or hypomenorrhoea. It may be stated that a great proportion of cases of genital tuberculosis is diagnosed by microabrasion of the endometrium in an endocrinological clinic rather than elsewhere. Obviously no endocrine condition is involved. The specific infection is transferred to the endometrium directly from the oviducts or by the haematogenic route from the lungs and causes sterility and disorders of the cycle. On histological examination we find multiple granulomas containing Langhans' giant cells surrounded by an infiltrate of lymphocytes.

Suspicion of a specific process is aroused by the clinical picture of amenorrhoea or hypomenorrhoea with a high basal temperature drawing attention to subfebrile temperatures. The histological finding from the microabrasion or curettage is supplemented by direct detection of mycobacteria by cultivation and inoculation of the obtained mucosa.

Causal therapy is focused on the basic disease. A combination of streptomycin, isoniazid and PAS is used. The prognosis of fertility in these women is poor.

## APLASIA OF THE VAGINA AND UTERUS
## (MAYER-ROKITANSKI-KÜSTER-HAUSER SYNDROME)

The authors of this syndrome described this unit as "uterus septus" or uterus bipartitus solidus cum vagina solida. The formal genesis of this syndrome has not been elucidated so far. Usually it is assumed that this developmental anomaly is caused by teratogenic noxious agents during the second month of embryonic development. Evidence on the genetic origin of this disorder, however, is also accumulating. This is suggested by dermatoglyphic studies and chromosome analyses which revealed rare mosaics with three and more X. As the Müllerian ducts fail to join, the vagina is absent. At the site of the uterus there is a transverse strip with peritoneal duplicature. On both sides there are non-canalized muscular rudimentary hemiuteri, normal ovaries and normal oviducts.

The reported incidence is 1:5,000 in all newborn infants. In our material they accounted for 24% of all cases of primary amenorrhoea. The main complaint is primary amenorrhoea. The chromosomal sex is female, the ovaries are functionally efficient and the gonadotropin and steroid levels are normal, which suggests ovulation; the basal temperature is biphasic. The external genitalia are of the female type, and so are the somatic development and secondary sex characteristics. Anomalies of the urogenital tract are encountered frequently (28%), less frequently inguinal hernias (13%). Rarely an associated Klippel-Feil anomaly is encountered which comprises a triad of symptoms: short neck, low line of hair and limited mobility of the neck due to fusion of some cervical vertebrae which form a bony block. Treatment of this syndrome is the artificial creation of a vagina (for review see 72). Among different procedures dissection of the rectouretral septum and insertion of a soft prosthesis covered by skin removed by a dermatome proved best.

## CRYPTOMENORRHOEA AND ISOLATED ATRESIA OF THE VAGINA

Hymen imperforatus causes primary amenorrhoea with haematocolpos and haematometra respectively and with menstrual molimina. In childhood and at the latest during puberty, women usually see a doctor about this disorder. By discision of the hymen normal menstruation is established.

The obstacle for the flow of menstrual blood need not be only a hymen imperforatus, isolated atresia of the vagina may be also involved: only a small space remains closely before the normally shaped portio vaginalis uteri. This finding is less frequent and more difficult to diagnose. It differs from cryptomenorrhoea by the fact that there is only slight haematocolpos and a bulging resistance in the vulva is not palpable. It differs from Rokitanski's syndrome by a normal shape of the uterus. For treatment we apply the same procedure as in aplasia of the vagina and uterus: dissection of the rectouretral septum up to the portio vaginalis uteri and then we join the margins of the residual part of the vagina in front of the portio vaginalis uteri with the distal parts of the mucosa. The therapeutic results are perfect. A prosthesis is not needed and pregnancy is possible.

# DISORDERS WITH NORMAL OVARIAN FUNCTION

## DYSMENORRHOEA

Dysmenorrhoea is gradated pain in the hypogastrium during menstruation accompanied by general complaints. Mild pain and complaints are described as molimina menstrualia. With regard to the time of development and for aetiological and therapeutic reasons we must differentiate between two main groups: primary dysmenorrhoea (idiopathic, functional) and secondary dysmenorrhoea (symptomatic, organic). The aetiology and pathogenesis have been discussed in another chapter (see p. 160) (for review see 548).

# PRIMARY (IDIOPATHIC) DYSMENORRHOEA

The clinical picture of dysmenorrhoea is dominated by intense pain during menstruation which in varying intensity is encountered in about 20% of all women. Milder pain is often tolerated without consultation with a physician. Sometimes the pain may be so intense that it makes the woman unable to work or even to move and confines her to bed rest. The local pain is concentrated mainly in the hypogastrium and low back and irradiates to the adjacent parts. It is described as a pulling, blunt, sometimes cutting pain. It persists throughout menstruation, though usually it is most intense on the first days. Sometimes it combines with premenstrual and postmenstrual pain.

General complaints are of different intensity and are perceived as increased nervous irritability, vertigo, headache, sickness,. vomiting, diarrhoea or colicky pains, urinary frequency. It is known that primary dysmenorrhoea frequently disappears or diminishes after marriage or after the first delivery. Conversely secondary dysmenorrhoea frequently deteriorates with advancing age. Ovarian function is normal in dysmenorrhoea and the cycle is ovulatory. Urinary oestrogens reach the peak in the middle of the cycle and in the secretory stage they are significantly lower. The pregnanediol levels are quite normal.

Diagnostically we must differentiate the condition from the mild one, described as molimina menstrualia. The difference is, however, only quantitative. It is differentiated from the premenstrual syndrome by the time of pain at the onset of menstrual bleeding, although sometimes the two syndromes combine. Secondary dysmenorrhoea with menorrhagia often suggests a submucous myoma.

Because the aetiology of this disease has not been adequately elucidated, treatment is varied and not always a success. It differs substantially, however, from treatment used in secondary dysmenorrhoea.

(1) Psychotherapy.

(2) General adjustment of the living regime with correct spacing of work and leisure, suitable diet, time spent outdoors, mild sports activity.

(3) Special gymnastics, remedial exercise, and hydrotherapy, warm baths or compresses.

(4) Hormonal treatment. Formerly progesterone, oestrogens and testosterone were recommended; however, they did not have a constant effect. Block of ovulation by preparations used in contraception from the 5th to the 25th day of the cycle for 3–6 months is effective. The effect often persists for prolonged periods.

(5) For symptomatic treatment often analgetics, spasmolytics and ataractics are used. It proves possible to inhibit the increased tonus and contractility by some stimulator of $\beta_2$-receptors, e.g. terbutalin or phenoterol, which act in particular on the uterus, bronchi and peripheral vessels.

(6) Recently recommended but not yet adequately evaluated preparations

include ε-aminocaproic acid, indomethacin and some of the retroprogesterones (dydrogesterone and trengestone).

ε-Aminocaproic acid is administered by mouth in 2 g doses on the first day and in 1 g doses on the subsequent days of menstruation. An effectiveness of 91% was reported in primary dysmenorrhoea as well as in premenstrual syndrome, although the mechanism of action in these cases is not clear.

The use of indomethacin, an inhibitor of prostaglandin synthesis, is based on the idea that prostaglandins participate in the pathogenesis of primary dysmenorrhoea either because their synthesis in the uterus is enhanced or because the sensitivity of the myometrium to their action is increased (for review see 312). The elevated endogenous concentration of the metabolite 15-oxo-13,14-dihydroPGF$_2$ has been actually found in women with dysmenorrhoea and in all investigated cases its decline has been confirmed as well as a reduced contractility of the uterus and regression of pain after indomethacin. For therapy $3 \times$ 50 mg indomethacin are administered by mouth daily from the day preceding the onset of menstruation. Another inhibitor of prostaglandin synthesis is flufenamic acid (a derivative of anthranilic acid), mefenamic acid or naproxen-sodium.

As to retroprogesterones, dydrogesterone is used, $3 \times$ 1 tablet à 5 mg per day from the 5th to 25th day of the cycle. This new gestagen caused disappearance of symptoms in 82% of all cases. The positive effect was confirmed also in a double blind experiment. Data that ovulation during this treatment is not blocked were confirmed only partly. When the hormonal parameters were investigated during treatment, in the minority of patients a reduced ovarian activity was observed. Trengestone, contrary to the previous substance, not only does not inhibit ovarian activity while exerting a progestation effect, but it stimulates the former. One tablet per day is administered from the 5th to the 24th day or from the 12th to the 24th day of the cycle.

(7) Finally presacral or parauterine block with 0.5% novocaine can be used or reflex dilatation of the cervix.

(8) In rare instances radical resection of the lower hypogastric plexus as described by Cott is used, combined sometimes with resection of the posterior ligaments according to Doyle.


## SECONDARY (SYMPTOMATIC) DYSMENORRHOEA

Dysmenorrhoea is included in this group where the pain is caused by organic disease in the minor pelvis. According to several authors this is the case in about 10% of all cases of dysmenorrhoea. The causes include: pelvic endometriosis, adenomyosis, hypoplasia of the uterus, inflammatory processes in the pelvis, stenosis of the cervical canal, fibromyomas, and abnormal position of the uterus.

**Pelvic endometriosis** is the most frequent and most reliably confirmed organic cause. In about 50% it takes a painless course. Frequently other symptoms predominate such as dyspareunia, rectal pain, tenesmus, or backache. In other instances associated adhesive processes with subsequent deviation of the uterus cause more intense dysmenorrhoea. Laparoscopy helps to establish the diagnosis, and in more extensive processes treatment is surgical. Conservative treatment by pseudopregnancy is partly successful but recently it was found that it did not fulfil the expectations of complete cure. Successful is the treatment with danazol.

**Adenomyosis** revealed on operation has as the most frequent symptom dysmenorrhoea and the causal relationship is obvious. The diagnosis is facilitated by the finding of an enlarged spherical, softer uterus associated with pain during menstruation. Treatment is surgical. Therapeutic pseudopregnancy does not cause relief.

As many as about 40% women with **hypoplasia of the uterus** suffer from dysmenorrhoea. The relationship is significant. It seems, however, that the cause is mediated. The main role is probably played by a dysplastic type of female with mental immaturity. Therefore attempts to influence dysmenorrhoea in uterine dysplasia by hormonal treatment are very frequently a failure.

**Uterine myomas** are only rarely associated with dysmenorrhoea, unless their localization is submucous. The diagnosis of submucous myoma is suggested by dysmenorrhoea and menorrhagia when the uterus is slightly enlarged. For confirmation hysterography is used.

**Inflammatory processes** in the pelvis, stenosis of the cervical canal and retroflexion of the uterus as causes of dysmenorrhoea have been formerly overestimated.


## PREMENSTRUAL SYNDROME

Sometimes also the term premenstrual tension is used. It is a group of psychic, somatic and vegetative symptoms which accompany in graded intensity the second half of the cycle up to menstruation; they are associated with the cycle and are unpleasantly perceived by the patient. The pathogenesis does not seem to be uniform and was discussed previously (see p. 163).

Data on the incidence vary greatly, because the perception of complaints is individual, their intensity differs, and thus the borderline between health and disease is not evaluated uniformly. About 40–85% women report certain complaints during the second half of the cycle, but only about 20% require treatment. Women in the third and fourth decade of life are affected more frequently.

The **symptoms** of the condition are very varied (for review see 512). The complaints can be divided into several groups: psychoneurotic, vegetative, somatic, metabolic and allergic. *Psychoneurotic complaints* most frequently comprise headache, sometimes even of a migrainous character, moodiness, increased irritability, the sensation of mental tension, affectability, aggressiveness, small concentrating capacity, fatigue, insomnia, and depression. *Vegetative complaints* develop in different systems of the organism. In the urogenital tract there is congestion in the minor pelvis, pain and tension in the hypogastrium, sacralgia, dysuria, and dyspareunia; in the gastrointestinal sphere it may be nausea, anorexia, diarrhoea, constipation, meteorism; in the cardiovascular system palpitations develop, hot flushes, acrocyanosis, or the subjective feeling of dyspnoea. *Somatic and metabolic manifestations* of the premenstrual syndrome include retention of water, the development of oedema, an increase of body weight on average by 1–2 kg and tension in the breasts and mastodynia. Frequently *allergic symptoms* develop such as pruritus, eczema or genital herpes, and asthma, if previously present, deteriorates.

The symptoms begin 5–14 days before menstruation and become more intense as menstruation approaches. On the last day before menstruation there is striking relief, and the complaints recede on the first day of menstruation. In the course of life premenstrual complaints increase with the approaching menopause. The premenstrual syndrome leads to deterioration of some other diseases such as epilepsy and hyperthyroidism. Frequently the premenstrual syndrome is considered a manifestation of hyperoestrinism. Objective assessment of oestrogens and their fractions in urine did not reveal differences from the normal ovulation cycle. However, in some cases immunoreactive plasma oestrogens were elevated, closely before menstruation, as compared with controls.

**Treatment** depends on the predominating symptoms. (1) General treatment and psychotherapy are indicated in women with a predominance of psychoneurotic complaints: adjustment of the working environment, physical therapy and hydrotherapy, climatic treatment. Aimed psychotherapy may eliminate contributing psychic factors. (2) Sedative and psychopharmacological preparations are used. (3) Dehydration treatment is used where oedema predominates: hydrochlorothiazide, 25–50 mg/day, is administered. (4) Best results are obtained by the combined administration of e.g. guaiphenesine 250 mg, dihydroergotamine 0.2 mg, caffeine 25 mg, and phenobarbital 20 mg in one tablet $3\times$ per day. (5) Hormonal treatment mainly with gestagens has been supposed to compensate the assumed relative hyperoestrinism. It has been recommended to administer 5–15 mg norethisterone for seven days before menstruation, in other instances a combination of diuretics, psychopharmaceutical preparations and gestagens. The success is, however, usually not permanent. Similar to dysmenorrhoea, it is frequently possible to eliminate premenstrual complaints, usually associated with the cycle, by blocking ovulation using an oral contraceptive combination.

# Hormonal Treatment of Disorders of the Menstrual Cycle

## SUBSTITUTION THERAPY OF MENSTRUAL DYSFUNCTION WITH OVARIAN STEROIDS

Treatment with ovarian steroids may be (a) substitutional, (b) inhibitory and (c) stimulatory. Inhibitory administration will be discussed in detail on p. 360 in the chapter on steroid contraception, and stimulatory treatment on p. 332 in the chapter dealing with treatment of anovulation.

### OESTROGEN SUBSTITUTION

The starting point are the known values of daily production in normal women, approximately 40–60 μg oestrone and 50–90 μg oestradiol in the follicular phase of the cycle and about three times as much during the luteal phase. The above data correspond roughly to a production of approximately 2.2 to 3.7 mg oestrone and 2.8 to 5.0 mg oestradiol in the course of the entire menstrual cycle.

Because of biological activity, the same steroid may differ diametrically in biological tests in animals and when used for clinical purposes (e.g. α-bis-dehydrodoisynolic acid is one of the most potent oestrogens in rats, while its effectiveness in women is very small). In subsequent paragraphs we quote (also for other steroids) only the clinical effectiveness of different hormonal preparations.

The amounts of oestrogens needed to achieve proliferation of the endometrium along with the assumed duration of action after a single dose are summarized in Table 19.

In clinical practice the proliferative dose of oestrogens must be assessed individually, mainly with regard to the length of previous amenorrhoea (see p. 115). Depending on the ability and will of the patient to cooperate, we decide for either oral or injection therapy. Injection is also used in case of intolerance to oral preparation (if it did not prove helpful to take the preparation after the last meal, before going to bed, or combined with anacid or with gastric-mucosa-protecting products before or after a meal).

*Table 19* Total proliferating doses of oestrogens and persistence of effect after a single dose of some oestrogen preparations

| Substance | Route of administration | Proliferating dose (mg) | Persistence of effect of single dose (days) |
|---|---|---|---|
| **Steroid oestrogens** | | | |
| Oestriol | p.o. | cca 600 | |
| Oestradiol | percutaneous | 150 | |
| Oestradiol | perlingual | 60–180 | 1 |
| Oestradiol benzoate | perlingual | 60–140 | 1 |
| Oestradiol benzoate | p.o. | | |
| Oestradiol valerate | p.o. | 80 | |
| Oestradiol benzoate | i.m. | 25– 30 | 6 |
| Oestradiol dipropionate | i.m. | 25– 30 | 6 |
| Oestradiol valerate | i.m. | 15–20– 30 | 10–12–14 |
| Oestradiol benzoate, microcrystalline suspension | i.m. | 20 | 21 |
| Ethinyloestradiol methylether | p.o. | 3 | |
| Ethinyloestradiol | p.o. | 1.5– 2 | 1 |
| Methyloestradiol | p.o. | 2 | |
| Conjugated equine oestrogens | p.o. | 80 | |
| Methallenoestril | p.o. | cca 400 | |
| **Non-steroid oestrogens** | | | |
| Trianisylchlorethylene | p.o. | over 100 | |
| Hexoestrol | p.o. | 70–110 | |
| Hexoestrol diacetate | perlingual | 45 | |
| Hexoestrol dipropionate | i.m. | 25 | |
| Dienoestrol diacetate | p.o. | 30 | |
| Dienoestrol diacetate, microcrystalline suspension | i.m. | 50 | |
| Diethylstilboestrol | p.o. | 20– 30 | |
| Diethylstilboestrol dipropionate | p.o. | 20– 30 | |
| Diethylstilboestrol dipropionate | i.m. | 12,5– 15 | |
| Diethylstilboestrol dipropionate, microctystalline suspension | i.m. | 5 | 21–28 |
| Diethylstilboestrol dimethylether | i.m. | 20– 40 | |

The criterion of effect is endometrial bleeding from the withdrawal of the circulating oestrogen level (*withdrawal bleeding, Entzugsblutung, Abbruchblutung*). For oral administration we use e.g. mestranol 0.15 mg/day for 21 days; if within one week pseudomenstruation does not develop, we repeat the administration in the same way. In amenorrhoea persisting for a long period, usually several substitutional cycles are needed to produce an effect, or we add daily 10 mg folic acid p.o.

After the effect has been achieved, we add during the last five days gestagen p.o. to the mestranol (see further); depending on the type of uterine bleeding, we reduce the oestrogen substitution during subsequent cycles using the same dose during 10 days, starting on the 17th day of the cycle (along with gestagen); 0.15 mg may be replaced by a daily p.o. dose of 1 mg diethylstilboestrol or by 0.075–0.1 mg ethinyloestradiol.

In case of amenorrhoea persisting for a long time, we can also start with injections of oestradiol valerate, 10 mg per week, for a period of 4–5 weeks. We do not wait for pseudomenstruation more than two weeks after the last injection, and possibly after 10 days we add the progesterone test. If bleeding from the endometrium occurs, we always reduce the administration period during subsequent cycles by one week and combine the last injection with gestagen. Subsequently we always administer on the 10th and 17th day of the cycle 10 mg oestradiol valerate and combine the second injection with gestagen. Depending on the nature of uterine bleeding, we can then in the majority of patients cut down medication to one combined injection of 10 mg oestradiol valerate with gestagen (see also further) on the 17th day of the cycle.

Excessive dosage of oestrogen is manifested on the endometrium mainly during prolonged and continuous administration of the oestrogen preparation. Depending on the period of administration and size of the dose, quantitatively and qualitatively different grades of proliferation occur, and subsequently also glandular cystic and in extreme cases also adenomatous proliferation with foci of foam-like lipid (cholesterol esters) containing cells in the stroma. *Breakthrough bleeding* occurs. A potential risk of prolonged oestrogen administration is carcinoma of the endometrium.

It is remarkable that by extremely high oestrogen doses in monkeys atrophy of the endometrium can also be induced. It cannot be explained by feedback inhibition of gonadotropic secretion with inhibition of ovarian oestrogens.

During the postmenopausal period we select oestrogens for substitution in doses which are clinically effective (the criterion is the regression of hot flushes), but do not complicate the situation by endometrial bleeding from the withdrawal of circulating steroids or breakthrough bleeding (*Durchbruchblutung*), when administered continuously (see p. 317). "Weak" oestrogens, i.e. those with a minimal effect on the endometrium, are best, particularly oestriol, and some non-steroid oestrogens.

A special chapter is **oestrogen treatment in pubertal girls with familial or constitutional excessive growth,** the incidence of which is reported as $25^0/_{00}$. Indication for intervention is a growth prognosis of 180 cm or more. We select some of the mentioned procedures. Treatment takes, as a rule, two years. In the first year growth is reduced to approximately one third and in the second year to one quarter of the anticipated value. The effect depends on the oestrogen dose (it is a function of oestrogenic biological activity). Effective doses are approximately five times higher than doses needed to block deficiency phenomena in adult women. Growth is frequently arrested long before closure of the epiphyseal plates. The cause is inhibited production of somatomedin; the plasma level of GH rises during treatment.

## GESTAGEN SUBSTITUTION

The daily production of progesterone in the follicular phase of the menstrual cycle is estimated to amount to 0.75–2.5 mg, and in the luteal phase 15.0–50.0 mg; in ovariectomized women 0.75 mg progesterone is produced per day. The corresponding value of the total amount of progesterone formed in the luteal phase is thus approximately 200–700 mg. In the literature we find most frequently the figure of 200 mg. For the prevention of endometrial bleeding from the withdrawal of the circulating progesterone level after extirpation of the corpus luteum, a substitution of 5 mg per day is sufficient in women. To reach the normal concentration of circulating progesterone in peripheral blood in the luteal phase usually 25 mg or more per day are needed.

Progesterone produced in the follicular phase of the cycle is probably of adrenal origin (after ACTH its concentration in the peripheral blood rises). However, the maturing follicles, no doubt, already produce progesterone during the first phase of the cycle. During substitution therapy we replace only progesterone secreted by the corpus luteum.

What has been said about oestrogens applies to the biological tests of the effectiveness of gestagen preparations. For gynaecological practice, clinical tests are conclusive which determine the dose necessary for (a) secretory transformation of the proliferated uterine mucosa after ten days administration (transformation dose), (b) retardation of menstruation whereby administration begins one week after the rise of the BBT and proceeds for another three weeks, (c) the induction of endometrial bleeding from the proliferated mucosa after discontinued five-day administration, (d) inhibition of ovulation, (e) inhibition of oestrogenic changes in the cervical mucus, (f) depression of the karyopyknotic index and (g) a rise of the BBT.

The same gestagen may exert a very different effect in the tests mentioned. Moreover, there are differences between different polyvalent ("impure") gestagen preparations as to their oestrogenic activity [which is either inherent to the molecule (e.g. in norethynodrel) or is secondary and develops as a result of a metabolic transformation (e.g. one of the metabolites of norethisterone is ethinyl oestradiol)] or androgenic activity, and among "pure" gestagens, as to their antiandrogenic effectiveness (e.g. it is marked in chlormadinone acetate and in particular in cyproterone acetate).

*Table 20*  Transformation doses of gestagens and doses required to retard menstruation

| Substance | Route of administration | Transformation dose (mg/cycle) | Dose retarding menstruation (mg/day) | Persistence of effect of single dose (days) |
|---|---|---|---|---|
| **Progesterone derivatives** | | | | |
| Progesterone | i.m. | 200 | 1000 | 2 |
| Progesterone microcrystalline suspension | i.m. | 200 | | 10–12 |
| 17α-Hydroxyprogesterone caproate | i.m. | 250 | | 8–10 |
| 17α-Hydroxynorprogesterone caproate | i.m. | 50 | | 8–10 |
| **Retroprogesterone derivatives** | | | | |
| Dydrogesterone | p.o. | 200 | | |
| Trengestone | p.o. | 50– 70 | | |
| **Derivatives of 17α-acetoxyprogesterone** | | | | |
| Medroxyprogesterone acetate | p.o. | 40– 70 | 20–30 | |
| Megoestrol acetate | p.o. | 35– 70 | 5–10 | |
| Chlormadinon acetate | p.o. | 20– 30 | 4 | |
| Cyproterone acetate | | 30 | | |
| **Derivatives of 17α-alkyl-19nor-androstane** | | | | |
| Allyloestrenol | p.o. | 300 | 30 | |
| Norethynodrel | p.o. | 150–200 | 14 | |
| Norethisterone (norethindrone) | p.o. | 100–150 | 10–15 | |
| Norethisterone acetate | p.o. | 40– 60 | 7,5 | |
| Norethisterone acetate micronized | p.o. | 12– 14 | | |
| Methylnortestosterone | p.o. | 150 | | |
| Lynoestrenol | p.o. | 35– 70 | 10 | |
| Ethynodiol diacetate | p.o. | 10– 15 | 1 | |
| Norgestrel | p.o. | 12 | 0,5 | |
| d-Norgestrel | p.o. | 5– 6 | | |

A suitable gestagen must be selected with regard to the situation which requires substitution (an obvious prerequisite is either sufficient production of ovarian oestrogens or replacement with oestrogenic products in proliferative doses). In common anovulatory disorders "pure" gestagen suffices; in concomitant hirsutism preparations with a more marked antiandrogenic effect are more suitable [possibly in combination with oestrogens (see p. 277)]. Polyvalent gestagens with an androgenic component are quite unsuitable. For cyclic prevention of anovulatory dysfunctional bleeding, on the other hand, polyvalent gestagenic preparations with an oestrogenic and androgenic action are suitable. The oestrogenic effect is, however, not welcome in late premenopausal dysfunctional bleeding, because it masks the decline of endogenous oestrogen formation [the oestrogenic action e.g. of norethisterone is so marked that it can induce bleeding from post-castration atrophic endometrium (205, 206)]. Therefore we administer on principle only "pure" gestagen during this period. For the same reason polyvalent gestagenic products with an oestrogenic activity are quite unsuitable for the oral variant of the progesterone test.

The gestagen doses needed for the secretory transformation of the proliferated endometrium and doses needed to delay menstruation are summarized in Table 20. These doses, similar to effective doses inducing uterine bleeding from the proliferated endometrium after five days administration, should be considered as an expression of the relative effectiveness of some gestagens rather than absolute values. We know that bleeding from the endometrium is also produced by a dose which does not suffice for the complete secretory transformation and that proliferation need not be complete (see p. 209).

Excessive doses of "pure" gestagen, i.e. a dose higher than the transformation dose, is manifested on the endometrium by marked oedema of the stroma with restricted physiological winding of the glandules and manifestations of secretory exhaustion (little secretion in the lumen, flattened cells); during administration extending over more than two weeks atrophy of the glands and decidualization of the stroma becomes more marked and the appearance of so-called rigid secretion develops which is explained usually by inhibited maturation of follicles and a decline of secretion of ovarian oestrogens. However, an antioestrogenic effect of progesterone has been demonstrated by interfering with the subcellular mechanism of oestrogen action (see p. 115).

The final result of the prolonged administration is endometrial atrophy which in extreme cases is irreversible (95). This antiproliferative effect of large doses, and in particular of prolonged continuous gestagen administration, is used in clinical practice in the treatment of endometriosis.

We decide to use oral or injection replacement therapy, similar to the case of oestrogen therapy, depending on the will and ability of the patient to cooperate. The criterion of effect, provided there are sufficient endogenous oestrogens or there is a concomitant adequate oestrogen administration, is the type of uterine bleeding caused by the withdrawal of the circulating gestagen level. We want it to resemble previous normal menstruation; therefore, we administer the full transformation dose of gestagen in the first cycles.

For oral substitution we use e.g. the Czechoslovak 17α-acetoxyprogesterone derivative (16-methylene-6-dehydro-17α-acetoxyprogesterone); at first we administer p.o. 15 mg/day for 10 days, starting on the 17th day of the cycle (in previously shorter cycles we start on the 14th day). Depending on the nature of endometrial bleeding, we can reduce the dose during subsequent cycles either to 10 mg per day, or we administer 15 mg per day but only for 5 days and we begin only on the 22nd (or 19th day respectively) of the cycle.

For injection treatment we use 17α-hydroxyprogesterone caproate, 250 mg on the 17th (or 14th) day of the cycle; again, depending on the nature of uterine bleeding, we can reduce the dose during subsequent cycles to 125 mg.

## OESTROGEN AND GESTAGEN SUBSTITUTION

Experience with complete combined oestrogen and gestagen substitution indicates that the condition of the endometrium depends on the total dose of the two steroids and on their mutual ratio. Deviations lead to atypical secretory transformation

*Fig. 40.* Dependence of the endometrial histology on doses (or production) of oestrogens and gestagens (175).

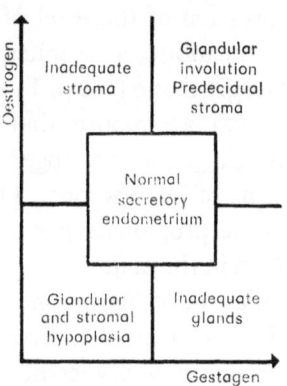

(Fig. 40). If insufficient amounts of the two hormones are administered, glandular and stromal hypoplasia develops. Gestagen deficiency or oestrogen excess lead to hypoplasia of the stroma with excessive proliferation of the glands (winding, dilatation and several rows of epithelium). Excess of gestagen or oestrogen deficiency lead to hypoplasia of the glands in the predecidual stroma. Excessive doses of both steroids cause predecidual stroma with involution of the glands (175). Defects in the secretory transformation of the endometrium may not only be due to specific progesterone deficiency, but rather to an unsuitable ratio of oestrogens and gestagens.

# TESTOSTERONE SUBSTITUTION

The daily plasmatic production of testosterone in females is roughly 150 to 300 µg/24 hours, i.e. 4.0–8.5 mg in the course of the whole menstrual cycle, which corresponds approximately to the total oestrogen production during the cycle. The physiological role of testosterone in females is so far quite obscure.

According to classical ideas, the physiological effect of testosterone on the endometrium is inhibition of growth and secretory activity of the glandular epithelium and inhibition of the development of spiral arterioles; it is assumed that not only the secretion of hypophyseal gonadotropins is reduced but also direct action on the uterine mucosa is suggested. On the other hand, endometrial bleeding has been observed after discontinued short-term testosterone administration in amenorrhoea with an adequate endogenous oestrogen production as well as in a castrated woman after oestrogen administration. Therefore, the assumption was expressed of a possible gestagenic or gestagen-like effect of testosterone. [Other variants interpreting uterine bleeding are (a) inhibition of FSH secretion and temporary depression of the level of circulating oestrogens, (b) feedback stimulation of LH release and (c) a peripheral antagonism and neutralization of the oestrogen effect in target tissue (see p. 115)].

There are reports that in an ovariectomized woman after endometrial priming with exogenous oestrogens it proved possible to induce secretory transformation by means of testosterone. The quoted transformation dose is at least 200 mg testosterone propionate per cycle. 200–300 mg testosterone per cycle is also the dose which in the majority of patients does not exert a masculinizing effect. Testosterone, similar to progesterone, delays endometrial bleeding caused by discontinued administration of oestrogens in ovariectomized women. Testosterone, however, does not prevent bleeding from the proliferated uterine mucosa which results from the withdrawal of the circulating progesterone level.

Since basic data on the role of androgens in the physiology of reproduction in the female are still lacking — except the assumed physiological stimulation of sexual activity (in ovariectomized monkeys they stimulate the sexual perceptivity and receptivity and in women a marked stimulation of sexual appetence is observed as a side-effect of androgen treatment) — it is difficult to speak of testosterone replacement therapy in women. We shall, however, discuss two indications for testosterone administration in women. These are: (a) secondary disorders of sexual appetence and (b) dyshormonal disorders of the mammary glands.

In secondary disorders of sexual appetence in women we administer methyltestosterone as an adjuvant, 10 mg per day p.o. for 10 days, starting on the 17th day of the cycle.

As to the differential diagnosis of dyshormonal diseases of the mammary glands, and in particular the frequently difficult differentiation from an initial malignoma of the mammary gland, we refer to special literature. In mastodynia (most frequently part of the premenstrual syndrome) and fibrous and cystic mastopathy we administer methyltestosterone in similar doses, for at least three consecutive cycles. The subjective relief is surprising, regression of morphological changes occurs. Unfortunately, in some patients the effect is not permanent and therapy must be repeated.

# HORMONAL THERAPY OF DYSFUNCTIONAL UTERINE BLEEDING

Regarding hormonal treatment we differentiate: (a) substitution treatment (oestrogens, progesterone, norsteroids and oestro-progestational combination), (b) stimulating treatment (choriongonadotropin, clomiphene citrate), and (c)

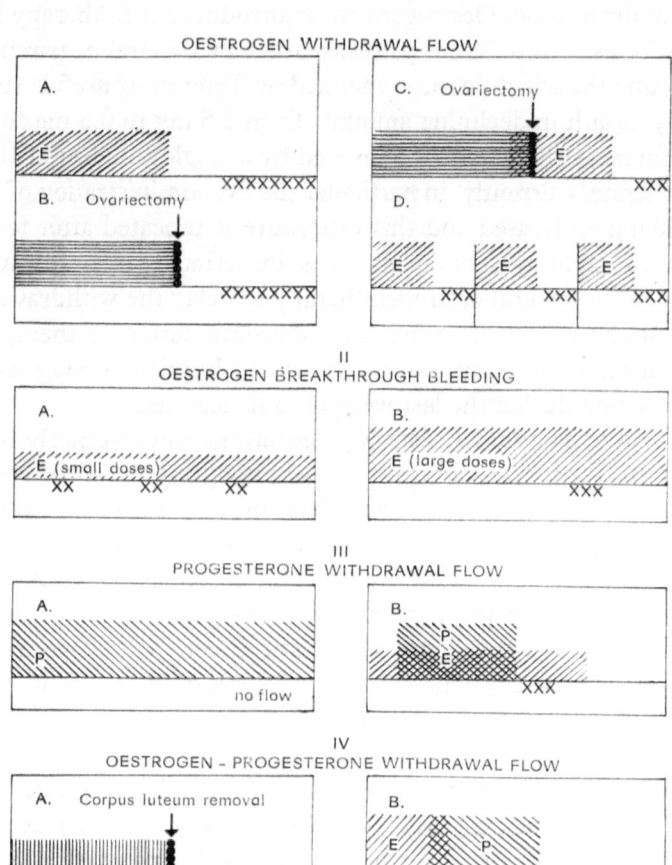

*Fig. 41.* Several basic axiomas in the endocrine physiology of uterine bleeding. (E — oestrogens, P — progesterone, XXX — uterine bleeding) (527).

inhibitory treatment (androgens). To the use of steroids for stopping or induction of haemorrhage certain basic rules of gynaecological endocrinology apply which were elaborated on the basis of empirical and experimental data (Fig. 41).

## SUBSTITUTION

Substitution treatment is basic. It has two stages. First we stop haemorrhage, then we prevent relapses.

## HAEMOSTASIS

**Oestrogens.** Since haemorrhage occurs when the plasma oestrogen level declines or during relative oestrogen deficiency, haemorrhage can be arrested by their administration. Oestrogens were introduced into therapy by Hamblen in 1936 and were used in different patterns either by the oral or parenteral route. Formerly we found the schedule recommended by Teter most useful: stilboestrol is administered by mouth in declining amounts from 2.5 mg to 0.5 mg for a period of four weeks. Haemostasis can also be ensured by a single i.m. dose of 10–20 mg depot oestradiol valerate. Currently, in particular the i.v. administration of conjugated oestrogens — 20 mg — is used and this procedure is repeated after four or six hours. It is the most rapid way of haemostasis in serious cases. Intravenous therapy must be followed by oral oestrogen therapy to delay the withdrawal bleeding and to induce a four-week cycle. Since after discontinuation of therapy bleeding due to withdrawal would occur, it is necessary to administer gestagens after having stopped the bleeding during the last week of oral treatment.

**Pure gestagens.** Although gestagens were formerly recommended for haemostasis, their use is not justified and pure gestagens alone (progesterone, 17-hydroxyprogesterone or oral derivatives of acetoxyprogesterone — Superlutin, chlormadinon and others) are a failure in haemostasis.

**Norsteroids.** These are potent gestagens, derived from testosterone, which are metabolized in the organism to oestrogens, and have therefore, contrary to pure gestagens, an excellent haemostatic effect. Nowadays they dominate in the treatment of dysfunctional bleeding. We administer 15 mg norethisterone acetate or other norsteroids by mouth (lynestrol, norethynodrel) for a period of 10 days. After 2–3 days bleeding stops but after termination of treatment we must foresee pseudomenstruation of the extent of normal menstruation.

**Oestrogen-gestagen combinations.** They are used in different mixtures. As to oral preparations for haemostasis, 0.15 mg mestranol can be used and 20 mg Superlutin for a period of 10 days or an injection of 10 mg oestradiol valerate and

250 mg hydroxyprogesterone caproate by the i.m. route in a single dose. A similar effect is exerted by 2–3 contraceptive pills/day taken for a period of 10 to 14 days. Combinations of oestrogens and gestagens are often available as mixed pharmaceutical preparations.

## PREVENTION OF RELAPSE

Since arrest of bleeding is not causal treatment, it does not suffice alone for the permanent cure of dysfunctional bleeding. Prevention of relapses is always necessary. For this either a pure gestagen or norsteroid is best suited. From the 17th day of the onset of bleeding, caused by a decline of oestrogens, either 5 times 20 mg progesterone i.m. on alternate days are administered, and haemorrhage occurs usually two days after the last injection, or else 17α-hydroxyprogesterone caproate is administered in a single dose of 125 mg. Equally suitable is oràl administration of Superlutin from the 17th day, 10–20 mg/day, for a period of 10 days. It is also possible to administer one tablet of a sequential contraceptive preparation from the 5th day for a period of 21 days. Nowadays we more frequently prevent relapses by use of norethisterone acetate from the 17th day, 15 mg per day for a period of 10 days for 3–6 months. If it is necessary to proceed, we reduce the doses and time of administration (to two tablets for five days from the 22nd day of the cycle).

## STIMULATION

For stimulation treatment choriongonadotropin sometimes is used. Its action on haemostasis is probably mediated by an increase of endogenous oestrogens. 1,000 IU per day are used until bleeding stops. It serves, however, rather to prevent relapses by inducing ovulation. It is administered from the 17th day of the cycle for 3 days à 1,500 IU. It is recommended in particular in young women or in juvenile bleeding. In sterile women who wish to become pregnant, after establishing regular pseudomenstruation, ovulation is induced by clomiphene citrate in the usual dose of 100 mg for a period of five days from the 5th day of the cycle.

## INHIBITION

Inhibition therapy by androgens is used only in elderly women. It is administered after curettage — for 10 days 25 mg testosterone propionate per day, and during the subsequent 2–3 cycles in the second half 10 mg for a period of 10 days. In older women we usually find an atrophic endometrium on histological examination during this therapy. In other instances it is possible to administer depot testosterone iso-butyrate (50 mg) on the 17th day of the cycle or oral methyl testosterone in the second half of the cycle, 10–20 mg for a period of 10 days. In view of the well known side-effects of androgens, they are used very little in women.

Because dysfunctional bleeding is one of the most frequent causes of work incapacity in women, its proper treatment is of great economic importance. From the above described therapeutic patterns, the best results were obtained with treatment and prevention with norethisterone acetate with subsequent induction of ovulation by clomiphene citrate. Analysis of results obtained in women followed up for prolonged periods revealed that practically in one third of women with dys-functional haemorrhage which started before the age of 38 years complete cure with spontaneous ovulatory cycles and pregnancy was achieved. In the remaining two thirds there were regular pseudomenstruations and only in 6% was there a failure and curettage was necessary.

# THERAPY OF ANOVULATION

Ovulation can be induced by several groups of substances: (a) gonadotropins (HPG, HMG), (b) antioestrogens (clomiphene citrate, cyclofenil etc.), (c) retro-progesterones, (d) gonadotropin-releasing substances (LH-RH and analogues), (e) wedge resection of the ovaries, and (f) other methods.

## GONADOTROPINS

**Heterologous gonadotropins.** Induction of ovulation by implantation of the pituitary or by gonadotropin from sera of pregnant mares (PMSG) in animals, stimulated attempts to induce ovulation in women. By a combination of PMSG and hCG this proved occasionally possible. Inconstant results and evidence of neutralizing antibodies against alien gonadotropins after short or repeated adminis-tration, led to a decline of interest in this treatment. Nevertheless, some authors were able to induce ovulation in women with purified extracts from hog or sheep pituitaries. We induced ovulation by means of animal preparations only in rare instances.

**Homologous gonadotropins.** Human gonadotropins do not induce antibody formation after repeated administration. They are obtained from human pituitaries (HPG) and from urine of menopausal women (HMG), they contain FSH and LH at a ratio of 1:1 and were introduced into clinical treatment in 1958–1960 by Gemzell and Lunenfeld.

320

The *selection of patients* for treatment is governed by certain rules. Above all ovarian tissue must be present which is able to produce an oestrogenic response to gonadotropic stimulation. Disorders are involved with (a) a normal response of the ovary, but low gonadotropin level, i.e. of hypophyseal or hypothalamic origin, (b) with a reduced response of the ovary to endogenous gonadotropins, but a normal gonadotropin level, and (c) with a selective areceptivity of certain ovarian elements to FSH or LH. Furthermore sterility and age under 35 years are the prerequisite conditions. The clinical picture in these patients comprises amenorrhoea, anovulatory oligomenorrhoea and an anovulatory cycle. The third condition is knowledge of the pathogenetic classification and examination of the husband.

*Therapeutic schedules* vary. If HPG or HMG alone are administered, follicular growth is induced but ovulation only sometimes. Therefore after these preparations hCG is always administered. Types of treatment are: (1) daily an injection of HPG or HMG from the fifth day for 9-11 days, whereby the hCG injections on the last 1-3 days overlap and proceed then alone for another 1-2 days; (2) HPG or HMG daily for 9-12 days and after 1-2 days without medication hCG is administered for 1-3 days; (3) HPG or HMG along with hCG, with a declining dose of the former two substances and with a dose of hCG overlapping or after their termination; (4)HPG or HMG is administered on the 1st, 4th and 8th day, and hCG on the 11th day; (5) finally it is possible to administer on the first day one large dose of HPG or HMG and on the 11th day one large dose of hCG. The pattern quoted sub (2) is used most frequently. The daily dose of HPG or HMG is individual, 75-450 IU (most frequently 150-225 IU, i.e. 2-3 vials), the total dose per treatment is 400 to 4,500 IU. The total dose of hCG varies from 5,000 to 25,000 IU (for review see 314, 319, 436). In many investigations the effect of different conditions on the success of treatment was compared. Frequently the ratio between FSH and LH was compared and values between 0.3-3.0 were considered best — because of the highest number of ovulations and the lowest incidence of hypersensitivity. Others conclude that the number of ovulations does not depend on the FSH/LH ratio. Some authors proved that daily administration results in a higher percentage of ovulations than one large dose (436).

The *therapeutic results* improved substantially since it proved possible to evaluate accurately the condition of the follicle at the onset of treatment and follicular maturation during stimulation. The basic finding is that the sensitivity of the ovary to gonadotropins differs not only in different patients but also in the course of time in the same woman. The administered doses must therefore be adjusted individually with regard to the immediate response of the ovary to avoid unnecessary treatment with small ineffective doses or to prevent the development of hyperstimulation syndrome. The range of sensitivity varies as much as eight times. For the assessment of the reactivity of the ovaries, either the gonadotropin test is used according to different patterns (see p. 213), or a complex of criteria is followed up after the administration of a low therapeutic dose. During treatment the following are evaluated: (1) cervical scoring or some of its components, in particular "Spinnbarkeit", (2) the karyopyknotic index, (3) total oestrogens, or pregnanediol in urine, or oestradiol or progesterone in plasma. The total urinary oestrogen levels should be 50–80 μg/24 hours during the preovulatory period; if they exceed 150 μg/24 hours or plasma oestradiol is above 600 pg/ml, the hyperstimulation syndrome may develop. Conversely a low or zero response makes us increase the dose in the same or subsequent cycle. Currently, when the therapeutic administration of gonadotropins is properly monitored, the number of hyperstimulations declined; however, hyporeactive cases and ovaries resistent to gonadotropin treatment have been detected. A new syndrome of amenorrhoea developed with elevated gonadotropins and with a morphologically normal follicular apparatus which does not respond even to HMG doses of the order of 10 thousand and to 15,000–25,000 IU hCG. There also exist hyposensitive ovaries which respond by ovulation and pregnancy only to 4 vials HMG per day and 25,000 IU hCG. When the response of the ovaries is normal, we recommend to the patient intercourse daily from the day preceding the first injection of hCG, as it is assumed that ovulation will occur 1–2 days after the first injection of hCG.

The results of gonadotropin therapy are very satisfactory. There is no difference between the results after administration of HPG and HMG. It must be emphasized, however, that this treatment is expensive. Therefore careful selection and regular check-up examinations are necessary. This treatment remains reserved in particular for substitution in hypogonadotropic patients and normogonadotropic ones if they do not respond to clomiphene citrate. Recent results of treatment are summarized in Table 21. Monitoring is one way how to improve therapeutic results and depends on the rate at which we obtain information. Automatic methods of oestrogen assessment meet this demand. Another way how to enhance the effectiveness of treatment involves the successive administration of clomiphene citrate, HMG and hCG, where 100% ovulation was achieved and 68% of the women became pregnant. Different clinical pictures have a different rate of successful therapy. The poorest results are recorded in primary amenorrhoea. In polycystic ovaries caution is indicated because hyperstimulation occurs more frequently.

**Complications of therapy** are of three types: hyperstimulation syndrome, multiple pregnancies and abortions.

The pathogenesis of the *hyperstimulation syndrome* has not been elucidated so far. It is, however, associated with the attained oestrogen level. There are three grades of hyperstimulation: mild, medium and severe. Mild degree: tension in hypogastrium, ovaries enlarged but not more than to 5×5 cm, weight increment up to 5 kg. Medium grade: pain in hypogastrium, sometimes nausea, vomiting or diarrhoea, ovaries enlarged up to 10×10 cm, cystic. Weight increment more than 5 kg. Severe grade: complicated in addition by ascites, hydrothorax and in the

*Table 21*  Results of gonadotropin therapy

| | Patients | Cycles | Pregnancies | Pregnancy rates % |
|---|---|---|---|---|
| Taymor 1967 | 101 | 343 | 62 | 61.4 |
| Lunenfeld et al. 1969 | 228 | 463 | 101 | 44.3 |
| Brown et al. 1969 | 45 | 222 | 43 | 95.5 |
| Butler 1970 | 134 | 438 | 31 | 23.1 |
| Bettendorf and Insler 1970 | 157 | 275 | 47 | 29.9 |
| Thompson and Hansen 1970 | 1190 | 2798 | 334 | 28.1 |
| Spadoni et al. 1974 | 62 | 225 | 26 | 41.9 |
| Ellis and Williamson 1975 | 77 | 322 | 43 | 55.8 |
| Jewellewicz 1975 | 142 | 262 | 89 | 63.0 |
| Oelsner et al. 1978 | 510 | 1897 | 278 | 54.5 |
| Tsapoulis 1978 | 320 | | 163 | 51.0 |

most severe cases by haemoconcentration, increased viscosity, coagulation and thrombosis, weight increment more than 10 kg. The symptoms develop 5–7 days after the onset of HMG therapy, 2–4 days after hCG. They persist for one to two weeks and disappear during the third week. The severe grade calls for hospitalization; treatment is conservative and care is taken to avoid rupture of the ovary. If during monitoring the oestrogen level is above 300 µg/24 hours during the pre-ovulatory period, treatment is discontinued. Data on the incidence of hyperstimulation differ. Formerly the incidence was higher. Nowadays when monitoring is used, severe cases are rare. The last major reviews report 5–7% mild cases, and 0.4% severe cases of hyperstimulation.

Another complication are *multiple pregnancies*. Fertilization of several ova is always involved. However, the reason proper is not known. No relationship with hyperstimulation has been proved. The preovulatory oestrogen values in three cases of quadruplets and quintuplets were 40–129 µg/24 hours. The rate of multiple pregnancies is reported as 20–36%, the majority being twins. Once heptaplets were reported, aborted during the 20th week.

Pregnancies after gonadotropin treatment must be considered risk pregnancies as 10–25% end by *abortion*. A relationship has been revealed between the preovulatory oestrogen level and the percentage of abortions. When the levels were lower than 150 µg/24 hours, 10.5% abortions have been recorded, when the levels were 500 to 800 µg/24 hours, 50% and when the levels were above 800 µg/24 hours, as much as 100%.

# ANTIOESTROGENS

## CLOMIPHENE

Clomiphene citrate is a derivative of triaryl ethylene and related to the weak oestrogen chlorotrianisene (TACE) and triparanol which is known as a cholesterol inhibitor. Chemically it is 2-[p(2-chloro-1,2-diphenyl vinyl)phenoxy] triethylamine dihydrogen citrate. It is an antioestrogen and in animals its antifertility action was first demonstrated, i.e. antigonadotropic, antiovulatory and antizygotic. It is, however, also a weak oestrogen. It was expected to be used clinically as an oral contraceptive. The reverse, however, is the case and it has become a drug stimulating ovulation very effectively (for review see 224).

The **mechanism of action** of clomiphene citrate is competition with natural oestrogens for the oestradiol cytoplasmic receptor in cells of oestrogen-sensitive tissues. This takes place in particular in the hypothalamus, in the adenohypophysis, ovary, uterus and cervix. The effect depends on the dose. Large doses of clomiphene citrate, by its inherent oestrogenicity, overshadow the competitive properties and the final effect is oestrogenic. In clinically used amounts, the mechanism by which ovulation is induced is approximately as follows: clomiphene citrate takes up the oestrogen receptor sites in the hypothalamus but is unable to generate and transmit the oestrogenic message to the nucleus; the hypothalamic cells thus record the false message on oestrogen deficiency and therefore release and produce LH-RH. Enhanced FSH and LH secretion follows which reaches its peak approximately on the 5th day of treatment. The raised FSH level stimulates the growth and development of follicles; in the presence of elevated LH, the oestradiol level rises more than during a normal cycle. This preovulation peak of oestradiol causes another LH peak leading to ovulation similar to a normal cycle (for review see 232, 314) (Fig. 42). During clomiphene therapy at the same time the testosterone and androstenedione secretion from the ovary rises. According to recent findings the antioestrogenic action of clomiphene is not explained by competition for the cytoplasmic oestrogen receptor, which would create a complex with a reduced stimulating capacity for growth, but by causing long-term depletion of cytoplasmic receptors for oestrogen, not only in the uterus but also in the pituitary (343).

**Indication for treatment** and selection of patients has its rules. The treatment is suited for women with an impaired cycle who want to become pregnant and where the husband has a normal spermiogram. The main indication is anovulation, while the amount of endogenous oestrogens is adequate, i.e. the woman is normogonadotropic. It must be proved in advance by a positive progesterone test, vaginal cytology, biopsy of the endometrium or the urinary or plasma oestrogen level. Slight oestrogen deficiency or a mild hypogonadotropic condition has less hope of success but does not rule it out. The following anovulation disorders are suited for treatment: dysfunctional bleeding, anovulatory cycle, syndrome of polycystic ovaries, normooestrogenic amenorrhoea or oligomenorrhoea, amenorrhoea with galactorrhoea. The other indications are luteal insufficiency with infertility. Hypergonadotropic conditions such as early climacteric, dysgenesis of the gonads, as well

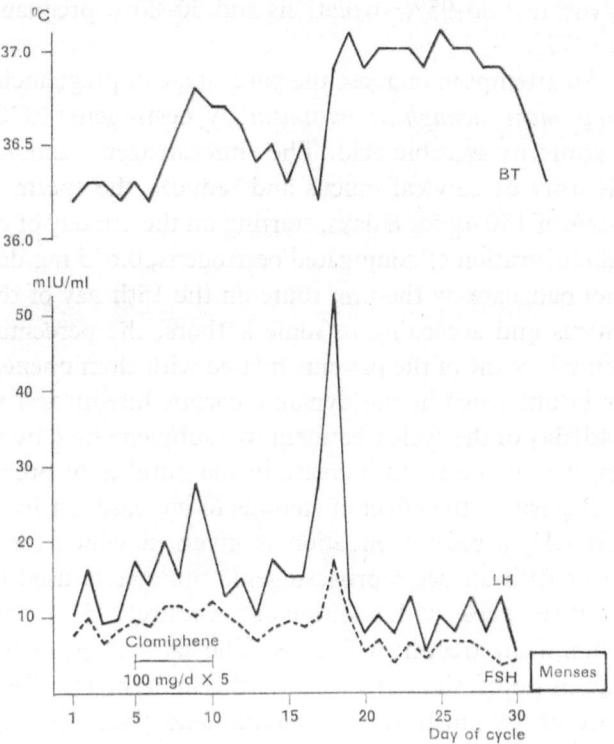

*Fig. 42.* Response of basal body temperature, LH and FSH plasma levels to clomiphene citrate.

as strongly hypogonadotropic conditions, namely panhypopituitarism or Sheehan's syndrome, are not suited for this treatment. The same is true for anovulations of adrenal or thyroid origin.

A **contraindication for treatment** in particular is pregnancy. During organogenesis clomiphene exerts a teratogenic action; the mistake of administering it at the onset of pregnancy can be avoided by investigating the basal temperature. Other contraindications are impaired hepatic function, impaired vision and ovarian cysts.

The **recommended dosage** of clomiphene in the first course of treatment is 50 mg per day for a period of 5 days, and during subsequent courses of treatment, 100 mg per day for a period of 5 days. A smaller dose is used at the beginning to prevent hyperstimulation, similar to gonadotropins. If there is a cycle, we start on the 5th day of normal bleeding or progesterone-induced bleeding, if there is no cycle, at any time, and if we fail to induce ovulation, we start again after 30 days. If after 3–6 cures ovulation is not induced, it is best to discontinue treatment and re-evaluate the indication.

Some authors, when the dose of 100 mg day fails, increase the clomiphene dose to 150–250 mg/day. This increasing dosage regimen is steadily gaining more advocates; 80–95% ovulations and 50–80% pregnancies are achieved (for review see 177).

An attempt to increase the percentage of pregnancies by treatment made authors *supplement clomiphene treatment* by oestrogens, hCG, an oestroprogestestational mixture or ascorbic acid. The antioestrogenic action of clomiphene increases the viscosity of cervical mucus and reduces the sperm cell penetration. EE in daily doses of 150 µg for 8 days, starting on the 4th day of clomiphene administration, or administration of conjugated oestrogens, 0.625 mg/day for 10 days or 1 mg oestradiol benzoate by the i.m. route on the 15th day of the cycle, improve the cervical mucus and according to some authors, the percentage of pregnancies increased. Since in some of the patients treated with clomiphene, a reduced progesterone level or insufficiency in the dynamic corpus luteum test were found, on the 13th and 14th day of the cycle treatment was supplemented by 5,000 IU hCG each day which apparently led to an increase in the number of pregnancies.

Regarding the effect of steroids to increase sensitivity of the adenohypophysis to LH-RH, a recommendation is given in which for three months cyclic pretreatment with an oestroprogestogenic mixture is used (oestradiol valerate 2 mg/day for three weeks with addition of norgestrel 0.5 mg/day during the last week). Then clomiphene treatment follows. The same effect is produced when the mixture is administered simultaneously with clomiphene. The last combination is the concurrent administration of clomiphene with 400 mg/day ascorbic acid and the presumed site of ascorbic acid action at the ovarian level. Views on some of these combinations are not clear so far. We administer them after failure of clomiphene alone, and we first start with a combination with hCG.

**Therapeutic results** can be evaluated on the basis of induced ovulations and the number of pregnancies. We can speak only of probable ovulation, as in most instances it is assessed by indirect tests. According to different authors, ovulation occurs in 50–90% of all cases. It depends on the selection of patients, and on the number of cures and doses. The difference between the percentage of probably induced ovulations and the percentage of pregnancies is striking; the latter occur only in about half the probable ovulations, i.e. in 30–40%. The reasons for this difference are explained in different ways: by a reduced permeability of the cervical mucus, by the occurrence of early unrecognized abortions, by pseudoovulation with luteinization of the unruptured follicle, or by the development of an inadequate luteal phase. We analyzed all cases where clomiphene treatment failed, i.e. patients who not only did not become pregnant but did not respond by probable ovulation. The reasons of pregnancy failure were a reduced fertility of the husband, conditions after adnexectomy, impaired structure of the endometrium and growing insufficiency of ovarian activity. Analysis of the remaining unknown causes by the LH-RH test alone revealed only that in all instances disorders of hypothalamic origin were involved and never disorders of hypophyseal origin.

Only a negative oestrogen amplification test (non-amplified response of LH in the LH-RH test after 2.5 mg oestradiol benzoate i.m. after 44 hours, as compared with the response before oestrogen administration) characterizes the group of non-responsors to clomiphene and is important for assessment of the indication for treatment (467).

We were also concerned with the problem of whether in clomiphene therapy only a single stimulation or repeated stimulation was involved. In a clinical trial arranged to obtain this answer, we demonstrated that in 30% we may foresee spontaneous biphasic cycles which occur repeatedly several times without treatment. This effect, where pregnancy occurred only during the next cycle after termination of clomiphene treatment, is described as a carry-over effect or rebound effect.

The majority of pregnancies occur after treatment during the first few cycles, about one third during the first cycle, the second third during the subsequent two cycles. In rare instances pregnancy occurs as late as after the 8th cycle or after repeating a series of cures with a longer interval in between. Pregnancy after clomiphene must be considered a risk pregnancy, since about 20–25% of women with these pregnancies have abortions or premature deliveries. The incidence of congenital anomalies is not raised and is reported to be about 2%. Multiple pregnancies are more frequent, formerly 10% were reported. Today it seems that, when short-term 5-day cures are used, where 100 mg/day are not exceeded, the percentage of multiple pregnancies declines.

Possible **side-effects** after clomiphene treatment include the following: (1) enlargement of the ovaries and formation of cysts as a sign of hyperstimulation, (2) vasomotor symptoms such as hot flushes, (3) abdominal pain, or (4) ocular symptoms such as blurred vision, black spots and flashes. When the recommended dosage is respected, signs of hyperstimulation are rare, however, and enlargement of the ovaries almost never calls for surgical operation and recedes after discontinuation of treatment and rest. In the polycystic ovary syndrome caution is indicated, as increased sensitivity to gonadotropins is frequently encountered there.

# CYCLOFENIL

The second non-steroid antioestrogen with a weak oestrogenic activity for induction of ovulation is cyclofenil. It is an asymmetrical diphenyl alkene, with the chemical formula: bis(*p*-acetoxyphenyl) cyclohexilidene methane which is related to stilboestrol and triphenyl ethylene.

The **mechanism of action** is based, similar to clomiphene, on the competitive inhibition at the level of hypothalamic and peripheral oestrogen receptors. It interferes with the negative feedback of oestrogens and renders possible the release of LH for ovulation by means of a positive feedback. When gonadotropin levels are investigated, LH and FSH already increase during administration, acting via LH-RH. The second rise which occurs most frequently on the 11th–15th day after the onset of treatment is the preovulation peak with subsequent ovulation. From animal experiments it seems that the direct action on peripheral receptors, i.e. enzymes of ovarian steroidogenesis in the theca interna, is greater than in clomiphene.

Distribution studies in the organism revealed accumulation of cyclophenil in the follicle, corpus luteum, pituitary, liver and kidneys. It is excreted within one hour from the circulation, and after 24 hours it disappears from all organs (except the liver and corpus luteum). It is a substance which even in large doses is not toxic.

**Indications for treatment** are the same as in clomiphene. Liver diseases are a contraindication.

The **recommended dosage** of cyclofenil tablets à 200 mg is three or four tablets per day for five days, starting on the 5th day of the cycle, i.e. doses of 600–800 mg per day.

The **clinical results,** i.e. induction of probable ovulation and pregnancy, resemble those of clomiphene treatment. Perhaps they are only somewhat lower. Ovulation occurs in 42–77%, pregnancy in 12–61%. We used a very strict criterion and selected women for treatment where previously clomiphene treatment failed and we recorded pregnancies in 7 of 40 patients. Thus when clomiphene fails, there are other therapeutic possibilities.

Pregnancy after cyclofenil must be considered a risk pregnancy and abortions and premature deliveries occur in about 20%, i.e. equally often as after gonadotropins or clomiphene. Similar to clomiphene, after cyclofenil the rebound effect is also encountered and pregnancy may occur also in a later cycle after therapy. Contrary to clomiphene and gonadotropin treatment, after cyclofenil multiple pregnancies do not occur. Some authors achieved substantially better result by adding 5,000 IU hCG on the 13th day of the therapeutic cycle.

Only a few authors compared the action of a major number of substances regarding their effect on induction of ovulation. Taking the percentage of pregnancies as a criterion, the order was as follows: gonadotropins 35, cyclofenil 22, clomiphene 17.3, epimestrol 16.9 (452, 452a). The number of therapeutic cycles needed to achieve ovulation was on average in cyclofenil 8–9, in gonadotropins 8–9, in clomiphene 16.3, and in epimestrol 13.6. The ratio of pregnancies to ovulations was approximately the same, 26–32%.

Side-effects are encountered in only about 2%: hot flushes, disturbed sleep, nausea, pain in the hypogastrium, in rare instances galactorrhoea.

The main advantage of cyclofenil is the absence of toxicity and consequently thus neither the hyperstimulation syndrome nor multiple pregnancies occur (for review see 326).

## TAMOXIFEN

Another antioestrogen for the induction of ovulation is tamoxifen (ICI 46,474). Chemically it is 1-(p-β-dimethyl amino ethoxyphenyl)-1,2-diphenyl-1-butene. Clinical experience with it is so far very limited. The dosage is 20 mg/day from the second day of the cycle for a period of four days, during subsequent courses of treatment the dose can be increased to 40–80 mg/day, depending on the response of the basal temperature and cervical mucus. In a group of sterile women where there were not only patients with anovulation but also with luteal insufficiency as many as 80% ovulations were achieved and 50% of the women became pregnant. Ovulation occurred in most instances on the 13th–24th day of the cycle. Here too the rebound effect is known and pregnancy occurs only during a later cycle after treatment. Multiple pregnancies do not occur but abortions are more frequent. As to complications, mild hyperstimulation develops when doses of 80 mg/day are used. However, it always improved spontaneously.

## RETROPROGESTERONES

Contrary to antioestrogenic stimulators of ovulation, **trengestone** is a steroid substance, a retroprogesterone (for review see 507). This group of synthetic substances has a nucleus which differs from progesterone by changing the hydrogen on the 9th carbon atom into the β-position and the methyl groups on the 10th carbon into the α-position. Trengestone is chemically 6-chloro-9β,10α-pregna-1,4,6-trien--3,20-dione. It has a strong progestogenic action and stimulating effect on the hypothalamo-hypophyseal system. It does not possess a direct oestrogenic or androgenic action. It indirectly stimulates the oestrogen production in the ovary, however, via the central nervous system.

The **mechanism of action** for induction of ovulation is not quite clear. According to animal experiments trengestone is very effective in the facilitation of ovulation, much more effective than progesterone or related gestagens, dydrogesterone and chlormadinon. The facilitation is implemented either directly or by potentiation of the positive feedback. The LH levels after administration did not provide a final conclusion, as according to some authors they did not change, according to others they increased. Trengestone is not toxic. It is rapidly absorbed and within seven days after administration the substance is completely excreted in urine and faeces. Contrary to progesterone, it does not raise the basal temperature and is not metabolized to pregnanediol but to $20\alpha$-hydroxy derivatives.

In clinical practice it is best to start with administration on the 14th day of the cycle and to administer 1–2 tablets à 4 mg for a period of 10 days. Treatment is continued during 3–6 cycles, sometimes longer. **Indications for this treatment** are, in particular, patients with normooestrogenic anovulation. It induces ovulation in 30–60%, depending on the type of disease, in 12–71% according to data reported in different papers, on an average in 52.4%. Pregnancy was achieved on average in 20%. Both results are lower than after clomiphene. The pregnancies were thus far not threatened. Ovulation occurs after trengestone administration either immediately after termination of treatment or much later. Usually so-called late ovulations are recorded where after termination of the course of treatment bleeding occurs fairly soon and only during the subsequent cycle, rather late (on the 20th–26th day) ovulation occurs. Ovulation can be explained by the rebound effect. After treatment the hyperstimulation syndrome was not encountered, there were no signs of virilization, and only about 6% of the women have side-effects such as mastalgia, headache and fatigue. Another indication for its administration are other functional disorders of the cycle (short luteal phase, haemostasis in dysfunctional bleeding) and treatment of imminent abortion. Due to its harmless character, but smaller effectiveness in promoting pregnancy, it is suited for regulation of the cycle in young women who do not wish to become pregnant.

## LH-RH

Due to its natural function to stimulate LH and FSH it was obvious to use LH-RH to induce ovulation. In animals this can be achieved reliably not only by LH-RH but also by its more potent analogues. In women ovulation can be also induced. However, the therapeutic procedure has not been standardized so far. The first ovulation and pregnancy in a woman was induced by Kastin in 1971. Since then more work has been published on the success of this treatment; however, the doses used differed greatly. The original recommendations with small single doses did not prove useful. It seems that treatment must be biphasic: first it is necessary to stimulate follicular maturation by means of LH or HMG or clomiphene and then to induce ovulation proper by LH-RH or hCG. Intravenous administration only has a short effect, therefore infusions after 4–6 hours and intramuscular administration are more satisfactory. After 50 µg doses of LH-RH in a daily infusion after clomiphene pretreatment, doses of 100 µg by the i.m. route on the 9th and 10th day of the cycle are now used after pretreatment with HMG. The Chilean group induced ovulation 13 times in a total of 28 treated cycles with doses of 50 to 500 µg and they conclude that smaller doses administered every 8–12 hours for a period of 10–20 days are more effective than large doses (0.5 mg) administered only less frequently. The Mexican group achieved ovulation 10 times in a group of 42 women by stimulating them for five days with doses of 200–500 µg LH-RH by the i.m. route. The Japanese group (355) recorded the most satisfactory results after clomiphene stimulation, followed after another 5–10 days by administration of 200 µg LH-RH by the i.v. route, and 200 µg by the s.c. route following insemination. Some authors using doses of 100–200 µg LH-RH by the s.c. route for 17–21 days did not achieve stimulation of the ovary assessed from a rise of oestrogens.

Up to 1976, in the literature 333 women were reported, treated with LH-RH in different amounts and combinations, where ovulation had been induced in 42% and pregnancy only in 14%. It was not clear, however, whether the effect had not been produced by combinations of other drugs than LH-RH (for review see 551). We achieved in 52 women, with anovulation not responding to clomiphene, by five different therapeutic procedures with LH-RH alone or in combination with clomiphene and hCG, stimulation of the follicle only in some, but never ovulation. Hitherto achieved results are thus disappointing.

Hopes were aroused by superactive analogues of LH-RH where the stimulating action on LH and FSH was many times higher and more persistent than in LH-RH and where perspectively also intranasal administration was possible. The following were used with alternating success — (D-Ala$^6$, des Gly-NH$_2$$^{10}$)-LH-RH EA, (D-Leu$^6$, des Gly-NH$_2$$^{10}$)-LH-RH EA in amounts of 25–200 µg/day as well as D-Ser(TBU$^6$-EA$^{10}$)LH-RH in doses of 10 µg/day (366) with no pregnancy. D-Trp$^6$-LH-RH was administered in an 8-hour i.v. infusion (40 µg) and at the end of the infusion 40 µg s.c. Some of the women were pretreated with 10 µg i.m. for 10 days, others with clomiphene or HMG in the usual therapeutic amounts. Three of nine women ovulated and three of them became pregnant (234). Acute single administration can stimulate the follicle. When daily doses are administered, however, plasma gonadotropin and oestradiol rise only for 2–3 days, then a permanent inhibitory effect sets in which persists up to the end of administration. LH-RH analogues used for inducing ovulation have not been very successful so far either.

## OTHER METHODS

**Oestrogens.** The effect of oestrogens in a positive feedback during the release of LH is beyond doubt. So far it has not proved possible to simulate this stimulating effect to induce ovulation in women, although various types of oestrogen treatment with large and small doses are recommended. Among oestrogens we also include anovulation treatment with epimestrol (Org 817). Chemically it is 3-methoxy-17--epioestriol. Doses of 5 mg for a period of 10 days induced ovulation according to different authors in 12–32$^{0}/_{0}$.

**Corticoids.** Corticoids suppress ACTH and hence also adrenal secretion of androgens. They are thus causal treatment in anovulation with an adrenal genesis. Success has been recorded in syndromes of polycystic ovaries and mild hyperplasia of the kidneys.

**Bromocryptine.** 2-Br-α-ergocryptine reduces the prolactin secretion and promotes gonadotropin secretion. It proves very useful in the treatment of hyperprolactinaemia; very frequently ovulation is induced and frequently also pregnancy follows (see p. 282).

**Substances acting on the CNS.** These substances, e.g. phenamine, can also induce ovulation.

The **ovarian wedge resection** and the effect of **prostaglandins** have been discussed in the appropriate chapters (see p. 277 and 116).

# Sterility and Infertility

It is expedient to differentiate in women between **sterility** (*impotentia generandi*) and **infertility** (*impotentia gestandi*) where the woman conceives but is unable to become pregnant and to bear a viable foetus. We shall therefore deal with the two disorders of the female reproductive function separately. [In particular in the Anglo--american literature, we find a wider concept of the term infertility which comprises also sterility. It is based on the wider term of **fertility** (*fecundability*) which covers the ability of a woman to deliver a live infant.]

## STERILITY

The rate of unwanted childless marriages in economically developed countries with a high standard of health care is estimated as 15% (USA 1968) to 20% (GFR 1969).

The probability of impregnation is influenced by (a) the age of the woman, (b) the age of the man, (c) the frequency of coitus and (d) the length of time when pregnancy was attempted.

*Table 22*  Dependence of conception on coital frequency (293)

| Average coital frequency (weekly) | No. of cases | Conception up to 6 months (%) |
|---|---|---|
| Less than 1 | 24 | 16.7 |
| Less than 2 | 109 | 32.1 |
| Less than 3 | 123 | 46.3 |
| Less than 4 | 100 | 51.0 |
| More than 4 | 72 | 83.3 |

The maximum fertility is reached by women at the age of approximately 24 years. Then the probability of conception declines relatively rapidly, in particular after the age of 30 years. The same applies to men. It seems that the optimal rate of coitus for the fertilization of women is not less than four times per week (Table 22).

From the relationship of impregnation and the duration of the period of unprotected intercourses (Table 23), it follows that gynaecological consultation should already be sought after 12–18 months of an unwantedly sterile marriage (Fig. 43) (534).

*Table 23* Dependence of conception on the duration of unprotected coital activity. I.(98); II.(27)

| Duration of coital activity (months) | Incidence of conception % I. | II. |
|---|---|---|
| 1 | | 25 |
| 3 | 50–60 | |
| 6 | 60–70 | 65 |
| 9 | | 75 |
| 12 | 75–80 | 80 |
| 18 | | 90 |

The cause of sterility is in as much as 80% of cases caused by the woman, in as much as 30% by the man, and in about 10–20% it is due to a combined subfertility of both partners, which in isolated cases may be compensated by increased fertility

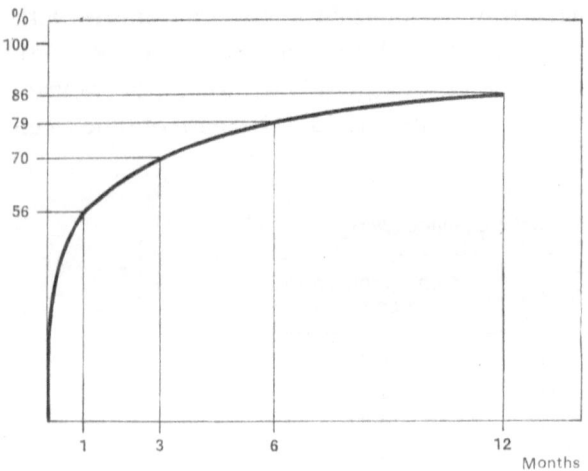

*Fig. 43.* Relationship between conception and period of unprotected intercourses in 850 primiparae (534).

of the other partner. In as many as 15–20% of unwanted childless marriages the causes of sterility are not detected.

Analysis of sterility in large groups indicates (Table 24) that in the foreground are disorders of the hypothalamo-pituitary-ovarian system. Disorders of tubular patency hold the second place. Fundamentally we may differentiate between two groups: (1) sterility due to impaired function of the reproductive system (functional sterility) and (2) sterility from anatomical causes which make it impossible for the sperm cells to encounter the ovum (anatomical sterility, most frequently due to

*Table 24*  Causal factors of sterility in 1160 (I. 118), 524 (II. 122) and 114 (III. 90) sterile women

| Factor | Incidence (%) | | |
|---|---|---|---|
| | I. | II. | III. |
| Ovarian*) | 41.9 | 46.4 | 44.5 |
| Tubal | 29.0 | 22.5 | 15.8**) |
| Uterine | 6.7 | 5.3 | |
| Cervical | 3.6 | 1.5 | |
| Vaginal | 4.9 | | |
| Psychogenic | 0.6 | 0.2 | |
| Other extragenital | 1.2 | 1.5 | |
| No obvious factor | 12.1 | 22.3 | 31.5 |

*) ovulatory disturbances (in I. inclusive uterine hypoplasia)
**) all organic factors

obstruction of the oviducts). Sterility may be *primary* if the woman was never pregnant, or *secondary*, when as a rule one pregnancy precedes.

## ANATOMICAL STERILITY

Anatomical sterility is most frequently the consequence of salpingitis which results in (a) chronic interstitial salpingitis, (b) sactosalpinx (hydrosalpinx or in rare instances pyosalpinx) or (c) chronic nodose salpingitis due to fusion of the endo-salpingeal mucosal folds. In particular the two latter forms of chronic inflammation of the oviducts are frequently complicated by obstruction.

In addition to this anatomical obstruction, there is also *"functional obstruction"* or incompetence of patent oviducts, i.e. a disorder of the normal tubal function, motor or secretory, which is essential for retaining the ovum, its migration through the tube and penetration through the uterotubal junction into the uterine cavity. It is the result of a previous inflammation, possibly despite successful surgical operation of the oviducts which were made patent (for review see 194). The reverse is obstruction caused by spasm of the uterotubal junction which on kymoinsufflation or hysterosalpingographic examination not only pretends anatomical obstruction but which may be a serious impediment of impregnation, e.g. in psychogenic sterility (for review see 346a).

Periampulloovarian adhesions may also, despite preserved patency of the oviducts, be the cause of anatomical block on the pathway of the ovum or may interfere with the physiological motor function of the tube. The cause of anatomical as well as functional tubal occlusion may also be *pelvic endometriosis* (for review see 265).


## FUNCTIONAL STERILITY

Functional sterility comprises those cases of female sterility where the result of examination of the partner's ejaculate was normal and the examination of the patency of the oviducts not only confirmed it but also ruled out periampulloovarian adhesions. Therefore, hysterosalpingography with a hydrosoluble contrast solution is essential (to eliminate uterotubal spasm an instillation of 2–4 ml 4% trimecaine chlorate 5 min. before the examination is effective). Kymoinsufflation of $CO_2$ gives too optimistic results; it may be falsely positive. In obscure cases we supplement the examination with pneumohysterosalpingography (a combination of hysterosalpingography and pneumopelvigraphy) and always with pelvic endoscopy (by laparoscopy or culdoscopy) with hydrotubation with a coloured solution or, in extreme cases, with explorative laparotomy, and also with pertubation. Only direct visualization of the oviducts with hydrotubation provides conclusive evidence of occlusion of the tubes; conversely, endoscopy with hydrotubation revealed in 11.5% of patients patency of the oviducts, although they appeared obstructed on hysterosalpingographic and kymoinsufflation examination (391a). Laparoscopy reduces the rate of the so-called unexplained sterility, most frequently by revealing pelvic endometriosis or peritubal adhesions (123).

The purpose of the differential diagnosis in functional sterility is above all the pathogenetic diagnosis—elucidation of the impaired function of the reproductive system.

With regard to the regulatory hierarchy we may differentiate:
A. central disorders
   (a) psychogenic disorders
   (b) hypothalamic disorders
   (c) hypophyseal disorders
B. ovarian disorders
C. uterine disorders (corporal)
D. cervical disorders
E. vaginal disorders.

## CENTRAL AND OVARIAN CAUSES OF STERILITY

These are manifested in particular by anovulation, either "isolated" in a complete anovulatory cycle, or as part of menstrual dysfunction.

Most frequent central causes of sterility are hypothalamic disorders of ovulation (data on the incidence of psychogenic disorders are rather controversial); hypophyseal and ovarian disorders are most frequently cases of extremely serious disorders of the menstrual cycle. However, even ovulation does not rule out the possibility of functional sterility.

Clinically we assess thus:

A. anovulation (or oligoovulation)

   (a) with a regular menstrual cycle (so-called complete anovulatory cycle)

   (b) in menstrual dysfunction

B. ovulation

   (a) with impaired function of the corpus luteum (so-called short and/or inadequate luteal phase)

   (b) with normal function of the corpus luteum
      (aa) with functional disorders of the internal genitalia

      (bb) without detectable functional disorders of the internal genitalia ("apparent" sterility in 15–20% of all cases)
         ($\alpha$) with systemic disorders (e.g. immunological or psychogenic)
         ($\beta$) without detectable disorders (true "unexplained" sterility).

Flow sheets for diagnosis in functional sterility are demonstrated in Fig. 44 and 45.

It must be stressed, however, that the decision trees presented in Fig. 44 and 45 are only a simplification of possible approaches and represent a starting point for selecting the appropriate procedures.


## UTERINE CAUSES OF STERILITY

Corporal uterine causes of sterility (for review see 528) include in particular **uterine hypoplasia** which, contrary to infertility, plays a greater part than uterine malformation. It has been described in detail along with the diagnosis in a previous chapter (see p. 183).

We assume that in sterility defects in the maturation of the endometrium may play a pathogenetic role. Although the part played by inadequate secretory transformation in sterility and infertility is beyond doubt, we must not omit the possibility of pathological implantation of the blastocyst in a quite unphysiological medium: on the tubal or cervical mucosa or on the peritoneum, in extreme cases with a completed pregnancy.

In *treatment of uterine hypoplasia* therapeutic pseudopregnancy is most successful. It simulates the steroid hormonal pattern in the first trimester of pregnancy.

For oral treatment a single-phase steroid contraceptive may be used (a combination of oestrogen and gestagen), during the first 20 days one tablet per day,

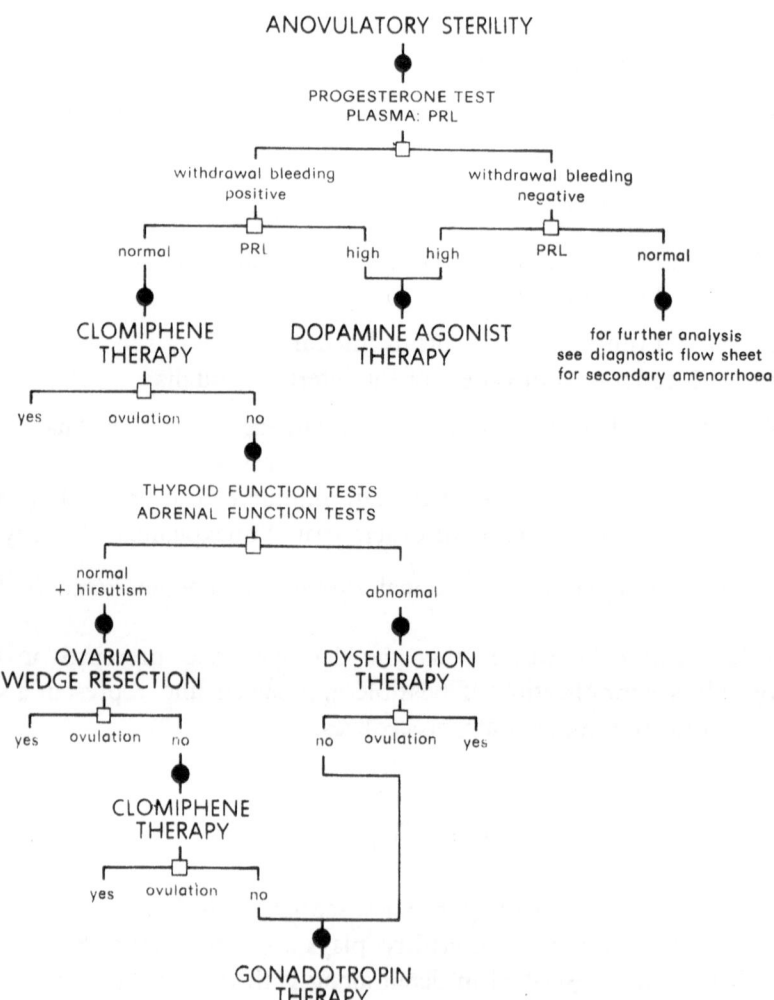

*Fig. 44.* A stepwise flow chart for the therapeutic approach to functional sterility with anovulation (● — decision nodes, ☐ — chance nodes).

during the subsequent 20 days 2 tablets, and finally three tablets per day. Breakthrough bleeding is an indication for an earlier increase of the daily dose if it does not call for discontinuation of administration.

For injection treatment we administer e.g. oestradiol valerate, 10 (to 20) mg i.m. per week, along with 250 mg 17α-hydroxyprogesterone caproate i.m. for 6 weeks, during the 7th week we increase the gestagen dose to 500 mg and during the 8th week we complete the cure by an injection of 500 mg gestagen without oestrogen.

We can also combine weekly i.m. administration of oestradiol valerate with oral norethisterone. The oestrogen dose does not change throughout the six-week period; during the first 2 weeks we administer 10 mg norethisterone per day, during the subsequent 4 weeks 15 mg per day and during the last 7th week only norethisterone, 20 mg per day.

During therapeutic pseudopregnancy the uterus becomes markedly enlarged, by approximately 1.5–2.0 cm; then regression occurs, a certain enlargement

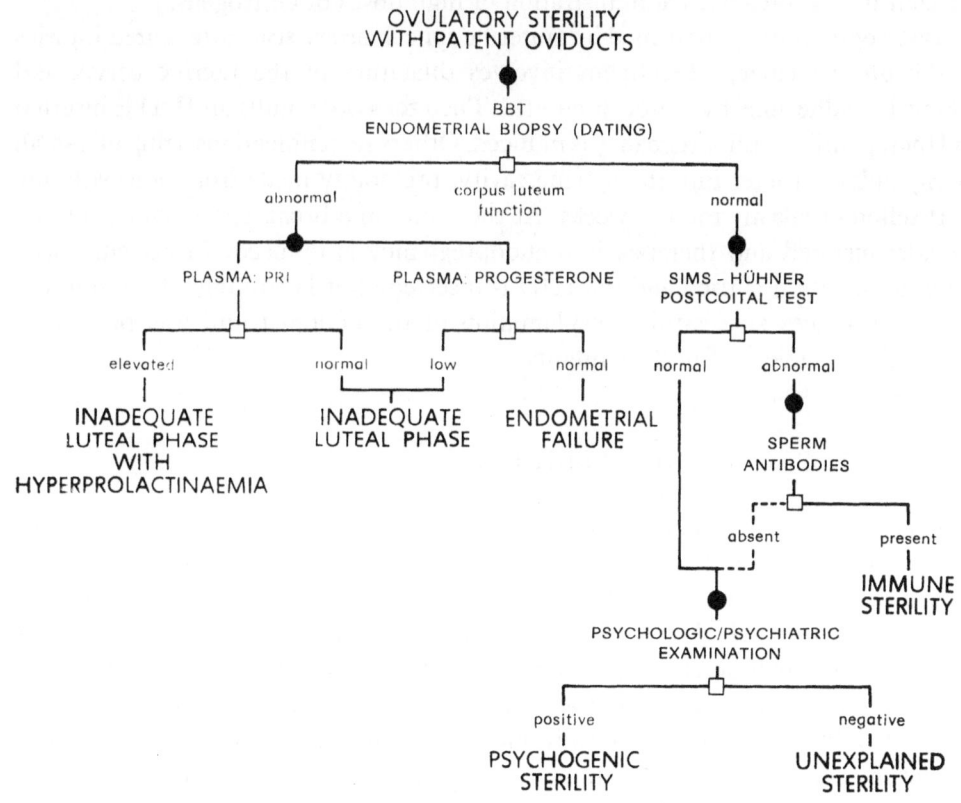

*Fig. 45.* A stepwise flow chart for the diagnostic approach to functional sterility with ovulation (● — decision nodes, ▢ — chance nodes).

(approximately by 1 cm) persists, however, even after 6 months. It is not clear what part this iatrogenic enlargement of the uterus plays in conception. Therapeutic pseudopregnancy, however, also plays a favourable role by its effect on anovulation, probably as a result of temporary block of ovulation, by the mechanism of the so-called *rebound effect* (*Rückpralleffekt, Desensibilisierungseffekt*). The incidence of ovulations after treatment is reported to be higher than before treatment.

We assume that **chronic endometritis** (see p. 302) and the **Fritsch-Asherman syndrome** (posttraumatic intrauterine synechiae or endometrial sclerosis) (see p. 299) should be included among less frequent causes of anatomic sterility; they interfere with the implantation of the blastocyst and the subsequent development of the ovum.

*Treatment* of confirmed chronic non-specific endometritis is very difficult, changes persist even after curettage. We recommend therefore the administration of broad-spectrum antibiotics before, during and after curettage, and to begin with the continuous long-term administration of high doses of oestrogens.

Hysterographically confirmed intrauterine synechiae are scars after cured injuries of the uterine cavity. Treatment involves dilatation of the uterine cervix and removal of adhesions by a tube or curette. Then for two months an IUD is inserted and therapeutic pseudopregnancy is induced. Others recommend inserting of a small (3 ml) Foley catheter into the uterine cavity, preferably made from non-irritating inert teflon or silastic for 1–2 weeks. At the same time broad-spectrum antibiotics are administered and therapeutic pseudopregnancy is induced. In extreme cases cervical dilatation is used and the IUD is inserted after laparotomic hysterotomy; in rare instances successful transplantation of the endometrium was performed followed by delivery of healthy infants.


## CERVICAL CAUSES OF STERILITY

The secretory activity of glands of the endocervical mucosa reaches its peak during the ovulation period. The amount and quality of cervical mucus which undergo typical changes in the course of the cycle (see p. 124) are most favourable during the period mentioned; they render possible the entry of sperm cells into the uterine cervix and its function as a receptacle where the sperm cells survive for a certain period. From there they can migrate into the internal genitalia, and thus increase the probability of meeting a fertilizable ovum during a relatively short period. The cyclic changes in the amount and properties of cervical mucus are so marked that they form the basis of a series of clinical tests of ovulation and for detection of the ovulation period (optimal period for conception) in women (for review see 45, 338).

The compatibility of sperm cells and cervical secretion is assessed by means of two basic tests, performed in different modifications:

A. Sims-Huhner postcoital test of sperm migration (*in vivo*)

B. Kurzrock-Miller test of sperm penetration (*in vitro*).

The **Sims-Huhner** test is unfortunately not standardized. It is performed during the ovulation period. The patient is recommended not to interrupt coitus immediately after ejaculation of the partner and to remain for some time on her back. The mucus from the lower part of the cervical canal is collected at different intervals after coitus. Comparison revealed that there is no substantial difference between tests performed after 5, 6–10 and 11–12 hours. After 24 hours, however, the sperm concentration in the cervical mucus declines. Collection as soon as possible after coitus is closest to the physiological conditions. When the test is negative or has failed, it is therefore recommended to repeat it after a shorter interval.

At the same time the amount of cervical mucus is evaluated, its macroscopic appearance, its "Spinnbarkeit" and pH. Part of the sample is used for microscopic examination for ferning (arborization) and cellularity.

Various arbitrary grades of possitivity of Sims-Huhner test are given. They agree that it is negative if not a single motile sperm cell is found, and that 20 and more motile sperm cells in one visual field at a $400 \times$ magnification means that it is clearly positive. The postcoital test within 12 hours after coitus is rated as "good" when more than 20 sperm cells/high power field are seen and when more than 50% of these show "purposeful" motility. At the other extreme, the test is qualified as "bad", when fewer than 5 sperm cells high power field are seen and when more than 50% of the sperm population do not move across the microscopic field. The intermediate range of test results is only of limited prognostic value (45).

Obviously, positive tests permit a delay in the examination of the partner's ejaculate when the husband refuses the examination. A negative or "bad" postcoital test implies that (a) the collection of cervical mucus was badly timed (outside the ovulation period), (b) the cervical mucus is abnormal from a quantitative or qualitative aspect, (c) the cervical mucus is incompatible (many immobilized sperm cells are seen in an otherwise normal mucus), or (d) sperm abnormality is involved. Differentiation is possible by examination of other parameters of cervical secretion, suitable timing of its collection and semen analysis.

In case of an inadequate amount of mucus, considerable viscosity and inadequate ferning (arborization) of cervical mucus, preovulatory oestrogen administration is recommended, however, to avoid block of preovulatory release of hypophyseal gonadotropins: ethinyloestradiol in daily doses of 0.01–0.04 mg or diethylstilboestrol 0.1–0.2 mg or mestranol 0.1 mg from the 9th to the 12th day or from the 5th to the 15th day of the cycle (in that case smaller doses).

The presence of leucocytes, more than 0–4 in the visual field during the ovulation period or a yellowish and turbid mucus, arouse suspicion of endocervitis and indicate a microbiological cultivation examination and appropriate therapy. Antibiotics are administered several days before and after ovulation or the mucosa of the endocervix is repeatedly treated with a 20% $ZnCl_2$ solution or it is destroyed by cryosurgery or "cold" electrocoagulation.

In incompatibility of cervical mucus an immunological examination is indicated. Where this examination is not possible, it is recommended, in order to differentiate whether the interfering factor is present in the cervical mucus or in the sperm, that a cross-match Kurzrock-Miller test of sperm penetration be performed *in vitro*. In case of confirmed or suspected immunological incompatibility, coitus condomatus is recommended for a period of two to six months in order to reduce the antibody concentration against sperm cells. In case of failure, high cervical artificial insemination with the first portion of the husband's ejaculate should be considered. Intrauterine artificial insemination involves a higher risk of allergic reactions due to sperm incompatibility (for review see 32).

Similarly, the **Kurzrock-Miller test** is not standardized. A drop of cervical mucus of the patient, collected during the ovulation period is applied to a slide at a distance of 2–3 mm from a drop of fresh ejaculate of the husband. By movement of the slide contact of the two drops is achieved and the borderline of contact is observed under the microscope. The sperm cells must overcome the barrier of surface tension between the two drops. A positive test implies a sperm concentration at the borderline between drops and finger-like phalanges of sperm penetrating the cervical mucus where they move.

In the cross-match test the cervical mucus of the patient and the ejaculate of a fertile man and conversely the ejaculate of the husband and cervical mucus of a fertile woman is used. The practical value of the cross-match Kurzrock-Miller test of sperm penetration is, however, reduced by organizational difficulties associated with obtaining suitable material.

## VAGINAL CAUSES OF STERILITY

During coitus the ejaculate is deposited in the posterior vault of the vagina. It is beyond doubt that the increased amount of vaginal secretion in colpitis dilutes the liquified ejaculate and reduces the sperm concentration. An adverse effect is also exerted by leucocytes which may phagocytize the sperm cells and interfere with their metabolism. The increased pH of the vaginal environment, observed in particular in trichomoniasis, but also in bacterial discharge, does not probably disturb the very rapid physiologic buffering effect of alkaline seminal plasma. (Conversely, the optimal medium in the uterine cervix and higher portions of the internal genitalia is alkaline, pH 7–9.5, promoting sperm motility and survival.)

Under normal conditions, at pH 4 the sperm cells do not survive in the vagina longer than 1–1.5 hours. The deterioration of conditions could be, analogously to cervical block, described as "vaginal block". Examination of the microbial pattern of the vagina in sterile women is equally indispensable as treatment focused on the normalization of the vaginal biocoenosis.

Sperm cells have an antigenic action (for review see 298, 329). The dominant antigen of the ejaculate is probably the component of seminal plasma which is absorbed on the surface of sperm cells (decapacitation factor), forming a "film" of sperm cells and probably protecting the sperm cells in the genital tract of the female. The term **capacitation of sperm cells** implies the change of sperm in the female genitalia which enables the sperm cells to penetrate into the ovum (for review see 201). This process comprises: (1) the gradual enzymatic removal or inactivation of the decapacitation factor; thus those components of the sperm cell membrane are exposed which react with the complementary receptive substances of the ovum; (2) in the activation of acrosomal enzymes; thus the sperm cells acquire the capacity to penetrate through the membranes of the ovum.

Carriers of antigenic activity include also sperm cells, in particular their acrosomes which cover the anterior portion of the head. Isoantigens act there as enzymes which render it possible for sperm cells to penetrate between cells of the cumulus oophorus and corona radiata (enzyme penetrating the corona and hyaluronidase) and through the zona pellucida (acrosomal proteinase, called also zonalysin or acrosin). The activation of the enzyme penetrating the corona and acrosin, i.e. splitting off the inhibitors of seminal plasma which bind with sperm cells during ejaculation, is ensured by a hitherto unidentified factor in the genital tract of the female. (Hyaluronidase seems to be present in the active form.) Oestrogens promote the capacitation of sperm cells. Progesterone inhibits it only in the uterus, however, not in the oviduct. Although there are some doubts, many authors are convinced that capacitation of sperm cells is also an essential prerequisite of fertilization in humans (for review see 201). Inhibition of capacitation is one of the promising trends of contraception.

Sperm cells apparently also carry antigens of blood groups. In this connection it is remarkable that in many instances of intractable sterility ABO incompatibility has been found. The prerequisite for the development of the disorder is a homozygous partner of blood group A or B and a woman with blood group O with a high titre of circulating antibodies in the cervical mucus.

Under normal conditions natural insemination does not immunize females, as the sperm cells do not penetrate into tissues of the genital tract but are phagocytized in the uterine cavity and removed within several hours from the uterus via the uterine cervix. At the same time enzymatic factors are involved which are able to break down seminal antigens before they can reach the system which forms antibodies. However, deep (subepithelial) penetration of sperm cells into the endometrium with intranuclear fragments of sperm cells has been found in decidual cells (so-called somatic fertilization) in the preimplantation area in rats. A similar possibility is also assumed in primates. Possible penetration of sperm cells into the epithelium of the ectopia of the uterine cervix is also taken into consideration. Deep penetration of sperm cells may lead to contact and sensitization of antigen--reactive T-lymphocytes. In this connection, the very frequent incidence (in more than 70% of all cases) of humoral antibodies in serum and antibodies fixed in tissue in the endocervical mucosa and in the endometrium, i.e. sites most exposed to antigenic stimulation, in prostitutes, is of interest. These muco-antibodies which are formed after local immunization, are probably of much greater clinical importance than humoral antibodies.

**Antispermatozoal immunity** may be manifested as follows (493):

(1) by the presence of humoral antibodies,
(2) by the presence of antibodies fixed in tissue,
(3) by enhanced phagocytosis of sperm cells by sensitized monocytes in the uterine cavity,
(4) by the reaction of delayed sensitization after contact of sperm cells with sensitized uterine tissue (the blastocyst is not implanted or is destroyed by a late allergic reaction),
(5) by intensive contraction of the uterus of the sensitized woman exposed to the action of the sensitizing antigen (Schultz-Dale reaction) which rejects the ejaculate.

At present we may use in clinical practice, e.g. the haemagglutination test [as antigen we use a pooled sample of a large number (several hundred) normospermal ejaculates] and the sperm-agglutination, sperm-immobilization or sperm-cervical mucus methods (as antigen the partner's sperm is used). The haemagglutination test can be only used for screening.

The incidence of humoral antibodies is relatively high in sterile women without a detectable anatomical or functional disorder; data vary between 20 and 50%. The results of the haemagglutination test, however, were consistent with the postcoital test of sperm cell migration in only 30% of these women. Lack of agreement included cases with a positive immunological test as well as cases with a negative postcoital test and vice versa.

Treatment of confirmed immunological incompatibility is again, as mentioned above, coitus condomatus. The purpose is to reduce the titre of antispermatozoidal antibodies. Treatment was successful even in cases where a drop of the concentration of circulating immobilization antibodies was not achieved; a reduction of its local formation is assumed (for review see 298). An alternative is artificial insemination (for review see 32).

# INFERTILITY

The term *infertility* comprises habitual abortion (i.e. three or more consecutive spontaneous abortions) as well as repeated premature deliveries, repeated prenatal or intranatal foetal deaths at term or deliveries of non-viable infants. In all instances pathological pregnancies are involved which are beyond the scope of the present monograph.

# Contraception

The main purpose of contraception is to prevent unwanted pregnancy and child-birth. It enables the woman herself and her family to decide on a suitable time of

*Table 25* Estimated number of couples using birth control, world--wide, by method, 1970 and 1977 (182)

|  | 1970 (millions) | 1977 (millions) |
|---|---|---|
| Voluntary sterilization | 20 | 80 |
| Oral contraceptives | 30 | 55 |
| Condom | 25 | 35 |
| IUD | 12 | 15 |
| Diaphragm, spermicides, rhythm, withdrawal, etc. | 60 | 65 |
| Total | 147 | 250 |
| Abortion (annual incidence) | 40 | 40 |

*Table 26* Contraceptive practice levels, 1976, world-wide (IPPF estimates, People 5, 3, 27, 1978)

|  | Practice % | Percentage of those practising | | |
|---|---|---|---|---|
|  |  | oral & IUDs | sterilization | other methods |
| Africa West | 2.9 | 87.5 | 0.1 | 12.4 |
| Africa East | 13.6 | 61.5 | 7.5 | 31.0 |
| Middle East & North Africa | 18.3 | 82.4 | 1.4 | 16.2 |
| Indian Ocean | 20.0 | 16.0 | 74.0 | 10.0 |
| E & SE Asia & Oceania | 20.9 | 75.1 | 8.1 | 16.8 |
| Latin America | 21.3 | 73.9 | 2.0 | 24.2 |
| Carribbean | 41.9 | 58.2 | 14.7 | 26.7 |
| West Pacific | 53.1 | 22.5 | 9.1 | 68.4 |
| Europe East | 56.0 |  |  |  |
| Europe West | 67.0 |  |  |  |
| North America | 80.0 |  |  |  |
| World (excl. China & USSR) | 34.0 | 38.0 | 19.0 | 43.0 |
| China | 37.0 |  |  |  |

Table 27 Contraceptive method (%) currently used by women aged 14–45 years in some developed countries (146a, 262, 294a)

| Country | Pill | IUD | Sterili-zation | Condom | Cap | Spermicide | Rhythm | With-drawal | Other | None | All using |
|---|---|---|---|---|---|---|---|---|---|---|---|
| England and Wales 1975 | 30 | 6 | 14 | 18 | 2 | 1 | 1 | 5 | | 24 | 76 |
| Denmark 1977/8 | 30 | 8 | | 37 | 5 | 6 | 1 | 1 | 4 | 8 | 92 |
| Sweden 1977 | 31 | 19 | 2 | 20 | | | | | 3 | 25 | 75 |
| Belgium 1975/6* | 32 | 3 | 6 | 7 | | | 16 | 33 | 1 | 13 | 87 |
| Italy 1976/7* | 22 | 3 | | 16 | 1 | 3 | 9 | 29 | | 30 | 70 |
| Poland 1972* | 2 | | | 10 | | 2 | 21 | 30 | | 43 | 57 |
| Finland 1975–8 | | 20 | | | | | | | | 29 | 71 |
| France 1978 | 28 | 9 | 4 | 5 | | | 6 | 17 | 2 | 25 | 75 |
| Hungary 1974 | | 2 | | | | | 6 → | | | 29 | 71 |
| Netherlands 1975 | 47 | 4 | 4 | 10 | → | | 6 → | | → | 40 | 60 |
| Japan 1977 | 2 | 7 | 2 | 47 | → | | 27 → | | 2 | 31 | 69 |
| United States 1976 | 23 | 6 | 20 | 7 | 3 | 3 | 3 | 2 | 2 | 31 | 69 |

Note: Some statistics indicate all women, some parents, some married resp. pregnant only; for Italy the age 18–64, for Poland 16–49 years are included; * the answer includes more than one method, therfore the sum is more than 100

pregnancy and the desirable number of children. It is the main constituent of family planning. The second, and in no way less important task of contraception, is in the population policy of countries. It is becoming a demographic factor which helps to resolve one of the most important world problems of recent times, the population explosion. Contraception is rapidly spreading in all parts of the world (Table 25). Contraception and population problems are the subject of many monographs to which we refer and we shall restrict our comments only to the contemporary state of female contraception (Table 26, 27).

There are several methods of female contraception.

They are of different reliability, their tolerance by the woman differs and so does their aptness for different conditions (Table 28). Therefore a greater choice of methods is needed, and the selection of the method is the result of the wishes of both partners and health demands. The reliability of contraceptive methods is evaluated in two ways. The pregnancy rate (Pearl's index) is the number of unwanted pregnancies per 100 woman years (100 $\times$ 12 months or cycles of use). Nowadays the method

*Table 28*  Reliability of contraceptive methods (pregnancy index)

|                          | Tietze 1962 | Borell 1966 | FDA 1969 | Tietze-Lewit 1968 | Kopera 1973 |
|--------------------------|-------------|-------------|----------|-------------------|-------------|
| No contraception         | 50          | 80–100      |          |                   | 61–117      |
| Irrigation               | 40.8        | 18–36       |          |                   | 21–41       |
| Ogino-Knaus              | 38.5        | 14–35       |          |                   | 0.3–47      |
| Spermicides              | 23.5        | 8–38        |          |                   | 8–43        |
| Coitus interruptus       | 16.8        | 3–38        |          |                   | 3–38        |
| Diaphragm                | 14.4        | 8–33        |          |                   | 2.4–25      |
| Condom                   | 13.8        | 11–28       |          |                   | 3–36        |
| Oral: combined           |             | 0–2.7       | 0.7      |                   | 0.003–0.1   |
|    sequential |         |             | 1.4      |                   | 0.4–1.4     |
|    minipills |          |             |          |                   | 0.4–4       |
| IUD:                     |             |             |          |                   |             |
|   Birnberg's bow (small) |   |             |          | 10.8              | 0.8–6       |
|   Lippes loop (large) |      |             |          | 2.6               |             |
| Surgical sterilization   |             |             |          |                   | 0.02–3      |

of cumulative data is being introduced (according to Tietze and Potter) which expresses data per 100 users during a certain period of time (see p. 355).

# BIOLOGICAL METHODS

The common principle of biological methods (periodic abstinence, postovulation infertile phase, calendar method, thermometer method, method of rhythms, natural family planning) implies that they permit intercourse only on infertile days after ovulation and after menstruation resp. The infertile period is assessed either by calculation based on the menstruation calendar or from basal temperature or other signs of accomplished ovulation. Assuming a stable ovulation time in the cycle — 14 ± 2days before the onset of the subsequent menstruation — and a three-day fertilizing capacity of sperm cells, Ogino defined the fertile period in a regular 28-day cycle as the 12th–19th day before the subsequent menstruation, i.e. the 10th–17th day of the cycle. In irregular cycles it is necessary to assess the shortest and longest cycles and to subtract from the shortest 18 and from the longest 11 days. Knaus assumed a shorter period of fertility (11th–15th day of the cycle), as he subtracted from the shortest cycle 17 days, from the longest one 13 days. At least 12 cycles had to be followed up, the calculation had to be done by a doctor and from practical evaluation all cycles were excluded which may have been influenced (closely after delivery, after an illness, operation etc.).

The postovulatory infertile phase is easier to assess by taking the basal temperature and unprotected intercourse is recommended after 2 days, and more recently after three days following its rise, or as late as on the 4th day after a rapid and on the 6th day after a slow rise. It is generally accepted that the preovulatory infertile phase is associated with a greater risk of failure. This was proved by a prospective investigation where during the preovulatory phase the pregnancy number was 19.3, while in the postovulatory phase it was 6.6. It seems that the unfavourable pregnancy number of the Ogino-Knaus method is due to permitting unprotected intercourse during the preovulatory phase.

Another way how the woman can assess her fertile and infertile days for periodic abstinence is the assessment of the peak symptom of cervical mucus described as Billings' ovulation method or natural family planning (42) (see p. 240). The last evidence that in 96.9% of 65 women, where by daily follow up of hormone levels the day of ovulation was assessed, the peak symptom was proved (209), makes it worthwhile to investigate the method further, although so far views based on the clinical application were controversial.

Contraception by periodic abstinence is a simple method which in more recent evaluations (for review see 439) achieves better results than formerly (0.3–47). Nevertheless, its criticism is focused quite rightly on the following points: (1)variability of the cycle and ovulation time, (2) inaccurate assessment of ovulation, (3) the fertilizing capacity of sperm cells lasting longer than three days, (4) hypermaturity of the ova leading to delayed ovulation and their fertilization with more frequent congenital malformations.

## MECHANICAL METHODS

Sometimes they are also called barrier methods. In women they include several types: cervical cap, Dumas vault cap, vimule cap and diaphragm. Sometimes the male condom is also included in this group. These methods alone would not be very reliable and therefore they are used in combination with a spermicide jelly or cream where half is spread on the inside and half on the outside of the cap. Selection and first insertion is made by a doctor, as it is important for the caps to fit closely the portio vaginalis or the vaginal vaults.

The *cervical cap* is made from rubber or plastic and after insertion adheres to the portio vaginalis uteri without reaching the vault. It is therefore suited only for portio vaginalis uteri which is sufficiently long and is not deformed.

The *Dumas vault cap* has thicker margins but a thin central portion and adheres by pressing the air into the vaults. It is suited for shorter types of the portio vaginalis uteri. The *vimule cap* is a combination of both previous ones, it has thin and widened margins and is suited for an amputated portio or women with decensus of the vagina.

Most widely used is a dish-shaped *diaphragm* with an elastic metal spiral. The latter maintains the diaphragm unfolded in a circle and fits between the posterior vaginal fornix and the symphysis pubis. All types of caps are manufactured in several sizes, the diaphragm with a diameter from 4.5–9.0 cm, cervical caps from 2.2–3.1 cm. It is important to give practical instructions to women on how to insert the diaphragm.

The mechanical method is suited mainly for women where there is a contra-indication of oral contraceptives or IUD. Its advantage is the simple manipulation when inserting it before intercourse. It is left *in situ* not more than 12 hours before intercourse and at least 6 hours afterwards. A complication is the frequent slipping during intercourse, when not properly inserted. The total effectiveness in women with good motivation (intelligence, will, living standard) are 2.6 pregnancies per 100 woman years, in the general population 17.9 with a mean of about 10 pregnancies per 100 woman years.

The *condom* is one of the barrier methods and is the oldest method of male contraception. It is estimated that 35 million families in the world use this method. In some countries it is the main regulator of family planning. It is most widely used in Japan where it accounts for 70% of all methods. In addition to modern oral contraception and IUD it has maintained its justification and its importance, which due to the original unreliability was pushed somewhat into the background, and is being re-evaluated again. The condom is becoming nowadays part of depopulation programmes in many developing countries. In India it is recommended under the name of Nirodh which means prevention in sanscrit. Its use increased between 1968–1973 four times. The advantages of the condom are its relative reliability, low price, no need for medical checking, no side-effects, postcoital control of effectiveness, simultaneous protection against venereal diseases. Condoms are manufactured from three types of material: mainly from latex (rubber), in small amounts from so-called skin (from the appendix of young lambs) and recently from plastic material (ethylene ethyl acrylate and polyurethane). A condom made from skin conducts heat better and is a luxury article; a plastic condom has advantages over a latex one regarding thinness (0.025 mm), heat conduction, smoothness, and unrestricted durability which is important in particular in tropic countries. The reliability of condoms has been improved due to electronic control of quality and elaboration of standard criteria, approved by the IPPF commission, which are used as national standards in many countries of the world. Sometimes all products are subjected to control examination. Failure of the method is reported currently as 0.8–1.6 pregnancies per 100 years exposure. The practical effectiveness formerly has been between 3–36 per 100 years exposure. The figures depended on motivation to such an extent that a British study of couples with several children where careful family planning was used had the lowest score (3.9), while older statistics from developing countries (India, Porto Rico) gave the highest figures (23–36). The results of a recently aimed investigation from 17 centres in England revealed again a high general effectiveness, 4.0 per 100 woman years (169). Among permanent users even the figure of 0.4 was achieved. It ensues from the fact that due to the present standard of condoms their effectiveness depends on the care of the user.

# WITHDRAWAL (COITUS INTERRUPTUS)

It is the oldest contraceptive method which has long been refuted but is still commonly used in practice. In some countries it is the most widely used method of contraception. In England it is used by 40% couples. In Hungary it accounted for 50–60% of all contraceptive methods and in Latin America it is also a common method of contraception. It is also very widely used in the Middle East in the muslim population. Frequently psychological and sexuological objections are raised against this method. Emotional disorders and fear lead according to some to male impotence and female frigidity, tension and neurotic conditions develop. Seen from more modern aspects it seems that these adverse effects were overestimated. It is rather the unreliability of the method which is a shortcoming, but in this respect too, data vary and depend on the experience of the couple. The pregnancy rate varies round 18, i.e. somewhat higher than for the condom. Nowadays it is recommended as a method for family planning, in particular in developing countries, where the goal is to implement rapid demographic changes by using the simplest means.

# CHEMICAL METHODS

Substances acting in the vagina are often described as *spermicides*. Contraceptives of this type are made of two components: an inert base which acts as a physical barrier for sperm cells and from an effective spermicide substance which immobilizes or kills the sperm cells. Their combined use with mechanical devices has been already mentioned, for separate application the following are available nowadays: jellies, creams and pastes, suppositories, foaming tablets and aerosol foams, and a soluble film.

Jellies and pastes have a water-soluble base such as gelatin and tragacanth gum which melt at body temperature and rapidly disperse the spermicides. 4–5 g are squeezed from the tube into the applicator. Creams have a water insoluble base such as stearates or glycerin, suppositories have as a base cocoa butter, stearin, soap, or glycerin. Foam tablets contain in the base polyethylene glycol, glycerin and foam-producing tartaric acid with sodium bicarbonate. In aerosol containers there is the same base but the foam is produced by carbon dioxide and freon under pressure. By means of an applicator they are introduced directly into the vagina. A soluble film has polyvinyl alcohol, glycerin, paper and carboxymethyl cellulose as its base. It is a square 4 × 4 cm which is folded and is inserted by hand into the vagina 30 minutes before intercourse.

The second component of all above forms of contraception is the active substance which may be of three types and is added either alone or in a mixture. Surface active substances, bactericide or strongly acid substances are used. The most frequently used surface active substances which inhibit oxygen consumption and fructolysis of sperm cells and destroy sperm cells by causing osmotic disbalances are: nonoxynol-9(nonyl-phenoxypolyethoxyethanol), *p*-diisobutylphenoxy-polyethoxyethanol, methoxypolyoxyethylene glycol-550-laurate and *p*-methanylphenylpolyoxyethylene-(8,8)-ether (TS-88). The most frequently used spermicides are: phenylmercuriacetate, oxychinoline sulphate, methylbenzethonium chloride. For acids, the following are effective: boric, tartaric, citric. Application of chemical substances is recommended 3–10 minutes before intercourse. The spermicide action persists for 10–60 minutes. IPPF elaborated uniform tests to check the total spermicide power.

The advantages of chemical methods are: simple application, no medical control, no systemic side-effects or contraindications. The disadvantages are the short spermicidal effect and the necessity of application shortly before intercourse, a smaller effectiveness and sometimes also unpleasant sensations when foam is formed. It is estimated that presently in the world chemical contraception is used regularly (data of IPPF) by some 10 million women. In different countries chemical methods account for 5–10% of all methods. In many countries a decline occurred after the introduction of oral contraceptives (Australia from 20% to 2–3%). In England about 1% of married women use the chemical method alone, about 5% in combination with a diaphragm or condom. Aerosols are very popular in the United States and are used nowadays by numbers equal to the IUD. The pregnancy number varies considerably in various surveys (35) from 2–40 per 100 women years. Here too a major part is played by motivation and care taken by the women, and not only the spermicide action. It seems that the lowest pregnancy rate (2–5) was recorded in those investigations with creams, foam tablets and aerosols which contained nonoxynol 9 and TS-88. Vaginal foams and creams belong thus among effective forms of contraception. Jellies and suppositories are less reliable. The soluble C-film can be evaluated only from sparse data which are controversial: one investigation from several centres reports a pregnancy rate of 5.3. The spermicide test in IPPF revealed, however, a pregnancy rate of 62. In future we must foresee the preparation of substances with a longer vaginal effectiveness, or possibly substances inhibiting acrosin, i.e. protease in sperm cells.

## INTRAUTERINE DEVICES

IUD (intrauterine devices) are nowadays one of the main methods of modern contraception. In 1976 they were used by 15 million women in the world, half of them in developed and half in developing countries. In at least 10 countries IUD are the main method of contraception. In South Korea and Taiwan they successfully helped to implement the depopulation programme. There are inert (non-medicated) types of IUD and biologically active (medicated) IUD.

# INERT IUD

Inert types have an infinite number of shapes. The most widespread and so to speak standard device is Lippes loop D (largest of four sizes). Others very widely used nowadays are Saf-T-Coil. Tatum's T, 7-shaped IUD, Yussei Ring, Spira Ring, Flower of Canton, Spring Coil, Ypsilon, Antigon-F, Ragab Ring, Dana Super Fix, Pharmatex, Om-ga, Beospir, Spiran W.

The great majority of IUD is made from polyethylene, alathon-20 polyethylene or ethylene vinyl acetate, always with addition of barium sulphate for X-ray control.

The **mechanism of action** of IUD despite extensive investigations is not quite clear (for review see 506). In women IUD interfere in some way with the implantation of the fertilized ovum in the endometrium. Currently it is assumed that this occurs by a non-specific inflammatory cellular reaction which takes place in the uterine cavity as the reponse to a foreign body. This is corroborated also by the finding of an immense number of macrophages in the uterine cavity after intercourse which phagocytize the intact sperm cells and are thus another defence reaction activated by the IUD. The hypothesis of the inflammatory reaction is opposed by the view that in the uterine fluid biochemical changes take place as a result of the IUD, and the idea is that these changes interfere with the blastocyst already before implantation. Moreover *in vivo* in women with IUD an increased uterine motility was proved which may make implantation difficult. The cause of increased uterine activity is, according to some – due to an increasing concentration of the prostaglandin level in the uterus, in particular as it proved possible by means of indomethacin, a prostaglandin inhibitor – to inhibit the motility as well as hypertrophy of the uterus which developed after IUD. Recently after IUD a rise of immunoglobulins G and M was recorded and an inflammatory response after IUD could prevent the nidation by suppressing immunological tolerance. Experimentally it has been possible by immunosuppresive drugs to suppress the antifertile action of IUD. From this it is concluded that the action of IUD is at least partly due to the capacity to produce antibodies. The question is still open of whether IUD suppresses the growth of the already implanted embryo, since some work using sensitive methods, detected in some cases, hCG or hCGβ in the second half of the cycle with IUD. Others, however, had negative results (449). It is possible that the action of IUD is combined and that several factors participate in it.

The clinical aspects of intrauterine contraception with inert IUD are sufficiently known (for review see 222, 400, 506) and therefore it is summarized only from the contemporary aspect.

**Indications and contraindications.** IUD are indicated: (1) in particular in women who have already accomplished their reproductive function and do not want merely to delay pregnancy, and (2) in women who for various reasons are unable to use other methods. Contraindications are: (1) acute and subacute inflammatory processes in the pelvis (a recent collaborative investigation using double blind tests revealed that no changes occurred when IUD was inserted after evacuation in an incomplete abortion when a certain danger of infection had to be assumed), (2) suspected pregnancy as in half the cases abortion occurs, (3) suspected carcinoma of the cervix and corpus uteri, (4) metrorrhagia, (5) malformation of the uterus and fibromyoma, since due to the irregulatory of the uterine cavity the protection is not sufficient, (6) severe dysmenorrhoea. IUD are considered unsuitable for nulliparae; in more recent models of copper-medicated devices this reason is eliminated.

**Insertion.** The most suitable time for insertion of an IUD is the end of menstruation when the cervix is still relaxed, but an IUD can be inserted on any day of the cycle. If this happens soon after childbirth, a large number of expulsions occurs. It is best to insert the IUD during the examination 6–8 weeks after delivery. According to the majority of authors an IUD can be inserted without an increased risk of expulsion or infection closely after induced abortion. A check-up examination should be made after 1, 3, 6 and 12 months and then after annual intervals.

**Side-effects and complications** are: (1) haemorrhage and pain, (2) pelvic inflammation, (3) perforation of the uterus, (4) a possible carcinogenic effect, and (5) effect on reproduction. Haemorrhage and pain may be transient after insertion. Syncopes, so-called cervical shock, are very rare (1:1,000). The first few menstruations after insertion may be associated with menorrhagia, frequently with pain, sometimes postmenstrual spotting. Usually the complaints disappear after several months. In rare instances the haemorrhage is more profuse, or occurs later as irregular metrorrhagia and the IUD must be removed. The mechanism of haemorrhage in conjunction with IUD is not clear and symptomatic treatment with ethamsylate and aminocaproic acid is not always satisfactory. The most serious complication after insertion of IUD are inflammations of the adnexa. This affects 2–3% of women, most frequently during the first months after insertion. It is assumed that this is a reactivation of a former chronic infection. It is, however, not clear how often a new infection is involved. As a rule the inflammation is mild and can be brought under control by antibiotics without removal of the IUD. If the antibiotics are not effective, the IUD must be removed. Unilateral tuboovarian abscesses and even fatal cases of septicaemia were described where an IUD was the probable cause. Perforation of the uterus and penetration of the IUD into the peritoneal cavity are rare and usually symptom-free. An incidence of 0–1.2% is reported in different investigations. It may occur during the insertion but also during the removal of IUD. Convincing evidence is lacking that IUD have a carcinogenic effect, no changes were detected in the exfoliative cytology. If pregnancy occurs despite the presence of an IUD, the incidence of spontaneous abortions increases (30–50%), and some pregnancies (5–10%) are ectopic. In term pregnancies, the incidence of malformations was not raised. Presently, there is, a tendency however, to remove IUD, if it has a tail, in case of pregnancy for fear of possible infection. After removal of IUD for a planned pregnancy the fertility did not deteriorate: 30% of the women become pregnant during the first month, 60% within three months, 90% within one year.

The evaluation of the effect of intrauterine contraception is made on the basis of several criteria of failure: (1) number of pregnancies, (2) number of expulsions, (3) number of necessary removals. Nowadays the effect of IUD is evaluated by the method of cumulative data elaborated by Tietze and Lewit (1973) (*life-table method*) which calculates the probability of each risk factor, for every month or year and gives cumulative data per 100 users for a given period. The sum of all risk factors then gives the cumulative termination rate of inserted IUD per 100 women for a given period. Also important is the continuation rate, the number who continue to use it (per 100 women) during a given period of time, i.e. 100 minus terminated cases. To eliminate the subjective factor, it is recommended that in comparative studies all insertions of IUD should be made in one centre, otherwise the data are very variable. The failure (pregnancy rate) of IUD varies between 0.1–5.6 per 100 women for the first year after insertion.

For Lippes loop the following cumulative figures are given: 1.5 per year, 3.0 per 5 years, 5.3 per 10 years.

The larger the surface of the IUD, the smaller the pregnancy rate, while the number of removals on account of haemorrhage and pain increases with the increasing surface. In older women the number of failures is smaller because their fertility is lower.

The *expulsion rate* varies from 0.7–19.3 for the first 100 insertions within one year of use. The expulsions decline with time and age. They occur most frequently during the first three months after insertion, in particular at the time of menstruation. For reinsertion, as a rule, a larger size of

IUD is used. About 20% expulsions remain unrecognized and about one third of pregnancies are accounted for by this fact.

The *necessity to remove* IUD on account of pain and haemorrhage or during infection is the greatest complication of this method. The removal rate varies between 3.6–34.8 per 100 users during the first year. The decision is made by the doctor, but subjective factors may play a part. In the majority of women the volume of menstrual blood is increased when they have an IUD.

The continuation rate of a method is the percentage of women who for a certain time use the same contraceptive method.

The average IUD continuation rates are 72% for one year, 58% at two years, and 42% at four years.

After evaluation of all criteria until recently Lippes loop was considered best. In 1974 the scientific committee at the 8th International Congress on Fertility and Sterility concluded that comparison of contemporary inert types of IUD did not reveal any significant differences.

## BIOLOGICALLY ACTIVE (MEDICATED) IUD

Biologically active (medicated) IUD are the result of further efforts to improve some less favourable indicators of effectiveness of inert IUD. They contain either trace elements or progesterone (for review see 400, 506).

## COPPER IUD

Intrauterine devices with copper were made after Zipper's finding in 1969 that copper wire wound on the device considerably increased the effectiveness of IUD. In 1975 there were already some promising one- and two-year investigations available. For the first test three conventional types of IUD were used: Tatum's T, 7 IUDs and Lippes loop (T-Cu 200, 7 Cu 200, Lippes Cu 200) where on the vertical branch of the polyethylene device two layers of copper wire 0.2 mm are wound covering an area of 200 mm sq. The former two types are currently permitted in many countries. Improvement of types takes place along two lines: the area of absorbable copper is increased and T-Cu 300 and T-Cu 380 are tested clinically, the second trend applies copper on their own types of IUD.

The mechanism of the contraceptive action of these devices involves, apart from the response to the device, the release of copper ions into the uterine cavity where these ions influence various biochemical reactions. Copper ions inhibit competitively the binding capacity of receptors for oestrogens and even more for progesterone and thus morphologically the progestational and oestrogenic action on the endometrium. Furthermore they act by competition with zinc in the important enzyme carbonic anhydrase, and thus interfere with implantation. They also influence, however, other enzyme systems, e.g. alkaline phosphatase and aryl amidase. Copper ions also interfere with cellular DNA in the endometrium and with the glycogen metabolism. It is also probable that copper toxicity influences the spermatozoa.

The effectiveness of copper IUD is at least that of inert (non-medicated) types.

The pregnancy rate varies between 0.6 and 3.0 per 100 women after one year. The expulsion rate is reported to be lower than in non-medicated IUD — 1.3–8.3 per 100 women after one year. The need of removal on account of haemorrhage and pain is markedly lower than in non-medicated IUD, the figure of 5.6–9.2 is reported. This better tolerance is, no doubt, an advantage and thus these IUD are also recommended nowadays for nulliparae. The number of women who continue to use them is also higher — 76–91 per 100 women after one year. All parameters improve slightly in IUD with a larger surface area of copper (T-Cu 300). One of the disadvantages of copper IUD is the need to exchange it after two years. By that time the copper has been absorbed to such an extent that the effectiveness of the IUD declines. The exchange involves problems, in particular in depopulation programmes in developing countries. Recently, therefore, the copper wire is replaced by a continuous layer of copper or several layers on the vertical and horizontal branch. Seven layers of copper in T-Cu 200 C will according to estimates extend the effectiveness of the device to more than 20 years. Less satisfactory results as compared with non-medicated IUD are reported when copper IUD are inserted after abortions.

## PROGESTERONE IUD

The second type of biologically active devices is based on the assumed local effect of progesterone on the endometrium, which is known from oral contraception. It has been assumed that much smaller doses without a general effect will suffice. The inhibitory effect of progesterone helped to reduce pain after insertion of the IUD. Usually Tatum's device was used which has a hollow space in the vertical branch containing progesterone: for a period of one year it releases 65 μg progesterone or 25 μg d-norgestrel per day and after one year the device is replaced. Clinical investigations confirmed that ovulation and menstruation are not affected and on the endometrium irregular changes (early decidual reaction, gland suppression) develop which prevent implantation. Subsequent analysis of gonadotropins and steroids revealed that no changes occur in hypothalamo-hypophyseal-ovarian relations (510). Clinical results report after one year a failure in 1 per 100 multiparous women and 1.4 per 100 nulliparous women.

Experience from subsequent years, and in particular parallel comparative studies of inert and medicated IUD, revealed, however, that the cumulative pregnancy rate did not differ significantly, contrary to initial data. The advantages of medicated IUD are smaller blood losses, for IUD with progesterone a better tolerance and thus also better continuation rate. Comparison of devices with copper and those with progesterone were very similar except for the period of effectiveness and blood losses. The pregnancy rates were 1.4 and 1.5 per 100 woman-years respectively; removal rates 2.8 and 3.0; expulsions 4.2 and 5.8; and continuation rates at 12 months 87.2% and 84.6% (401).

# HORMONAL METHODS

Depending on the route of administration we differentiate between oral, injection, subcutaneous implantation and intravaginal methods.

## ORAL CONTRACEPTION

Oral methods are mostly mono-phasic (classical, combined) or biphasic (sequential) and to a smaller extent there is luteal supplementation (so-called minipills), once-a-month methods or once-a-week methods. In 1956 clinical tests were started and in 1976 it was estimated that oral contraception is used by 55 million women in the world including 13–20 million in China. In at least five developed countries (Australia, Belgium, F.R.G., Holland and New Zealand) more than 25% of all women between the ages of 15 and 44 years used oral contraception in 1977 regularly (Table 29). Pills are currently the most effective method, although they are not the ideal or safest method. Their health hazards are, however, substantially smaller than the risks associated with pregnancy.

## SUBSTANCES USED FOR ORAL CONTRACEPTION

The oestrogenic constituent is formed by synthetic ethinyl oestradiol (EE) and 3-methyl ether ethinyl oestradiol or mestranol (MEE). The ratio of effectiveness in the test on the vaginal epithelium of the castrated female mouse is 2:1, and on the endometrium of women also 2:1; in the negative feedback, i.e. inhibitory effect the difference is slight in favour of EE. Their metabolism differs from natural oestrogens. The ethinyl group restricts usual transformations and mainly 2-hydroxy- to 2-methoxy-EE are formed and to a lesser extent $16\beta$-hydroxy-$6\alpha$--hydroxy-EE and traces of D-homoestradiol-$17\beta$. The majority is excreted in the urine and bile. For once-a-month oral administration quinoestrol is used. Recently the use of micronized oestradiol was introduced.

The progestogenic component is now formed by some 13 synthetic gestagens which are divided into three series: the norsteroid series, acetoxyprogesterone series and testosterone derivatives. These preparations include the following: norethisterone, norethisterone acetate, norethynodrel, lynestrenol, ethinodioldiacetate, d-norgestrel, quingestanol acetate, norgestrienon. Derivatives of acetoxy-progesterone are megestrol acetate, medroxyprogesterone acetate, chlormadinone

*Table 29*  Minimum percentage of women aged 15–44
supplied with oral contraceptives through commercial
channels in selected areas, 1970 and 1977 (432)

| Developed areas | 1970 | 1977 |
|---|---|---|
| Australia | 20.2 | 28.0 |
| Austria | 11.8 | 21.0 |
| Belgium | 12.1 | 28.7 |
| Canada | 23.9 | 18.7 |
| Denmark | 27.5 | 22.2 |
| Finland | 11.9 | 12.5 |
| France | 6.1 | 24.6 |
| Germany, Fed. Rep. | 18.9 | 26.8 |
| Greece | 0.9 | 1.6 |
| Ireland | 2.2 | 7.7 |
| Italy | 1.2 | 5.6 |
| Japan | 0.3 | 0.9 |
| Netherlands | 18.6 | 40.8 |
| New Zealand | 21.5 | 23.9 |
| Portugal | | 15.8 |
| South Africa | | 2.7 |
| Spain | 1.9 | 7.8 |
| United Kingdom | 9.9 | 20.3 |
| United States | 12.7 | 12.2 |
| Asia | | |
|   Indonesia | | 0.2 |
|   Iran | | 1.6 |
|   Pakistan | | 0.1 |
|   Philippines | 1.0 | 0.6 |
|   Saudi Arabia | | 1.9 |
|   Turkey | 1.0 | 3.7 |
| Latin America | | |
|   Argentina | 4.9 | 4.7 |
|   Brazil | 2.7 | 8.7 |
|   Colombia | 1.9 | 4.4 |
|   Ecuador | | 2.6 |
|   Mexico | 2.1 | 4.3 |
|   Peru | 1.0 | 2.7 |
|   Puerto Rico | 2.9 | 9.3 |
|   Venezuela | 2.0 | 5.6 |

acetate and 16-methylene chlormadinone acetate (chlorsuperlutin). A derivative of testosterone is dimethisterone (for systematic names of steroids see Fig. 15 and 16). The majority of these gestagens is prepared from diosgenin, a plant steroid obtained from the roots of the Mexican wild yam (*Dioscorea mexicana* and *D. composita*). Only d-norgestrel and norgestrienon are completely synthetic. The metabolism of norsteroids is not clear. Not more than 0.6% of norethisterone are aromatized to 17α-ethinyloestradiol. However, the alkyl group on $C_{17}$ remains, and therefore the metabolic change to 17-oxosteroids does not occur, nor does the metabolic change to pregnanediol or pregnanetriol. 40–70% of norsteroids are excreted in the urine as glucuronides and sulphates. Some norsteroids have also androgenic, others also oestrogenic activity. Synthetic substances of the acetoxy-progesterone series are not metabolized to pregnanediol, but they do not possess oestrogenic and androgenic effects.

## MECHANISM OF ACTION OF CONTRACEPTIVE STEROIDS

Steroids act in contraception by (1) impairing the feedback which controls hypothalamo–hypophyseal–ovarian relations and inhibits ovulation, (2) they induce changes in the reproductive system (cervical mucus, endometrium, myometrium, oviducts) which exert an adverse effect on the transport of the ovum, spermatozoa and implantation. The changes depend on the type of the method, the amount and type of substance. Oestrogens and gestagens act synergically.

Ovulation is inhibited in particular by oestrogens but also in larger amounts by gestagens. They inhibit the release of LH-RH in the hypothalamus and thus suppress LH, in particular, needed for ovulation. The classical oestroprogestational combination thus has a contraceptive action on ovulation as well as on the reproductive system which explains the smaller number of failures. Sequential preparations inhibit the gonadotropic function but do not act sufficiently on the cervical mucus and endometrium and therefore their effect is smaller. Small doses of gestagens alone inhibit ovulation only rarely, they have the smallest effectiveness. To ensure rapid elimination of steroids, constant intake is necessary; tablets therefore must not be skipped because after terminated oral contraception, ovulation occurs again after 3–4 weeks.

Changes of the cervical mucus, made use of in contraception, are caused in particular by gestagens. They cause the formation of highly viscous, sparse mucus which prevents the penetration of spermatozoa through the cervical canal. Both hormones act on the endometrium. Oestrogens cause proliferation, but alone they cannot maintain the rhythm of bleeding. Together with gestagens they ensure regular pseudomenstruation after discontinued therapy. Gestagens, in particular norsteroids, cause early or incomplete transformation, depending on the dose, and induce asynchronous changes on the endometrium in stroma and glands. The stroma is oedematous, displays pseudodecidual changes, and the glands are atrophic. This endometrium, which is beyond the phase, prevents implantation. The effect on the myometrium and tubes has been less explored. It is, however, assumed, that steroids interfere with the motility of smooth muscles, transport of spermatozoa, and the progress of the fertilized ovum into the uterus. Oestrogens as well as gestagens exert an adverse effect on the function of the corpus luteum and reduce the serum progesterone level. The influence on the enzymatic system of the ovary and on the reduction of the reactivity of the ovary to gonadotropins is also discussed.

## ADMINISTRATION

The daily doses of oestrogens and gestagens in contraceptive preparations have been gradually reduced. In EE the doses are mostly 0.05 mg, in mestranol from 0.05 mg to 0.08 mg, and in exceptional cases 0.1 mg. Recently EE doses were reduced in combined methods as much as to 0.03 mg or 0.02 mg respectively, while their full contraceptive effectiveness is preserved. Contemporary doses of gestagens vary between 0.15 and 2.5 mg, depending on the effectiveness of the preparation. Norethynodrel is used in a dose of 2.5 mg, norethisterone acetate 1.0–2.5 mg, ethynodioldiacetate 0.5–1.0 mg, dl-norgestrel 0.5 mg, d-norgestrel (levo-norgestrel) 0.15–0.25 mg, chlormadinone 2.0 mg, chlorsuperlutin 1 mg, dimethisterone 25 mg, ethynodiol diacetate 0.5–1 mg, lynestrenol 2.5 mg. In the course of time the gestagen doses have been reduced gradually to one quarter of the original amount. Some commercial preparations, however, still retain several types of dosage. Derivatives of acetoxyprogesterone are withdrawn from the market in some countries. Preferentially low-dose combined contraceptives with 0.03 mg ethinyl oestradiol and 0.15–0.25 mg levo-norgestrel are recommended which still block ovulation; we have to foresee, however, some bleeding irregularities in some women during initial cycles.

In the combined (classical, monophasic) method pills containing both substances are administered from the 5th to the 24th or 25th day respectively, and then again on the 5th day of the subsequent cycle. A variation of this method is supplementation by seven placebo tablets (21 and 7), and thus there is no need to count days. Another modification is to protract the dosage of active pills to 25 days and thus the cycle lasts 30 to 31 days, begins always on the same day of the month and there are only 12 cycles per year. The inert placebo tablets are sometimes supplemented with iron. Pseudomenstruation occurs, as a rule, 48 hours after termination of the active tablets. In this method omission of one pill does not influence the effectiveness as it is in the sequential method.

In sequential (two-phase) methods pills are also taken from the 5th to the 25th day of the cycle. They contain only oestrogen, however, during the first two weeks, and during the third week gestagen and oestrogen. This type (14 + 7) was gradually modified by increasing the number of days when both gestagen and oestrogen was administered (11 + 10 etc.). Sometimes oestrogen is already administered sooner, on the third day.

Sequential methods are no longer used in many countries because in unopposed action of oestrogens, there is an enhanced risk of carcinoma of the endometrium.

A transition to classical combined methods is the pattern where during the first 14 or 11 days oestrogen is administered with a lower dose of gestagen (e.g. one quarter) from the onset, and then the gestagen dose is increased. There are also three-phase methods.

The effectiveness of the two oral methods is high, although it is lower in the sequential method. The so-called theoretical effectiveness where the error of the woman is eliminated and only the failure of the method is considered, is expressed as pregnancy rate 0–0.1 per 100 women per year in the combined method, and 0.5 in the sequential method. The so-called total or practical effectiveness (use-effectiveness) best expresses the clinical effect and roughly 0.7 pregnancies per 100 women per year are reported for the combined method and 1.4 for the sequential method. Another criterion is the number of women proceeding with the method (continuation rate) per year. The reported rates of 65–80 per 100 women after one year are somewhat lower than for IUD users; the so-called pregnancy index (Pearl's) is the figure which gives the number of pregnancies per 100 women per year. So-called cumulative data are, however, more useful (see p. 355).

## SHORT-TERM SIDE-EFFECTS

Side-effects can be divided into two groups: **symptoms of pseudopregnancy** which imitate pregnancy or lactation and **symptoms related directly to the cycle.** The first group comprises nausea, vomiting, headache, enlargement and tension of the breasts, oedema and fluid retention in the body, increase of body weight. They are as a rule ascribed to oestrogen excess. Gestagen excess is reflected in the first group by an increasing appetite, fatigue, depressions and also a weight increment (108).

An effort to eliminate these side-effects by changing progestational potency of preparations is difficult and there are critical voices that it is not possible to obtain satisfactory clinical results (128). The frequency of different symptoms in this group varies between 3–16%. Comparison with placebo (173) revealed that in the first therapeutic cycle only nausea and vomiting, headache and nervousness differed significantly which was due to the high oestrogen doses (MEE 0.1 mg). All other symptoms after the usual doses (MEE 0.05 mg) as well as all symptoms in subsequent cycles were within the range of the placebo effect and after adaptation they disappeared as a rule. Therefore it is better to wait rather than change from one preparation to another. Tolerance of pills is improved when they are taken at night or after the evening meal.

The second group of symptoms is related to menstrual bleeding. Reduced blood losses during menstruation are the most frequent phenomenon in oral contraception and are encountered in 50–70% of women. In some women there may be slight breakthrough bleeding or spotting before all the pills are taken. In more serious cases, and if the disorder of the cycle does not improve after the first few months, we recommend first to increase the dose by half a tablet in the second phase of the cycle when spotting and breakthrough bleeding are imminent, and only when this fails to change to another preparation. In most instances, however, a formerly irregular cycle becomes regular because artificial pseudomenstruations are involved. Oral contraception exerts a favourable effect on two other diseases: premenstrual tension and endometriosis. According to different data 40–95% of these conditions improve after pills, and thus contraceptive patterns are, in these pathological conditions, therapeutic procedures at the same time. Blocking ovulation is also well known treatment of dysmenorrhoea.

# LONG-TERM SIDE-EFFECTS

More serious than short-term side-effects are those which develop after prolonged use of tablets (Fig. 46). Evidence on side-effects is extensive, but without comparative data on the incidence in the normal population which does not use the oral method, conclusions are difficult, if not impossible. Many controlled retrospective studies revealed a higher incidence of thromboembolic disease and high blood pressure, and a lower incidence of benign breast tumours and functional ovarian cysts. A higher incidence of carcinoma of the mammary gland and the uterine cervix has not been revealed. Recently three extensive prospective investigations were organized: in Great Britain the Royal College of General Practitioners Study — 23,000 women and the Oxford FPA Study — 17,000 women and in the USA the Walnut Creek Contraceptive Drug Study, California — 21,000 women. Control groups were formed by the same number of women. So far only preliminary results have been published (for review see 437, 524).

According to these investigations **thromboembolic disease** in women using

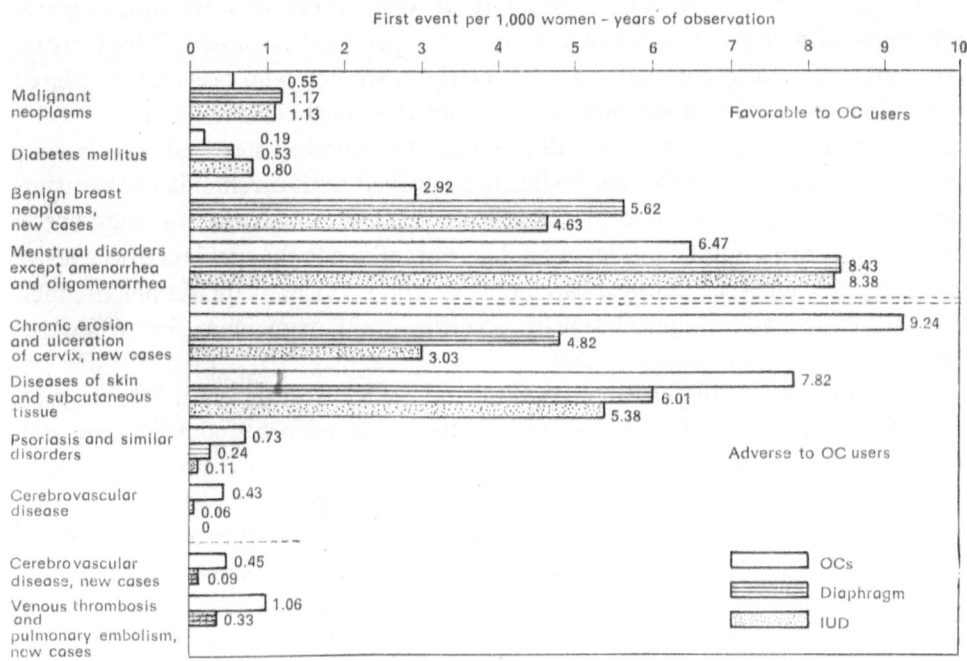

*Fig. 46.* Rates of various conditions in users of oral contraceptives (OCs), diaphragms and IUD in the Oxford/FPA Study (1968–1975). All conditions of OCs users differed significantly (p < 0.05) from rates for diaphragms or IUD; n: OC group = 31,076, diaphragm group = 14,739, IUD group = 10,014 women-years of observation (432).

oral contraception is 5–10 times more frequent. Less serious types (superficial thromboses) are more frequent than dangerous cerebral thromboses (the ratio is similar also for mortality figures). The risk depends on the oestrogen content of the pill, age and smoking. It is assumed that for disorders in blood coagulation oestrogen is responsible and not the gestagen. The dosage of oestrogen, 0.05 mg instead of the former 0.1 mg, reduced the incidence of thromboses by one quarter.

In women aged 35–44 years using oral contraceptives the mortality from circulatory disorders was 4–5 times higher than in controls. In smokers the mortality was 3 times higher than in controls. Therefore it has been recommended that women after the age of 30 using the oral method for 5 years who are smokers should consider abandoning either smoking or the oral method. Women after the age of 35 should consider an alternative method.

Evidence has also been provided of a slight increase in blood pressure. Former investigations recorded an average increase of the systolic pressure by 5–7 mmHg (0.6–0.9 kPa) and of the diastolic pressure by 1–3 mmHg (0.1–0.4 kPa). The results of aimed investigations revealed that the blood pressure of users probably rises one and a half times more often above 140/90 mmHg (18.7/12 kPa) than in women in the control group. In the course of three years there is a six times greater probability of a rise (0.9 as compared with 6.2 per 1,000 women). The increase is reversible after discontinued use. Conversely in women who previously suffered from hypertension the blood pressure declines after oral contraception.

Many investigations have been devoted to the **development of carcinoma** after contraception. No relationship has been proved with carcinoma of the mammary gland. Large prospective studies revealed that the incidence of benign breast tumours is reduced. Oral contraception does not influence the incidence of invasive carcinoma of the cervix, cervical carcinoma *in situ*, cervical dysplasia nor the incidence of abnormal cytological smears according to Papanicolau (for review see 124).

The position regarding carcinoma of the endometrium is different. The register of this disease in the USA revealed recently that of 26 women under 40 years with the diagnosis of carcinoma of the endometrium 17 used oral contraceptive pills, and of these 15 the sequential method. It is assumed that the risk is not due to the dose but to the pattern of oestrogen administration, the oestrogen being administered alone in the first half of the cycle without gestagen. Several new publications have drawn attention to the increased risk of the development of carcinoma of the endometrium in elderly women using oestrogens after the menopause (see p. 147). Epidemiological work revealed a steep rise of carcinoma of the endometrium during 1969–1974 in women above 50 years. The practical conclusions drawn from these findings in the USA are as follows: Mead-Johnson and Syntex Co. withdrew their sequential preparations and the Advisory Commission of the FDA recommends restrictions to be imposed on the sequential method of contraception (this applies to the original type of the first generation). However, the problem has not been yet closed and there is some criticism of statistical results (509).

**Metabolic changes** were observed during oral contraception in particular in the lipid and carbohydrate metabolism. They include hypertriglyceridaemia, hypersecretion of STH, hyperpyruvataemia, hyperphospholipidaemia, a rise of serum Fe, Zn, Cu, an increase of circulating macroglobulin, transferrin, albumin, IgG, cryofibrinogen, transcortin and free non-conjugated cortisol. The glucose tolerance is reduced. These diabetogenic changes resemble those during pregnancy. They are more frequent in predisposed women and after discontinuation of contraception they are reversible.

**Hepatic disorders** are another frequently reported side-effect. The bromsulphthalein clearance deteriorates in as many as 40%; frequently abnormal SGOT values are found. Since sex steroids reduce bile excretion from the gallbladder, cholelithiasis is twice as frequent $(1.6^0/_{00})$ and cholecystitis is also recorded more often. The changes increase with the period of use but are reversible after discontinuation.

In women using a strong preparation for a prolonged period, benign tumours, hepatocellular adenomas which involve the danger of rupture and malignancy, are more frequent.

As to other side-effects, about $50^0/_0$ more infections of the urinary pathways and some dermal changes (photosensitization $4 \times$, rosacea $3 \times$ more often, eczema and chloasma) are recorded.

**Foetal malformations.** Exposure to contraceptive steroids (in particular gestagens) during pregnancy may increase the incidence of some malformations (reduction of extremities, anomalies of the digestive and cardiovascular system). Norsteroids cause manifestations of masculinization more frequently, but only in doses of 10 mg, not the dosage used at present. An effect on the foetus from subsequent pregnancies which occurred after discontinuation of contraception has not been proved, although this problem has been investigated in many comparative studies.

The concomitant administration of some drugs may reduce the effectiveness of contraception (e.g. the antituberculotic antibiotic rifampicin or barbiturates).

**Amenorrhoea after contraception.** Many investigations were devoted to amenorrhoea and anovulatory cycles after discontinued contraception. They are sometimes described as hypersuppressive syndrome. The frequency of amenorrhoea after contraception differs between 1 to $10\%$ according to different authors. Comparison of the group of functional secondary amenorrhoea with post-contraceptive amenorrhoea did not reveal any differences in the basal gonadotropin levels nor in the response to LH-RH.

Nowadays doubts are increasing on the causal relationship between oral contraception and prolonged secondary amenorrhoea after its discontinuation (362). It is found that it is more frequent in women with a formerly irregular cycle and that it is possible to diagnose clear pathogenetic units of disorders of the cycle such as stress situations, drastic changes of body weight with anorexia etc. A milder form of hypersuppressive syndrome is sterility manifested by an anovulatory cycle or a short luteal phase. Work by Australian authors provides evidence of a rise of anovulations from 3 to $19\%$ after contraception was introduced, and a prospective comparative study revealed an incidence of $9\%$ in women using contraception as compared with $4\%$ in the control group. In disorders of the cycle with inadequate bleeding therefore oral contraception is not suitable. For the treatment of this complication clomiphene citrate is used.


## CONTRAINDICATIONS

The following are absolute contraindications for oral contraception: (1) carcinoma of the mammary gland and uterus, (2) pregnancy, (3) liver disease, (4) hyperlipid-aemia and previous gestational diabetes, (5) a past history of thromboembolic disease (phlebothrombosis, cerebral and coronary form). Relative contraindications are: depressions, migraine, uterine myoma, hypertension, epilepsy, disorders of the cycle due to hormone deficiency.


## RECENT METHODS OF ORAL CONTRACEPTION

### SMALL DOSES OF GESTAGENS (LUTEAL SUPPLEMENTATION, MINIPILLS)

In an effort to avoid systemic side-effects of oestrogens since 1960 the method of using permanently small doses of gestagens has been developed. The mechanism of this action is multiple: (1) a change of physical and chemical properties of the cervical mucus, with inhibited transport of spermatozoa, (2) slight disorders of the hypothalamo-hypophyseal-ovarian relations and suppression or change of the LH and FSH peak, (3) sometimes inhibited ovulation, in other instances only inter-ference with steroid synthesis in morphologically normal corpora lutea, (4) changes in the endometrium, (5) changes of tubar motility. The action is complex. None of these factors alone would suffice for adequate contraception. The following gestagens are used: chlormadinone acetate (0.5 mg), megestrol acetate (0.5 mg), d,l-norgestrel (0.075 and 0.05 mg), d-norgestrel (0.03 mg), norethisterone (0.35 mg), quingestanol acetate (0.3 mg) and lynestrenol (0.5 mg) per day. The practical effect-iveness in clinical investigations varied between 1.1 and 9 pregnancies per 100 women per year. Comparative studies of four gestagens gave the following results: megestrol acetate (0.7 mg) 13, norethisterone (0.3 mg) 2, chlormadinone acetate (0.5 mg) 4, d,l-norgestrel (0.075 mg) 2 per 100 women per year. The effectiveness is in all instances lower than in the two previous oral methods. A *disadvantage* is irregularity of the cycle, the length of which varies between 25–35 days in 70% of the cases. Sometimes the cycles last only 21 days and in some investigations as many as 60% of the women have breakthrough bleeding or spotting. This leads frequently to discontinuation of this method of contraception. It seems that there is a narrow limit of tolerance: reduction of the dose leads to more frequent failure, larger doses to a cumulation of disorders of the cycle. Although small gestagen doses do not produce systemic side-effects, they can be recommended only to those women where there is a contraindication for the combined method, to lactating women, elderly women or smokers.

## ONE-PILL-A-MONTH METHOD

Since one of the causes of failure in some women is the difficulty of taking the pills daily, so that sometimes they miss taking them, use has been made of the depot effect of quinoestrol and quingestanol acetate for a new pattern of administration, once a month only. After absorption both substances are deposited in adipose tissue. Quinoestrol is excreted from the depot as EE for a period of one month. Quingestanol acetate has a brief depot effect and thus withdrawal bleeding occurs only after $10 \pm 4$ days. Dosage pattern: 2 mg quinoestrol on the 1st or 2nd day of the cycle, after three weeks 2 mg quinoestrol, and 5 or 2.5 mg quingestanol; then the same dose $2 + 2.5$ mg is always repeated after four weeks, regardless of haemorrhage. The mechanism of action is block of ovulation similar to the combined methods. The endometrium during the interval between haemorrhage and taking of the pill is proliferative; after administration of the pill, it is secretory for a short time. In the ovary there are no corpora lutea and inhibition of late stages of follicular maturing is proved histochemically. The clinical effect is very satisfactory. The first month is, however, uncertain regarding its effect and the protection must be supplemented, e.g. by a mini-dose of 0.3 mg quingestanol. During the first months bleeding is protracted by one day, and spotting or breakthrough bleeding are frequent. Disorders of the cycle recede and the length of the cycle becomes normal. The effectiveness is expressed by a pregnancy number of 0–4, most frequently 1–2 per 100 women per year. *Side-effects* are, in the first cycles, in 12–29%, nausea, vomiting, fluor, headache; in the 5th cycle these complaints are recorded only in 0.4–6%.

## ORAL ONE-PILL-A-WEEK METHOD

Clinical tests are under way with the one-pill-a-week method where norgestrienone — 5 mg — is administered once a week. In half the cases the LH peak disappears as well as the postovulation rise of progesterone. The contraceptive mechanism depends thus not only on inhibition of ovulation but probably also on similar factors as in minipills. The endometrium is mostly proliferative. *Side-effects* are analogous to small gestagen doses: irregular bleeding, oligomenorrhoea. The theoretical effectiveness is 3.7, the practical effectiveness 8.7 per 100 women per year.

## ORAL POSTCOITAL METHOD (INTERCEPTION, MORNING-AFTER PILL)

First oestrogens were used, later also gestagens and other preparations.

**Oestrogens.** The daily dose of 50 mg diethylstilboestrol or 30 mg conjugated oestrogens or 5 mg EE for a period of 5 days has a reliable antifertile effect if administered, according to some authors, within 36, and according to others within 72 hours after unprotected intercourse. There are two mechanisms of action proved so far: (1) reduced function of the corpus luteum, apparent from reduced serum progesterone and urinary pregnanediol, and (2) arrest of the secretory development of the endometrium. The effectiveness of the method originally seemed very satisfactory; several extensive investigations revealed a 100% effect. The first authors who originally reported zero failures, however, report now after extending their experience a pregnancy number of 0.4. The Dutch series, which is the second largest, gives a pregnancy number of 0.15. Among other results the figure of 2.4 is the least favourable one. *Side-effects* associated with the use of these large doses are considerable: nausea in 36–50%, vomiting in 16–20%. Retarded or irregular menstruation is also frequent. This method will be suitable only in some exceptional cases (rape, failure of another method detected immediately such as of a condom, diaphragm or unobserved expulsion of IUD).

**Gestagens.** Contrary to considerable side-effects of major doses of oestrogens, gestagens are tolerated well. It has been revealed that the antifertility effect rises with the dose. First quingestanol acetate in a single dose of 0.8 mg was used and produced an almost 100% effect when taken within 24 hours after intercourse. It seems that here the same effect of a protractedly acting gestagen was involved as in minipills. Side-effects were changes in the cycle. More extensive experience in non-selected groups of women gave a less favourable number of effectiveness (20–23). Doses raised to 1.5–2.0 mg increased the effectiveness but disorders of the cycle were recorded in 25–30% of the cycles. An effective gestagen is also a single dose of d-norgestrel, 0.4 mg, if administered within 12 or preferably 3 hours after intercourse. Only this 13 times larger dose, as compared with the daily dose of minipills, has a complete antifertility action with a theoretical effectiveness of 1.7 and practical total effectiveness of 3.5. The main *side-effects* are shorter cycles (33%) and breakthrough bleeding. However only 5% of women abandoned the method because of these symptoms.

In a comparative study of doses of 0.6–1.0 d-norgestrel administered within three hours after coitus the pregnancy index improved from 2.1 to 0.7 and the use-effectiveness from 6.0 to 3.4. Tablets of d-norgestrel, 0.6 mg, are available as a commercial preparation and are recommended for women with infrequent intercourse.

As to other postcoital gestagens, a favourable effect has been recorded with nor-gestrienone, 0.5 mg, clogestone acetate, 1.0 mg and retroprogesterone 30–40 mg. Among non-steroid substances in India the antioestrogen centchromate is tested on a clinical scale.

**Combined oestrogens and gestagens.** Postcoital administration of a combination of oestrogens and gestagens also proved to have a satisfactory antifertile effect. Two tablets, each containing 0.05 mg EE and 0.5 d,l-norgestrel, and another two after 12 hours administered in the course of three days after coitus, in a Canadian survey of 189 women proved to be safe protection with a pregnancy number of 0. *Side-effects* such as nausea and vomiting were rare. Only 9.5% of the women had short bleeding ( < 5 days) (484). The method needs further clinical testing.


## ORAL POSTOVULATION METHOD

It is based on the principle of postovulation block of the corpus luteum activity. Experimentally this can be produced by gestagens, which reduce the progesterone and oestrogen serum level while hCG eliminates this action. Consistent with this, the clinical administration of norethisterone (10 or 25 mg per day) from the 15th–22nd day of the cycle failed; the pregnancy number was 29. Much better results were achieved with ethylnorgestrienone (R 2323). This substance blocks the action of progesterone on receptors and is thus an antigestagen. In clinical practice 50 mg by mouth administered for three days from the 14th to the 16th day of the cycle had an antifertility effect with a theoretical effectiveness of 4.4 and a total practical effectiveness of 9.6 per 100 women per year. The only *side-effect* is vomiting; disorders of the cycle are not encountered.

## CONTRACEPTION BY INJECTION

The principle of the combined oral method was also applied by using the parenteral route, administering depot gestagens and oestrogens. One i.m. injection of 150 mg 16α, 17α-dihydroxyprogesterone acetophenide and 10 mg oestradiol enanthate proved most suitable. This was the first once-a-month method by the i.m. route. As the depot effect persists for about three weeks, the injection is administered on the 8th day of the cycle. The mechanism of action is above all a block of ovulation, but it also affects the endometrium and cervical mucus, as in the combined method. The excellent effectiveness is apparent from the pregnancy number 0. The cycle is shortened in 13% of women, with usually protracted bleeding. The main *side-effects* are tension in the breasts in 46%, dysmenorrhoea in 62%, nausea 35% and irregular bleeding in 22%. Spontaneous menstruation after discontinuation occurs within 5–13 weeks.

Much more widespread is the once-in-three-months injection method using gestagens only. The dose is 150 mg medroxyprogesterone acetate (DMPA) by the i.m. route/90 days or 200 mg norethisterone enanthate by the i.m. route/84 days. There are also doses of 300 mg DMPA for six months. Combinations with depot oestrogens oestradiol cypionate and oestradiol undecylate were also tested. Administration is started between the 3rd and 5th day of the cycle. The mechanism of action is: inhibition of ovulation, increased viscosity of cervical mucus, effect on the transport of the ovum through the oviduct, an endometrium less suited for implantation. Both contraceptive substances are manufactured on a commercial scale (Depo Provera, Norigest) and they are highly effective: Depo Provera on average 0.31 (0–1.2), Norigest 0–5.2. In some countries, however, Depo Provera is not permitted for contraceptive use because in experiments with beagle dogs it causes tumours of the breasts. In women, however, such tumours were not found and the reported association with the development of cervical carcinoma *in situ* is not clear.

The main *disadvantage* is complete discoordination of the cycle. About one third of the women have no bleeding during the first few months, one third 1-7-day bleeding and one third prolonged irregular bleeding. Later almost three quarters of the women suffer from amenorrhoea and the remainder from irregular bleeding. Improvement occurs after oestrogen supplementation, either regular or as required. For a period of 7 to 10 days DES is added, 1 mg/day or EE 0.1 mg/day always from the first day of the month or — in developing countries — from full moon. Most of the women put on weight (0.7 to 5 kg). The other side-effects are similar to other oral methods. It seems that norethisterone enanthate has fewer side-effects and disorders of the cycle. The acceptability of the injection method is not very great, 40–60% abandon it during the first year. The second striking phenomenon is the long period needed after discontinuation to restore a regular cycle. Normal ovulation and regular menstruation is re-established on average after 5.7 months, fertility returns 13 months after the last injection. In women where oestrogen supplementation was used, regular menstruation occurs immediately after discontinuation in 71% and fertility returns on average after 9 months.

The advantages of the method can be characterized as follows: (1) the effectiveness is the same as in oral methods, (2) it does not depend on intercourse, (3) simple administration, (4) long-term effect — injections 2–4 times per year, (5) it does not suppress lactation — it is suitable for lactating women, and (6) suitable for older women. It cannot be recommended to young women, not even for a short period. Currently this method is used by about 1 million women and has become part of depopulation programmes.

## SUSTAINED RELEASE SYSTEM METHODS

Attempts to simplify contraceptive methods by the development of depot substances proceeded with the aim of ensuring for a prolonged period even release of the substance into the organism without an excessive effect at the beginning. With the assistance of extensive investigations of bioengineers synthetic substances were found which form a container for the steroid and are capable of releasing small amounts of the steroid into the organism for a period of one year, and perhaps longer, and are tolerated by the organism. It must be emphasized that in this way it is possible to produce the same peripheral effect by a many times smaller steroid dose. So far the most suitable substance is polydimethyl siloxan (Silastic 382). Since 1966 four different forms of administration, using this substance, are being developed: subcutaneous capsules, vaginal rings, intrauterine devices and microcapsules. As to other substances the following come into consideration — polylactic acid, hydrophil polyacrylamide gels and other substances. So far these methods are being developed or clinically tested. Only the intrauterine device with gestagen exists already as a commercial preparation (see p. 357).

Subcutaneous capsules, i.e. tubes about 1.5–2 cm long with a wall 0.4–0.6 mm thick are implanted under sterile conditions into the lateral side of the thigh, either one capsule or several capsules (4–6). Clinically about six gestagens are tested including megestrol acetate, chlormadinone acetate, norgestrienone, norethisterone acetate, norgestrel. Megestrol acetate — 25 mg and 50 mg — proved to have a low effectiveness: the pregnancy number was 8–37. However, as many as 3 and 4 implanted tablets (i.e. 1,000 mg) did not lead to any pregnancy, but the effect persisted only for six months. Increasing the thickness of the silastic tube to 0.6 mm and the use of 40 mg norethisterone acetate in one dose with a release of 128 µg/day gave excellent results during a period of one year. No pregnancy was recorded, none of the women abandoned the method and there were no side-effects.

80% of the women had ovulation and normal bleeding, the remainder mostly polyhypermenorrhoea. Six capsules with a total dose of 180 mg d-norgestrel maintained the level sufficiently high to block ovulation in the majority of cases on average for a period of one year. Bleeding was, however, unpredictable.

A polylactate film with d-norgestrel is another clinically tested system for implantation as well as for IUD. One dose should be sufficient for 2–3 years.

Vaginal rings are made from silastic and impregnated with some new gestagens. The most suitable diameter seems to be 60 mm and a thickness of 9 mm. They are inserted into the vagina as a diaphragm but on the fifth day of the cycle; they are removed after 21 days and after another three days pseudomenstruation occurs. A frequent *side-effect* is breakthrough bleeding and spotting, while the rings are in place. Bleeding was slightest after 100 mg medroxyprogesterone acetate in the ring (2%), in the others (norethisterone acetate, norgestrienone and d-norgesterel) it was recorded in 33% and thus was not suitable for a clinical contraceptive method. In the mechanism of action ovulation block was involved, as concluded from the absence of LH and progesterone peaks in serum. In an attempt to reduce the amount of breakthrough bleeding clinical trials were started with a combination of d-norgestrel (39–77 mg) and oestradiol (29–66 mg) with a mean daily release of 288 μg/day and 212 μg/day respectively. Reduction of breakthrough bleeding to 0.3% of medicated cycles seems very promising (335). An advantage of this method, as compared with oral contraception, would be: effectiveness for one year, no adverse metabolic effects, regular withdrawal bleeding without breakthrough bleeding. Now vaginal rings releasing levonorgestrel (20 μg/day) proved to be satisfactory and acceptable.

Microcapsules, i.e. small beads with a diameter of 5–1,400 μm contain a steroid emulsion coated with different material such as gelatin, polyethylene oxide, polyvinyl alcohol etc. They release steroids for prolonged periods. Clinical experience so far is lacking.


## STERILIZATION OF WOMEN AND MEN

Sterilization is presently the most widely used method of contraception in the world. It is used by 80 million couples. *Voluntary sterilization of women* during the last decade has become a widely used method of planned parenthood in many countries. In England it is practiced more frequently than vasectomy, the reverse applies in India. The rate of all sterilizations in women from 18 to 39 years is estimated as 10%. Mostly surgical sterilization is used. The approach is as follows: (1) by laparotomy, (2) by colpotomy, (3) by laparoscopy or (4) by culdoscopy. The **laparotomic route** uses many techniques. The Commission of IPPF experts recommends Pomeroy's or Uchid's technique of minilaparotomy where the failure rate is lowest and which permits in about 50% restitution, if required. The **colpotomic approach** is frequently preferred on account of the slight morbidity (1.6%). The **laparoscopic technique** of sterilization is increasing in popularity since the introduction of cold light, the operation proper is made by electrocoagulation or special tubal clips or bands. Major complications are recorded in 0.6%, failure in 0.1–0.2%. Possible complications are damage of the intestine and haemorrhage. **Culdoscopy sterilization** is usually performed by ligature according to Pomeroy or by means of a clip. Sterilization is frequently combined with delivery by Caesarean section or abortion. In surgical sterilization where Pomeroy's technique is used a failure is foreseen in about 0.3%, Madlener's technique being less reliable. The mortality associated with laparoscopic and other techniques is $0.1–0.3^0/_{00}$. Laparoscopic and vaginal sterilization simplified surgical procedures and reduced peritoneal irritation (for review see 182).

Further progress is expected from two procedures which are experimental so far: transuterine sterilization and chemosterilization. **Transuterine sterilization** where formerly blind cauterization of the orifice of the oviduct was used has been a success only in 50%. Today, using hysteroscopy, accurate cauterization of the orifice is possible without anaesthesia and without contact with the abdominal cavity. With respect to **chemosterilization,** two groups of substances are investigated: non-specific sclerotizing substances such as ethanol formalin, methyl-cyano acrylate and gelatin-resorcinol-formaldehyde, which create an occlusion in the intramural orifice of the oviduct by a scar. The second group of highly specific substances is represented by quinacrine. Quinacrine causes occlusion by its bond with epithelial DNA in the orifice of the oviduct only where no zinc is present, inhibiting its effect, as e.g. in the endometrium. In clinical studies occlusion was achieved so far in 90% of cases and this rate must be further improved (for review see 231).

*Vasectomy* is one of the simplest, cheapest and safest methods of birth control. It is easier and safer than sterilization in women. The most widely used technique is removal of part of the vas deferens, ligature and anastomosis of the ends. In other instances electrocoagulation of the vas deferens is recommended or two clips with or without resection. So far only on an experimental scale there are three other techniques which render easier reversibility of the obstruction possible, if needed. Into the lumen an intravasal nylon fibre (1–2 cm) is inserted, or reversible intravasal bodies are used made from propylene and finally a miniature T-shaped phaser was developed which is applied to both ends of the severed vas deferens and renders occlusion or patency possible, as desired. These techniques have not met expectations so far. Chemical substances for non-surgical sterilization are being developed. Among others, most frequently the sclerotizing action of ethanol is used. Complications after vasectomy are very rare (2–4%) and depend on the technique. They include: haematoma, infection, epididymitis, spermatic granuloma, recanalization.

Half to two-thirds of vasectomized men develop antibodies against spermatozoa but these do not influence the health status. Vasectomy is popular in particular in the USA and India and gradually it is being introduced elsewhere. The effectiveness is evaluated by the number of sperm cells 3 months after operation. Failure was recorded in less than 1%. The cause is usually spontaneous recanalization. It can be prevented by separating the ligatured ends of the fascia. The results of vasectomy improve gradually, and it holds its place also in depopulation programmes of some countries.

## IMMUNOLOGICAL METHODS

For a number of years immunological research has concentrated on methods on how to interfere by means of antibodies with different sections of the reproductive process, with the aim to elaborate an immunological method to suppress fertility (by contraception or interception). So far the results have not passed the stage of animal experiments. There are, however, further possibilities.

The first group is formed by **antihormonal substances.** Antisera were prepared against releasing hormones (anti LH-RH) which block ovulation in rabbits and rats. In sheep, active immunization against LH-RH prevents ovulation. Work is under way on specific antibodies against FSH and LH. However, many obstacles still remain to be overcome. Despite this, it proved possible to terminate pregnancy in the rat and in monkeys by antiserum against the β-sub-unit of sheep LH (348). Effective antisera were also prepared against 17β-oestradiol and by active immunization of sheep and cows ovulation was blocked (420). In immature rats ovulation can also be inhibited by anti-progesterone antiserum (341).

The formation of antibodies against hCG has advanced furthest. Antibodies against the whole molecule had a crossed reactivity with LH, and the antibodies against the β-sub-units were not sufficiently specific either. A group of workers headed by Talwar in India therefore prepared a vaccine against pregnancy by eliminating the non-specificity (crossed reactivity) by purifying the β-sub-unit of hCG by means of immunoabsorption and increased the antigenicity by covalent conjugation of the β-sub-unit with tetanic toxoid (processed β-hCG-TT). Thirty-three thus immunized women are being followed up for three years so far, their clinical finding is quite normal, and the same applies to laboratory findings and the ovulatory cycle. More extensive clinical trials, in the second stage in 57 women, are under way (503). Furthermore Stevens was able to make use of the difference between the β-sub-unit of hCG and hLH, which is in 30 amino acids at the carboxyl end, and by means of synthetic peptides with the same end structure, conjugated to a protein carrier specific antibodies against hCG were formed. Thus immunized monkeys had a reduced fertility and after administration of specific antisera, pregnant animals aborted (496).

The second group is formed by **antispermatic substances** in women. Circulating antibodies against human spermatozoa are investigated (229). A new antigen was detected which immobilizes human sperm cells in human seminal plasma and milk. In human cervical mucus in sterile women antibody activity against spermatozoa was detected (481). In a group of volunteers by immunization with testicular homogenate, the formation of antibodies against spermatozoa was stimulated in men and by immunization with human sperm cells antibodies in women. In healthy women these procedures were not used.

The third group is formed by **antiembryonic substances.** The immunology of the placenta and embryo is being studied. In rats pregnancy can be interrupted by passive immunization with serum against the mouse placenta. In rabbits pregnancy is interrupted by anti-HPL serum. After active immunization with HPL in rabbits death of the foetuses or their reabsorption is observed. It has been found that the enzyme neuraminidase in some way influences the immunity system and causes rapid abortion in rats.

Many factors are known by now but so far we cannot foresee a practicable immunological method of contraception in the near future. Talwar's vaccine is closest to it.

# PROSTAGLANDINS IN CONTRACEPTION AND INTERCEPTION

As has been already mentioned (see p. 118), prostaglandins act at many sites of the reproductive process. Investigations concerned with their possible use in contraception have been focused on four areas: the effect on the hypothalamus and pituitary, the effect on the mechanism of ovulation in the ovary, the luteolytic effect, and the effect on the smooth muscles of the uterus.

(1) $PGE_2$ causes the release of LH *in vitro* and *in vivo*. $PGF_{2a}$ stimulates the release of LH *in vivo*. Inhibitors of prostaglandin synthesis – indomethacin and aspirin – block ovulation at a central level according to some experimental work, and according to other work directly at the level of the ovary. According to the former groups of investigations prostaglandins are possible mediators of oestrogen action for the release of LH.

(2) Some work with inhibitors provides evidence that ovarian prostaglandins are essential for rupture of the follicle but not for maturation or luteinization of granulosa cells. Administered prostaglandins imitate some effects of LH including stimulation of cAMP, but act as mediators of the LH effect only as regards rupture of the follicle. It is probably a direct effect on smooth muscle fibres which ensures the contractility of the ovary.

Thus for contraception in humans the use of indomethacin is promising, as the results in subhuman primates where ovulation was induced by means of HMG and hCG revealed that doses of 10 mg/kg/day for a period of 8 days blocked ovulation in 8 out of a total of 9 cycles. Since only rupture of the follicle did not occur, while the plasma levels of progesterone and oestradiol corresponded to a normal cycle and either a luteinized mature follicle or a corpus luteum was present, it may be assumed that local action of prostaglandins on the ovaries was involved. A method practicable in women has not been elaborated so far. The required doses calculated for humans would be too high with preparations available so far.

(3) The luteolytic action of prostaglandins is obvious in many animal species. It is even possible to synchronize by means of prostaglandins rut in animal breeding practice. In humans, however, luteolysis cannot be induced by prostaglandins available so far.

(4) The other trend which suggests a practicable method in women is the action of prostaglandins on the uterine musculature at the onset of pregnancy. It is a post-conception effect, i.e. interception. The original method of Czapo, using intra-uterine instillation of $PGF_{2a}$, attained satisfactory results (90%) but it was necessary to administer sedatives and the method was not suitable for clinical practice. Another investigation, however, was successful only in 65%. Using vaginal administration the results were not uniform and specific. The effect was manifested not only on the uterine muscles but also on those of the gastrointestinal tract. Only the vaginal use of new analogues, i.e. 15(S)15-methyl $PGF_{2a}$, methylester 16,16--dimethyl $PGE_2$ or 16,16-dimethyl-trans $\Delta^2$-$PGE_1$ methylester gave the first results which could be applied clinically. In out-patients total doses of 2.5–5.0 mg of the first substance were used in suppositories à 0.5 or 1.0 mg after three hours. Three to six hours after the onset of treatment haemorrhage began in all women corresponding as to its volume to menstrual bleeding or sometimes the haemo-rrhage was more abundant. The women had missed menstruation for 3 to 14 days and by means of the RIA method for hCG in all pregnancy had been diagnosed. The procedure was successful in all instances, in other series in 93% of cases. Side-effects were minimal. It seems that this will be a suitable post-conception method with simple ambulatory administration of vaginal suppositories by the woman herself (197). Other forms used are: single insertion of 3 mg substance in a long-acting base in suppository or 5 mg in a silastic device.

# CONTRACEPTION IN ADOLESCENTS

Contraception in adolescent girls and young women under 20 years is a separate problem of increasing importance. We are witnessing the fact that the frequency of premarital sexual relations and the number of pregnancies in teenagers is rising. This trend seems permanent because:

(1) The period of sexual maturity between menarche and marriage is increasing due to the known declining trend of the age of menarche.

(2) The socioeconomic conditions for entering marriage decline only little as regards age and in some countries marriage shifts even to an older age.

(3) Urbanization and the living pattern in developed countries give greater opportunities for sexual relations to young people under 20 years. Demographic data from all parts of the world indicate in the years from 1963–1972 a higher percentage of childbirths in young women under 20 years.

However, pregnancy at too early a stage of the reproductive period involves health risks as well as social risks. During this period the maternal mortality is inversely proportional to the woman's age, obstetric and gestational complications are more frequent. Social risks include discontinuation or late termination of training, premature marriage, problems of unmarried mothers, etc. Legalized abortions are not the best solution, in particular as regards possible adverse effects on future fertility. Thus sex education and correct contraception are of major importance.

The selection of the method is not unequivocal and it is important to keep in mind the specific conditions of young people: frequently unplanned intercourse, small frequency or irregular character of intercourse, the narrow cervix of the nullipara and the preservation of future fertility.

*Periodic abstinence* is often applied, it is simple but assumes a regular cycle and proper motivation (careful acquisition of knowledge of the method and its practising). Otherwise the method is not sufficiently reliable.

*Condoms* are also a widely used method, suitable in particular for irregular and infrequent intercourse. Its safety is enhanced by combinations with infertile days or the use of spermicide substances.

*Oral contraception* is the most reliable method. Among different forms minipills containing gestagens only can be recommended most. The combined oral method assumes a regular and stabilized menstrual cycle, since in disorders of the cycle after discontinuation, there is a greater risk of the development of amenorrhoea. The oral method is not suitable when intercourse is rare or irregular. With minipills sometimes gastrointestinal disorders must be foreseen, obesity or irregularities of the cycle, factors which for many women make this form of contraception unacceptable.

*Intrauterine devices* of the inert types are reserved for older women and are less suitable for nulliparae, in particular because they are more difficult to insert, there are more frequent expulsions and possible inflammatory complications. Only medicated IUDs such as T-Cu 200 seem suitable also for young women as they are reliable and the expulsion rate is low.

The *diaphragm with spermicide substances* is also a suitable method for young women. It requires, however, training to ensure proper insertion and a certain preparation and planning before intercourse, which makes it unacceptable for some women.

*Postcoital interception* is not suited for regular contraception. It can be used only in exceptional cases e.g. after rape, etc.

*Withdrawal* is not suited for sexually inexperienced couples and is not reliable.

In the conclusion of the chapter on contraception, it must be mentioned that so far none of the discussed methods meets all criteria expected from an ideal method. Such a method should be: effective, harmless, acceptable, simple, fully reversible and cheap. The most effective method today is, no doubt, the oral method with reduced steroid doses, its harmlessness is, however, only relative. Its risks can be considered minimal in relation to the risks of pregnancy or risks ensuing from modern life (e.g. motor car crashes). We cannot omit, however, the known sequelae of many years use of steroids. A final answer will probably be provided by extensive prospective studies extending over many years which have been conducted in some countries and which are still under way. Emphasis on the risk in particular in older women in recent years led to a slight decline of oral contraception in favour of sterilization which has become the most widely used method in the world, suited in particular for couples with fulfilled desire of parenthood. Least harmless are combinations of several methods which alone are not quite effective, such as a combination of periodic abstinence with a condom or diaphragm and spermicide substances. Then they match, as to their reliability, oral methods, the disadvantage is, however, the complexity and low acceptability. The simplest method is insertion of an intrauterine device, the disadvantage is, however, the lower reliability and the possible complications for a subsequent wanted pregnancy.

Therefore further development of contraceptive methods is proceeding intensely to improve old methods (biologically active IUD, prolonged release from subcutaneous or vaginal depots), and new ways are being sought. Possible approaches are inhibitors acting at different sites of the reproductive process such as competitive inhibitors of LH-RH, antibodies against gonadotropin sub-units, anti-embryonic substances and prostaglandins.

# References

1. *Abraham, G. E.:* Ovarian and adrenal contribution to peripheral androgens during the menstrual cycle. J. clin. Endocr., *39*, 340–346, 1974.
2. *Abraham, G. E., Maroulis, G. B., Marshall, J. R.:* Evaluation of ovulation and corpus luteum function using measurements of plasma progesterone. Obstet. and Gynec., *44*, 522–525, 1974.
3. *Abramson, D., Driscoll, S. G.:* Endometrial aspiration biopsy. Obstet. and Gynec., *27*, 381–391, 1966.
4. *Adamopoulos, D. A.:* Endocrinological studies in women approaching the menopause. J. Obstet. Gynaec. Brit. Cwlth., *78*, 62–79, 1971.
5. *Adler, R. A.:* The evaluation of galactorrhoea. Amer. J. Obstet. Gynec., *127*, 569–571 1977.
6. *Advis, J. P., Hall, T. R., Hodson, C. A., Mueller, G. P., Meites, J.:* Temporal relationship and role of dopamine in short-loop feedback of prolactin. Proc. Soc. exp. Biol. (N.Y.), *155*, 567–570, 1977.
7. *Aksel, S., Jones, G. S.:* Etiology and treatment of dysfunctional uterine bleeding. Obstet. and Gynec., *44*, 1–13, 1974.
8. *Aksel, S., Tyrey, L.:* Luteinizing hormone – releasing hormone in the human fetal brain. Fertil. and Steril., *28*, 1067–1071, 1977.
9. *Aksel, S., Schomberg, D. W., Hammond, C. B.:* Prostaglandin F$_2$α production by the human ovary. Obstet. and Gynec., *50*, 347–350, 1977.
9a. *Apter, D., Vihko, R.:* Serum pregnenolone, progesterone, 17-hydroxyprogesterone, testosterone and 5α-dihydrotestosterone during female puberty. J. clin. Endocr. *45*, 1039–1048, 1977.
10. *Arronet, G. H., Arrata, W. S. M.:* Dysfunctional uterine bleeding. A classification. Obstet. and Gynec., *29*, 97–107, 1967.
11. *Aschheim, P.:* Function of the aging ovary: Comparative aspects. Europ. J. Obstet. Gynec. reprod. Biol., *9*, 191–202, 1979.
12. *Aschoff, J.:* Circadiane Rhythmen im endokrinen System. Klin. Wschɪ., *56*, 425–435, 1978.
13. *Askalani, H., Wilkin, P., Schwers, J.:* Serum progesterone in non pregnant women. II. Correlation between serum progesterone and some other luteinization parameters. Amer. J. Obstet. Gynec., *118*, 1064–1068, 1974.
14. *Auletta, F. J., Agins, H., Scommegna, A.:* Prostaglandin F mediation of the inhibitory effect of oestrogen on the corpus luteum of the Rhesus monkey. Endocrinology, *103*, 1183–1189, 1978.
15. *Axelrod, J.:* Relationship between catecholamines and other hormones. Recent Progr. Hormone Res., *31*, 1–35, 1975.

16.  *Backman, G.:* Die beschleunigte Entwicklung der Jugend. Acta anat. (Basel), *4*, 421–480, 1948.

17.  *Bäckström, T.:* Oestrogen and progesterone in relation to different activities in the central nervous system. Acta obstet. gynec. scand., *56*, Suppl. 66, 1–17, 1977.

18.  *Bahner, F., Schwarz, G., Hienz, H. A., Walter, K.:* Turner-Syndrom mit voll ausgebildeten sekundären Geschlechtsmerkmalen und Fertilität. Acta endocr. (Kbh.), *35*, 397–404, 1960.

19.  *Bahr, J., Kao, L., Nalbandov, A. V.:* The role of catecholamines and nerves in ovulation. Biol. Reprod., *10*, 273–299, 1974.

20.  *Bailey, K. V.:* Ovarian changes concerned with gonadotrophic dysfunction and associated with amenorrhoea and infertility. J. Obstet. Gynaec. Brit. Emp., *66*, 556–565, 1959.

21.  *Baird, D. T., Horton, R., Longcope, C., Tait, J. F.:* Steroid dynamics under steady-state conditions. Recent Progr. Hormone Res., *25*, 611–664, 1969.

22.  *Baird, D. T., Burger, P. E., Heavon-Jones, G. D., Scaramuzzi, R. J.:* The site of secretion of androstenedione in nonpregnant women. J. Endocr., *63*, 201–212, 1974.

23.  *Baker, T. B.:* Gametogenesis. Acta endocr. (Kbh.), Suppl. 166, 18–47, 1972.

24.  *Banks, J. A., Freeman, M. E.:* The temporal requirement of progesterone on proestrus for extinction of the oestrogen-induced daily signal controlling luteinizing hormone release in the rat. Endocrinology, *102*, 426–432, 1978.

25.  *Barraclough, C. A., Yrarrazaval, S., Hatton, R.:* A possible hypothalamic site of progesterone in the facilitation of ovulation in the rat. Endocrinology, *75*, 838–845, 1964.

26.  *Barraclough, C. A., Wise, P. M., Turgeon, J., Shander, D., Depaulo, L., Rance, N.:* Recent studies on the regulation of pituitary LH and FSH secretion. Biol. Reprod., 20, 86–97, 1979.

27.  *Barrett, S. A., Brown, J. B.:* An evaluation of the method of Cox for the rapid analysis of pregnanediol in urine by gas-liquid chromatography. J. Endocr., *47*, 471–480, 1970.

28.  *Barry, J.:* Immunofluorescence study of LRF neurons in man. Cell Tiss. Res., *181*, 1–14, 1977.

29.  *Bass, F.:* L'amenorrhée au camp de concentration de Terezin (Theresienstadt). Gynaecologia (Basel), *123*, 211–219, 1947.

30.  *Baulieu, E. E., Robel, P.:* Catabolism of testosterone and androstenedione. In: The androgens of the testis. Eik-Nes, K.B. (ed.). New York, M. Dekker Inc., 1970, p. 49–71.

31.  *Beardwood, C. J., Russell, G. F. M.:* Gonadotrophin excretion at puberty. J. Endocr., *48*, 469–470, 1970.

32.  *Behrman, S. J.:* Artificial insemination. Clin. Obstet. Gynec., *22*, 245–253, 1979.

33.  *Behrman, S. J., Kistner, R. W.:* A rational approach to the evaluation of infertility. In: Progress in infertility. Behrman, S. J., Kistner, R. W. (eds). Boston, Little, Brown, 1968, p. 1–18.

34.  *Bell, J., Benveniste, R., Spitz, I., Rabinowitz, D.:* Isolated deficiency of FSH: Further studies. J. clin. Endocr., *40*, 790–794, 1975.

35.  *Belsky, R.:* Vaginal contraceptives. A time for reappraisal? Popul. Rep., Ser. H, 37–56, 1975.

36.  *Benker, G., Windeck, R., Hackenberg, K., Reinwein, D.:* Heterogenität von Peptid- und Proteohormonen. Dtsch. med. Wschr., *102*, 970–976, 1977.

37.  *Berger, M. J., Taymor, M. L., Patton, W. C.:* Gonadotropin levels and secretory patterns in patients with typical and atypical polycystic ovarian disease. Fertil. and Steril., *26*, 619–626, 1975.

38.  *Bergman, P.:* Sexual cycle, time of ovulation and time of optimal fertility in women. Acta obstet. gynec. scand., *29*, Suppl. 4: 1–139, 1950.

39. *Bergman, P.:* Menarche or spontaneous remission of primary amenorrhoea at 38 years of age. Obstet. and Gynec., *19*, 108–110, 1962.
40. *Bergqvist, N.:* The gonadal function in female diabetics. Acta endocr. (Kbh.), *15*, Suppl. 19: 3–20, 1954.
41. *Bidlingmaier, F., Wagner-Barnack, M., Butenandt, O., Knorr, D.:* Plasma oestrogens in childhood and puberty under physiologic and pathologic conditions. Pediat. Res., *7*, 901–907, 1973.
42. *Billings, E. L., Billings, J. J., Brown, J. B., Burger, H. G.:* Symptoms and hormonal changes accompanying ovulation. Lancet, *1*, 282–289, 1972.
43. *Björntorp, P.:* Fettsucht. Ingelheim/Rhein, Boehringer, 1972.
44. *Blanco, R.:* Human ovarian transplantation. In: Recent Progress in Obstetrics and Gynecology. Eds.: Persianinov, L. S., Chervakova, T. V., Presl, J. Amsterdam/Prague, Excerpta Medica/Avicenum, 1974, p. 583.
45. *Blasco, L.:* Clinical approach to the evaluation of sperm-cervical mucus interactions. Fertil. and Steril., *28*, 1133–1145, 1977.
46. *Blecha, J.:* Biologie dospívání. (Biology of puberty. – in Czech) Praha, Stát. zdravot. naklad., 1966.
47. *Bleha, O., Küchel, O.:* Klinická endokrinologie v praxi. (Clinical endocrinology. – in Czech) Praha, Stát. zdravot. naklad., 1967
48. *Bleu, G., Roberts, K. D., Chapdelaine, A.:* The in vitro and in vivo uptake and metabolism of steroids in human adipose tissue. J. clin. Endocr., *39*, 236–246, 1974.
49. *Blüm, V.:* Prolaktin: Phylogenetische Aspekte. Gynäkologe, *10*, 51–61, 1977.
50. *Bogdanove, E. M., Nolin, J. M., Campbell, G. T.:* Qualitative and quantitative gonad-pituitary feedback. Recent Progr. Hormone Res., *31*, 567–626, 1975.
51. *Bogolepova, I. N.:* Strojenije i razvitije gipotalamusa čeloveka. (Structure and development of the human hypothalamus    in Russian.) Leningrad, Medicina, 1968.
52. *Bogumil, R. J., Ferin, M., Van de Wiele, R. L.:* Mathematical studies of the human menstrual cycle. II. Simulation performance of a model of the human menstrual cycle. J. clin. Endocr., *35*, 144–156, 1972.
53. *Böhm, P., Fenske, M., Häffele, R., König, A.:* Limited significance of the LRH test in the diagnosis of ovarian dysfunction. Acta endocr. (Kbh.), *89*, 438–444, 1978.
54. *Borreman, E., Wyman, H., Van Campenhout, J.:* The responses to synthetic LH-RH in patients with primary deficiency in gonadotropins. Amer. J. Obstet. Gynec., *123*, 580–589, 1975.
55. *Boschann, H. W.:* Gynäkologische Zytodiagnostik für Klinik und Praxis. 2nd ed. Berlin/ New York, De Gruyter, 1973.
56. *Botella-Llusia, J.:* Le but de la menstruation. Rev. franç. Gynéc., *46*, 197–206, 1951.
57. *Bowman, A.. Dilley, S. R., Keverne, E. B.:* Suppression of oestrogen-induced LH surges in social subordination in talapoin monkeys. Nature, *275*, 56–58, 1978.
57a. *Boyar, R. M., Finkelstein, J. W., David, R., Roffwarg H., Kapen, S., Weitzman, E. D., Hellman, L.:* Twenty-four hour patterns of plasma LH and FSH in sexual precocity. N. Eng. J. Med., 289, 282–284, 1973.
58. *Boyar, R. M., Katz, J., Finkelstein, J. W., Kapen, S., Weiner, H., Weitzman, E. D., Hellman, L.:* Anorexia nervosa. Immaturity of the 24-hour LH secretory pattern. N. Engl. J. Med., *291*, 861–865, 1974.
59. *Brandau, H., Mestwerdt, W.:* Vergleichende enzymologische, endokrinologische und elektronenoptische Untersuchungen über die Funktion des Ovars in der Postmenopause. Endokrinologie, *62*, 150–174, 1973.
60. *Brandl, E., Mettler, L. ·* Timing of ovulation in a sterility clinic. Int. J. Fertil., *19*, 13–16, 1974.

61. *Brody, S.:* Protein hormones and hormonal peptides from the placenta. In: Foetus and placenta. Klopper, A., Diczfalusy, E. (eds.). Oxford, Blackwell, 1969, p. 299–411.
62. *Brown, E., Barglow, P.:* Pseudocyesis. Arch. gen. Psychiat., *24*, 221–230, 1971.
63. *Brown, J., Matthew, G. D.:* The application of urinary estrogen measurements to problems in gynecology. Recent Progr. Hormone Res., *18*, 337–385, 1962.
64. *Bugnon, C., Bloch, B., Fellmann, D.:* Cytoimmunological study of the ontogenesis of the gonadotropic hypothalamo-pituitary axis in the human fetus. J. Steroid Biochem. *8*, 565–575, 1977.
65. *Bulbrook, R. D., Greenwood, F. C., Hadfield, G. J., Scowen, E. F.:* Oophorectomy in breast cancer. An attempt to correlate clinical results with oestrogen production. Brit. med. J., *2*, 7, 1958.
66. *Burger, H. G., Baker, H. W. G., Hudson, B., Taft, H. P.:* Gonadotropic and gonadal function in the normal adult male. In: Gonadotropins. Saxena, B. B., Beling, C. G., Gandy, H. M. (eds.). New York, Wiley & Sons, 1972, p. 569–592.
67. *Bürgi, H., Labhart, A.:* The thyroid gland. In: Clinical Endocrinology. A. Labhart. (ed.). Berlin/Heidelberg/New York, Springer Verlag, 1974, p. 135–284.
68. *Burns, R. K.:* Role of the hormones in the differentiation of sex. In: Sex and Internal Secretions. Young, W. C., Corner, G. W. (eds.) 3rd ed. Baltimore, Williams and Wilkins, 1961, p. 76–158.
69. *Butcher, R. L.:* Changes in gonadotropins and steroids associated with unilateral ovariectomy of the rat. Endocrinology, 101, 830–840, 1977.
70. *Butt, W. R., Leeson, S., Robinson, W., Shirley, A.:* Bioassay and immunoassay of gonadotrophins: Routine procedures. Endocr. exp., 7, 43–48, 1973.
71. *Cantor, B., Kalra, P. S., Buhi, W. C., Birk, S. A., Spellacy, W. N.:* Factors influencing the dynamics of gonadotropin response following bolus infusion of luteinizing hormone-releasing factor in women with menstrual abnormalities. Fertil. and Steril., *28*, 526–530, 1977.
72. *Capraro, V. J., Gallego, M. B.:* Vaginal agenesis. Amer. J. Obstet. Gynec., *124*, 98–107, 1976.
73. *Carlsen, R. B., Bahl, P. O., Swaminathan, N.:* Human chorionic gonadotropin. Linear amino acid sequence of the ᵦ-subunit. J. biol. Chem., *248*, 6810–6827, 1973.
74. *Carmel, P. W., Araki, S., Ferin, M.:* Pituitary stalk portal blood collection in Rhesus monkeys: Releasing hormone (GnRH). Endocrinology, *99*, 243–248, 1976.
75. *Catt, K. J., Dufau, M. L.:* Basic concepts of the mechanism of action of peptide hormones. Biol. Reprod., *14*, 1–15, 1976.
76. *Catt, K. J., Dufau, M. L., Vaitukaitis, J. L.:* Appearance of hCG in pregnancy plasma following the initiation of implantation of the blastocyst. J. clin. Endocr., *40*, 537–540, 1975.
77. *Cavazos, F., Lucas, F. V.:* Ultrastructure of the endometrium. In: Uterus. Norris, H. J., Hertig, A. T., Abell, M. R. (eds.). Baltimore, The Williams & Wilkins Co., 1973, p. 136 to 174.
78. *Chan, L., O'Malley, B. W.:* Mechanism of action of the sex steroid hormones. New Engl. J. Med., *294*, 1322–1328, 1372–1381, 1430–1437, 1976.
79. *Chang, R. J., Jaffe, R. B.:* Progesterone effects on gonadotropin release in women pretreated with oestradiol. J. clin. Endocr., *47*, 119–125, 1978.
80. *Channing, C. P., Kammerman, S.:* Effects of hCG asialo-hCG and the subunits of hCG upon luteinization of monkey granulosa cell cultures. Endocrinology, *93*, 1035–1043, 1973.
81. *Channing, C. P., Kammerman, S.:* Binding of gonadotropins to ovarian cells. Biol. Reprod., *10*, 179–198, 1974.
82. *Chappel, S. C., Barraclough, C. A.:* Hypothalamic regulation of pituitary FSH secretion. Endocrinology, *98*, 927–935, 1976.

83. *Chiazze, L., Brayer, F. T., Macisco, J. J., Parker, M. P., Duffy, B. J.:* The length and variability of the human menstrual cycle. J. amer. med. Ass., *203*, 377–380, 1968.

84. *Collip, P. J., Kaplan, S. A., Boyle, D. C., Plachte, F., Cogut, M. D.:* Constitutional isosexual precocity. Amer. J. Dis. Child. *108*, 399–405, 1964.

85. *Collu, R., Ducharme, V. R.:* Role of the adrenal steroids in the regulation of gonadotropin secretion at puberty. J. Steroid Biochem., *6*, 869–872, 1975.

86. *Comfort, A.:* Likelihood of human pheromones. Nature (London), *230*, 432–434, 1971.

86a. *Connaughton, J. F., Garcia, C.-R., Wallach, E. E.:* Induction of ovulation with cisclomiphene and a placebo. Obstet. and Gynec., *43*, 697–701, 1974.

87. *Constam, G. R.:* The pancreas. In: Clinical Endocrinology. Labhart, A. (ed.). Berlin, Springer Verlag, 1974, p. 798.

88. *Conte, F. A., Grumbach, M. M., Kaplan, S. L.:* A diphasic pattern of gonadotropin secretion in patients with the syndrome of gonadal dysgenesis. J. clin. Endocr., *40*, 670–674, 1975.

89. *Cooke, I. D., Anderton, K. J., Lenton, E., Burton, M.:* Hormone patterns at the climacteric. Postgrad. med. J., *52*, Suppl. 6: 12–16, 1976.

90. *Cooke, I. D., Lenton, E. A., Adams, M., Pearce, M. A., Fahmy, D., Evans, C. R.:* Some clinical aspects of pituitary-ovarian relationships in women with ovulatory infertility. J. Reprod. Fertil., *51*, 203–213, 1977.

91. *Corbin, A., Beattie, C. W., Tracy, J., Jones, R., Foell, T. J., Yardley, J., Rees, W. A.:* The anti-reproductive pharmacology of LH-RH and agonistic analogues. Int. J. Fertil., *23*, 81–92, 1978.

92. *Corner, G. W.:* The histological dating of human corpus luteum of menstruation. Amer. J. Anat., *98*, 337–401, 1956.

92a. *Coulam, C. B., Ryan, R. J.:* Premature menopause. 1. Etiology. Amer. J. Obstet. Gynec. *133*, 639–643, 1979.

93. *Coy, D. H., Schally, A. V.:* Gonadotrophin releasing hormone analogues. Ann. clin. Res., *10*, 139–144, 1978.

94. *Crosignani, P. G., Robyn, C.* (eds.): Prolactin and human reproduction. London, New York, San Francisco, Acad. Press, 1977.

94a. *Cudmore, D. W., Tupper, W. R. C.:* Induction of ovulation with clomiphene citrate. A double--blind study. Fertil. and Steril. *17*, 363–373, 1966.

94b. *Cutler, G. B., Glenn, M., Bush, M., Hodgen, G. D., Graham, C. E., Loriaux, D. L.:* Adrenarche: A survey of rodents, domestic animals, and primates. Endocrinology, *103*, 2112–2118, 1978.

95. *Dallenbach-Hellweg, G.:* Endometrium. Pathologische Histologie in Diagnostik und Forschung. Berlin, Springer, 1969.

96. *Dallenbach, F. D., Vonderlin, D.:* The innervation of the human endometrium. Arch. Gynäk., *215*, 365–376, 1973.

97. *Dalton, K.:* The Premenstrual Syndrome. Springfield, Thomas, 1964.

98. *Daniel, P. M., Prichard, M. M. L.:* Studies of the hypothalamus and the pituitary gland. Acta endocr. (Kbh.), *80*, Suppl. 201: 1–210, 1975.

99. *Daume, E., Chari, S., Hopkinson, C. R. N., Sturm, G., Hirschhäuser, C.:* Nachweis von Inhibin-Aktivität in der Follikelflüssigkeit menschlicher Ovarien. Klin. Wschr., *56*, 369–370, 1978.

100. *David, M. A., Fraschini, F., Martini, L.:* Control of LH-secretion. Role of a short feedback--mechanism. Endocrinology, *78*, 55–60, 1966.

101. *Davies, I. J., Naftolin, F., Ryan K. J., Siu, J.:* A specific, high-affinity, limited-capacity oestrogen binding component in the cytosol of human fetal pituitary and brain tissue. J. clin. Endocr., *40*, 909–912, 1975.

102. *Davis, M. E., Friedrich, E. H.:* Diagnosing the amenorrhoeas — survey of causes and means of detection. In: Textbook of Gynecologic Endocrinology. J. J. Gold (ed.). New York, Harper and Row, 1968, p. 215–238.

103. *DeKretser, D. M., Burger, H. G., Dumpys, R.:* Patterns of serum LH and FSH in response to 4-hour infusions of luteinizing hormone releasing hormone in normal women during menstrual cycle, on oral contraceptives and in postmenopausal state. J. clin. Endocr., *46*, 227–235, 1978.

104. *Dencla, W. D.:* Pituitary inhibitor of thyroxine. Fed. Proc., *34*, 96, 1975.

105. *Denef, C., DeMoor, P.:* Sexual differentiation of steroid metabolizing enzymes in the rat liver. Further studies on predetermination by testosterone at birth. Endocrinology, *91*, 374–384, 1972.

106. *Dewhurst, C. J., Cowell, C. A., Barrie, L. C.:* The regularity of early menstrual cycles. J. Obstet. Gynaec. Brit. Cwlth., *78*, 1093–1095, 1971.

107. *Dickerman, Z., Prager-Lewin, R., Laron, Z.:* Response of plasma LH and FSH to synthetic LH-RH in children at various pubertal stages. Amer. J. Dis. Child., *130*, 634–638, 1976.

108. *Dickey, R. P., Stone, S. C.:* Progestational potency of oral contraceptives. Obstet. and Gynec., *47*, 102–106, 1976.

108a. *Diczfalusy, E.:* Steps in the human reproductive process susceptible to immunological interference. Acta endocr. (Kbh.), *78*, Suppl. 194: 13–36, 1975.

109. *Diczfalusy, E.:* Interrelations between plasma levels of biologically active LH and ovarian and adrenal steroids in the normal menstrual cycle. J. Reprod. Fertil., *51*, 193–201, 1977.

110. *Diczfalusy, E., Lauritzen, Ch.:* Oestrogene beim Menschen. Berlin/Göttingen/Heidelberg, Springer, 1961.

111. *Diedrich, K., Leidenberger, F., Lehmann, F., Bettendorf, G.:* Klinisch experimentelle Studien zur Therapie ovarieller Funktionsstörungen mit 2-Br-α-Ergocryptin (Pravidel^R). Geburtsh. u. Frauenheilk., *38*, 716–725, 1978.

112. *Dierschke, D. J., Karsch, F. J., Weick, R. F., Weiss, A., Hotchkiss, J., Knobil, E.:* Hypothalamic-pituitary regulation of puberty: Feedback control of gonadotropin secretion in the Rhesus monkey. In: Control of the onset of puberty. Grumbach, M.M., Grave, G. D., Mayer, F. E. (eds.). New York, John Wiley and Sons, 1974, p. 104–114.

113. *Dilman, V. M.:* Age-associated elevation of hypothalamic threshold to feedback control and its role in development, ageing, and disease. Lancet, *I*, 1211–1219, 1971.

114. *Doepfmer, R.:* Sterilität und Infertilität. Störungen von seiten des Mannes. In: Gynäkologie und Geburtshilfe, Bd. 1. O. Käser et al. (eds.). Stuttgart, Thieme, 1969, p. 596–627.

115. *Döring, G. K.:* Über die relative Sterilität in den Jahren nach der Menarche. Geburtsh. u. Frauenheilk., *23*, 30–36, 1963.

116. *Döring, G. K.:* Über die relative Häufigkeit des anovulatorischen Cyclus im Leben der Frau. Arch. Gynäk. *199*, 115–123, 1963.

117. *Döring, G. K.:* Die Aufwachtemperatur. In: Gynäkologie u. Geburtshilfe Bd. I. Käser, O., Friedberg, V., Ober, K. G., Thomsen, K., Zander, J. (eds.). Stuttgart, Thieme, 1969, p. 832–841.

118. *Döring, G. K.:* Über die Häufigkeit der verschiedenen Sterilitätsursachen bei der Frau und die Erfolgsaussichten ihrer Behandlung. Geburtsh. u. Frauenheilk, *30*, 302–307, 1970.

119. *Dörner, G.:* Sexualhormonabhängige Gehirndifferenzierung und Sexualität. Jena, Fischer, 1972.

120. *Dörner, G., Staudt, J.:* Vergleichende morphologische Untersuchungen der Hypothalamusdifferenzierung bei Ratte und Mensch. Endokrinologie, *59*, 152–155, 1972.

121. *Donovan, B. T., Van den Werff ten Bosch, J. J.:* Physiology of puberty. London, Edward Arnold, 1965.

122. *Dor, J., Homburg, R., Rabau, E.:* An evaluation of etiologic factors and therapy in 665 infertile couples. Fertil. and Steril., *28*, 718–722, 1977.

123. *Drake, T., Tredway, D., Buchanan, G., Takaki, N., Daane, T.:* Unexplained infertility. A reappraisal. Obstet. and Gynec., *50*, 644–646, 1977.

124. *Drill, V.:* Oral contraceptives: Relation to mammary cancer, benign breast lesions and cervical cancer. Ann. Rev. Pharmac., *15*, 367–385, 1975.

125. *Dufau, M. L., Dulmanis, A., Catt, K. J., Hudson, B.:* Measurement of plasma oestradiol-17β by competitive binding assay employing pregnancy plasma. J. clin. Endocr., *30*, 351–356, 1970.

126. *Dunbar, H. F.:* Emotions and bodily changes. 2nd ed. New York, Columbia University Press, 1938, p. 404.

127. *Earley, C. J., Leonard, B. E.:* GABA and gonadal hormones. Brain Res., *155*, 27–34, 1978.

128. *Edgren, R. A., Sturtevant, F. M.:* Potencies of oral contraceptives. Amer. J. Obstet. Gynec., *125*, 1029–1038, 1976.

129. *Edmonds, M., Molitch, M., Pierce, J. G., Odell, W. D.:* Secretion of α-subunits of luteinizing hormone (LH) by the anterior pituitary. J. clin. Endocr., *41*, 551–555, 1975.

130. *Egger, H.:* The representability of laparoscopic ovarian biopsies for the cellular structure and production of the ovaries. Arch. Gynäk., *218*, 323–329, 1975.

131. *England, B. G., Niswender, G. D., Midgley, Jr., A. R.:* Radioimmunoassay of oestradiol-17β without chromatography. J. clin. Endocr., *38*, 42–50, 1974.

132. *Epstein, Y., Lunenfeld, B., Kraiem, Z.:* The effects of testosterone and its 5α-reduced metabolites on pituitary responsiveness to gonadotrophin-releasing hormone (Gn-RH). Acta endocr. (Kbh.), *86*, 728–732, 1977.

133. *Erikson, L. E.:* Light-dark periodicity and the Rhesus-monkey menstrual cycle. Fertil. and Steril., *15*, 352–365, 1964.

134. *Escomel, E.:* La plus jeune mère du monde. Press méd., *47*, 875, 1939.

135. *Eskay, R. L., Warberg, J., Mical, R. S., Porter, J. C.:* Prostaglandin E₂-induced release of LH-RH into hypophyseal portal blood. Endocrinology, *97*, 816–824, 1975.

136. *Espey, L. L.:* Ovarian proteolytic enzymes and ovulation. Biol. Reprod., *10*, 216–235, 1974.

137. *Ettinger, B.. Golditch, I. M.:* Medroxyprogesterone acetate for the evaluation of hypertestosteronism in hirsute women. Fertil. and Steril., *28*, 1285–1288, 1977.

138. *Farber, M., Millan, V. G., Turksoy, R. N., Mitchell, G. W.:* Diagnostic evaluation of hirsutism in women by selective bilateral adrenal and ovarian venous catheterization. Fertil. and Steril., *30*, 283–288, 1978.

139. *Feng, L. J., Rodbard, D., Rebar, R., Ross, G. T.:* Computer simulation of the human pituitary-ovarian cycle: Studies of follicular phase oestradiol infusions and the mid-cycle peak. J. clin. Endocr., *45*, 775–787, 1977.

140. *Ferin, J., Thomas, K., Johansson, E. D. B.:* Ovulation detection. In: Human Reproduction. Conception and Contraception. Hafez, E. S. E., Evans, T. N. (eds.). Hagerstown, MA, Harper & Row, 1973, p. 260–283.

141. *Ferin, M., Bogumil, J., Drewes, J., Dyrenfurth, I., Jewelewicz, R., Vande Wiele, R. L.:* Pituitary and ovarian hormonal response to 48 gonadotrophin releasing hormone (GnRH) infusions in female Rhesus monkeys. Acta endocr. (Kbh.), *89*, 48–59, 1978.

142. *Figarová, V., Presl, J., Pospíšil, J., Wagner, J., Horský, J.:* Limited number of hCG-binding sites in the ovaries of immature rats. Physiol. bohemoslov., *20*, 59–60, 1971.

143. *Figarová, V., Presl, J., Krabec, Z.:* hCG-like activity in the cytosol of the target cells in immature female rats. IRCS med. Sci., *2*, 1168, 1974.

144. *Fiorindo, R., Justo, G., Motta, M., Simonovic, I., Martini, L.:* Acetylcholine and the secretion

of pituitary gonadotropins. In: Hypothalamic Hormones. Motta, M., Crosignani, P. G., Martini, L. (eds.). London, New York, San Francisco, Acad. Press, 1975, p. 195–204.

145. *Fishman, J.:* The catechol oestrogens. Neuroendocrinology, *22*, 363–374, 1976.

146. *Flowers, C. E., Wilborn, W. H.:* New observations on the physiology of menstruation. Obstet. and Gynec., *51*, 16–24, 1978.

146a. *Ford, K.:* Contraceptive use in the United States, 1973–1976. Family Plan. Perspectives, *10*, 264–269, 1978.

147. *Foster, D. L.:* Luteinizing hormone and progesterone secretion during sexual maturation of the Rhesus-monkey: Short luteal phases during the initial menstrual cycles. Biol. Reprod., *17*, 584–590, 1977.

147a. *Fotherby, K.:* Excretion of pregnanetriol during the normal menstrual cycle. Brit. med. J. *1*, 1545–1546, 1960.

148. *Franchi, L. L., Mandl, A. M., Zuckerman, S.:* The development of the ovary and the process of oogenesis. In: The Ovary. Vol. 1. Zuckerman, S., Mandl, A. M., Eckstein, P. (eds.). New York/London, Academic Press, 1962, p. 1–88.

149. *Franchi, L. L.:* The ovary. In: Scientific Foundations of Obstetrics and Gynecology. Philipp, E. E., Barnes, J., Newton, M. (eds.). London, William Heinemann, 1970, p. 107–131.

150. *Franchi, L. L., Baker, T. G.:* Oogenesis and follicular growth. In: Human Reproduction. Conception and Contraception. Hafez, E. S. E., Evans, T. N. (eds.). Hagerstown, Harper & Row, 1973, p. 53–83.

151. *Franchimont, P., Becker, H., Ernould, Ch., Thys, Ch., Demoulin, A., Bourguignon, J. P., Legros, J. J., Valcke, J. C.:* The effect of hypothalamic luteinizing hormone releasing hormone (LH-RH) on plasma gonadotrophin levels in normal subjects. Clin. Endocr., *3*, 27–39, 1974.

152. *Franchimont, P., Legros, J. J.:* Modification of LH-RH response under the influence of endocrine equilibrium. In: Hypothalamic Hormones. Motta, M., Crosignani, P. G., Martini, L. (eds.). London, New York, San Francisco, Academic Press, 1975, p. 311–324.

153. *Frantz, A. G.:* Prolactin. New Engl. J. Med., *298*, 201–207, 1978

154. *Fraser, I. S., Michie, E. A., Wide, L., Baird, D. T.:* Pituitary gonadotropins and ovarian function in adolescent dysfunctional uterine bleeding. J. clin. Endocr., *37*, 407–414, 1973.

155. *Fridrich, F., Holzner, H., Golob, E., Caucig, H., Laube, E.:* Die Diagnose der insuffizienten Gelbkörperphase durch Endometriumbiopsie, Pregnandiolserienbestimmung und Basaltemperaturmessung. Z. Geburtsh. Gynaek., *175*, 27–43, 1971.

156. *Friedrich, E., Etzrodt, A., Becker, H., Hanker, J. P., Keller, E., Kleisl, P., Pinto, V., Schindler, A. E., Schneider, H. P. G., Vanderbeke, O., Werder, H., Wyss, H. I.:* Dose-response study with a new LH-RH analogue D-Ser (TBU)⁶ LH-RH 1–9(EA)¹⁰ during the follicular phase of the menstrual cycle. Acta endocr. (Kbh.), *87*, 19–27, 1978.

157. *Fries, H., Nillius, S. J., Pettersson, F.:* Epidemiology of secondary amenorrhoea. II. A retrospective evaluation of etiology with special regard to psychogenic factors and weight loss. Amer. J. Obstet. Gynec., *118*, 473–479, 1974.

158. *Frisch, R. E., Revelle, R.:* Height and weight at menarche and a hypothesis of critical body weights and adolescent events. Science, *169*, 397–399, 1970.

159. *Frisch, R. E., Revelle, R.:* Height and weight at menarche and hypothesis of menarche. Arch. Dis. Childh., *46*, 695–701, 1971.

160. *Frisch, R. E., McArthur, J. W.:* Menstrual cycles: Fatness as a determinant of minimum weight for height necessary for their maintenance and onset. Science, *185*, 949–951, 1974.

161. *Fuxe, K., Löfström, A., Eneroth, P., Gustafsson, J.-A., Skett, P., Hökfelt, T., Wiesel, F.-A., Agnati, L.:* Involvement of central catecholamines in the feedback actions of 17β-oestradiol-

benzoate on luteinizing hormone secretion in the ovariectomized female rat. Psychoneuro-endocrinology, 2, 203–225, 1977.

162. *Fuxe, K., Pérez de la Mora, M., Agnati, L., Eneroth, P., Gustafsson, J.-A., Skett, P., Ögren, S.-O.:* Possible involvement of central aminergic, histaminergic, cholinergic and GABA ergic mechanisms in the central control of gonadotrophin secretion. A pharmacological analysis. Acta endocr. (Kbh.), 85, Suppl. 212: 15, 1977.

163. *Gallagher, J. C., Nordin, B. E. C.:* Estrogens and calcium metabolism. In: Aging and Estrogens. Front. Horm. Res. Vol. 2. Van Keep, P. A., Lauritzen, Ch. (eds.). Basel, S. Karger, 1973, p. 98–117.

164. *Garcia, C.-R.:* Detection and diagnosis of ovulation. Clin. Obstet. Gynec., 10, 380–389, 1967.

165. *Geynet, C., Millet, C., Truong, H., Baulieu, E. E.:* Oestrogens and antioestrogens. Gynec. Invest., 3, 2–29, 1972.

166. *Gilbert, C., Galton, D. J., Kaye, J.:* Triglyceride storage disease: A disorder of lipolysis in adipose tissue in two patients. Brit. med. J., 1, 25–27, 1973.

167. *Gilmore, D. P., Dobbie, H. G., McNeilly, A. S., Mortimer, C. H.:* Presence and activity of LH-RH in the mid-term human fetus. J. Reprod. Fertil., 52, 355–359, 1978.

168. *Givens, J. R., Andersen, R. N., Umstot, E. S., Wiser, W. L.:* Clinical findings and hormonal responses in patients with polycystic ovarian disease with normal versus elevated LH levels. Obstet. and Gynec., 47, 388–392, 1976.

169. *Glass, R., Vessey, M., Wiggins, P.:* Use-effectiveness of the condom in a selected family planning clinic population in the United Kingdom. Contraception, 10, 591–598, 1974.

170. *Goldenberg, R. L., Grodin, J. M., Vaitukaitis, J. L., Ross, G. T.:* Withdrawal bleeding and LH secretion following progesterone in women with amenorrhoea. Amer. J. Obstet. Gynec., 115, 193–196, 1973.

171. *Goldzieher, J. W.,* Polycystic ovarian disease. In: Advances in Obstetrics and Gynecology. Vol. I. Marcus, S. L., Marcus, C. L. (eds.). Baltimore, William and Wilkins, 1967, p. 354–371.

172. *Goldzieher, J. W.:* Polycystic ovarian disease. Clin. Obstet. Gynec., 16, 82–105, 1973.

173. *Goldzieher, J. W., Moses, L. E., Averkin, E., Scheel, C., Taber, B. L.:* A placebo-controlled double-blind crossover investigation of the side effects attributed to oral contraceptives. Fertil. and Steril., 22, 609-623, 1971.

174. *Gonzales-Barcena, D., Kastin, A. J., Coy, D. H., Nikolics, K., Schally, A. V.:* Suppression of gonadotrophin release in man by an inhibitory analogue of LH-releasing hormone. Lancet, 2, 997–998, 1977.

175. *Good, R. G., Moyer, D. L.:* Oestrogen-progesterone relationships in the development of secretory endometrium. Fertil. and Steril., 19, 37–49, 1968.

176. *Goodman, R. L.:* Site of positive feedback action of oestradiol in rat. Endocrinology, 102, 151–159, 1978.

177. *Gorlitsky, G. A., Kase, N. G., Speroff, L.:* Ovulation and pregnancy rates with clomiphene citrate. Obstet. and Gynec., 51, 265–269, 1978.

178. *Gorski, R. A.:* Gonadal hormones and the perinatal development of neuroendocrine function. In: Frontiers in Neuroendocrinology, 1971. Martin i,L., Ganong, W. F. (eds.). New York, Oxford University Press, 1971, p. 237–290.

179. *Graesslin, D., Leidenberger, F. A., Lichtenberg, V., Glismann, D., Hess, N., Czygan, P. J., Bettendorf, G.:* Existence of big and little forms of luteinizing hormone in human serum. Acta endocr. (Kbh.), 83, 466–482, 1976.

180. *Graves, W. P.:* Some observations on the etiology of dysfunctional uterine bleeding. Amer. J. Obstet. Gynec., 20, 500–505, 1930.

181. *Greeley, G. H., Nicholson, G. F., Nemeroff, C. B., Youngblood, W. W., Kitzer, J. S.:* Direct evidence that arcuate nucleus — median eminence tuberoinfundibular system is not of primary importance in feedback regulation of LH and FSH secretion in castrated rat. Endocrinology, *103*, 170–175, 1978.

182. *Green, C. P.:* Voluntary sterilization: World's leading contraceptive method. Popul. Rep., Spec. Topic Monographs, M 37–71, 1978.

183. *Greenblatt, R. B., Stahl, N. L.:* Classification of ovarian disorders. In: Gonadotropin Therapy in Female Infertility. Rosenberg, E. (ed.). Amsterdam, Excerpta Medica, 1973, p. 23–43.

184. *Grodin, J. M., Siiteri, P. K., McDonald, P. C.:* Source of oestrogen production in post-menopausal women. J. clin. Endocr., *36*, 207–214, 1973.

185. *Groll, M.:* Gonadotropic patterns in psychogenic amenorrhoea. Int. J. Gynaec. Obstet., *16*, 53–55, 1978.

185a. *Groom, G. V.:* The measurement of human gonadotrophins by radioimmunoassay. J. Reprod. Fertil., *51*, 273–286, 1977.

186. *Grumbach, M. M., Roth, J. C., Kaplan, S. L., Kelch, R. P.:* Hypothalamic-pituitary regulation of puberty in man: Evidence and concepts derived from clinical research. In: Control of the Onset of Puberty. Grumbach, M. M., Grave, G. D., Mayer, R. E. (eds.). New York, John Willey, 1974, p. 115–166.

187. *Guerrero, R., Aso, T., Brenner, P. F., Čekan, Z., Landgren, B.-M., Hagenfeldt, K., Diczfalusy, E.:* Studies on the pattern of circulating steroids in the normal menstrual cycle. I. Acta endocr. (Kbh.), *81*, 133–149, 1976.

188. *Guillemin, R.:* The expanding significance of hypothalamic peptides, or, is endocrinology a branch of neuroendocrinology. Recent Progr. Hormone Res., *33*, 1–28, 1977.

189. *Hagen, C., McNatty, K. P., McNeilly, A. S.:* Immunoreactive α- and β-subunits of luteinizing hormone in human peripheral blood and follicular fluid throughout the menstrual cycle, and their effect on the secretion rate of progesterone by human granulosa cells in tissue culture. J. Endocr., *69*, 33–46, 1976.

190. *Hagen, T. C., Guansing, A. R., Sill, A. J.:* Preliminary evidence for a human prolactin releasing factor. Neuroendocrinology, *21*, 255–261, 1976.

191. *Hagen, C., McNeilly, A. S.:* The gonadotrophins and their subunits in foetal pituitary glands and circulation. J. Steroid Biochem., *8*, 537–544, 1977.

192. *Hagino, N., Coy, D. H., Schally, A. V., Arimura, A.:* Inhibition of release in the baboon by inhibitory analogs of luteinizing hormone releasing hormone. Horm. metab. Res., *9*, 247–248, 1977.

193. *Hafez, E. S. E.:* Anatomy and physiology of the mammalian uterotubal junction. In: Handbook of Physiology. Sect. 7. Endocrinology. Vol. II. Female Reproductive System. Part 2. Greep, R. O. (ed.). Washington, D. C., American Physiological Society, 1973, p. 87–95.

194. *Hafez, E. S. E.:* Function of the Fallopian tube in human reproduction. Clin. Obstet. Gynec., *22*, 61–79, 1979.

195. *Hall, P. E.:* The World Health Organization's Programme for the standardization and quality control of radioimmunoassay of hormones in reproductive physiology. Hormone Res., *9*, 440–449, 1978.

196. *Haller, J.:* Increase of platelets and basal body temperature rise as indication of ovulation: A comparison. Acta endocr. (Kbh.), *40–41*, Suppl. 67: 131, 1962.

197. *Hamberger, L., Nilsson, L., Björn-Rasmussen, E., Atterfelt, P., Wiquist, N.:* Early abortion by vaginal prostaglandin suppositories. Contraception, *17*, 183–194, 1978.

198. *Hamberger, L., Hillensjö, T., Ahrén, K.:* Steroidogenesis in isolated cells of preovulatory rat follicles. Endocrinology, *103*, 771–777, 1978.

388

199. *Hamerton, J. L.:* Human Cytogenetics. Vol. I. and II. New York, London, Academic Press, 1971.

200. *Hammerstein, J.:* Die Ausscheidung von Steroiden und Gonadotropinen im anovulatorischen Cyclus der Frau. Arch. Gynäk. *200*, 638–658, 1965.

201. *Hamner, C. E., McLaughlin, K. C.:* Capacitation of sperm: As a function of the oviduct. In: The Oviduct and its Functions. Johnson, A. D., Foley, C. W. (eds.). New York/London, Academic Press, 1974, p. 161–192.

202. *Hardy, W. R., Lewis, L., Little, V., Swyer, G. I. M.:* Use of a spot test for chloride in cervical mucus for self-detection of the fertile phase in women. J. Reprod. Fertil., *21*, 143–152, 1970.

202a. *Harwood, J. P., Clayton, R. N., Catt, K. J.:* Ovarian gonadotropin-releasing hormone receptors. I. Properties and inhibition of luteal cell function. Endocrinology, *107*, 407–413, 1980.

203. *Hayes, A., Johanson, A.:* Excretion of follicle-stimulating hormone (FSH) and luteinizing hormone (LH) in urine by pubertal girls. Pediat. Res., *6*, 18–25, 1972.

204. *Hayward, J. N.:* Functional and morphological aspects of hypothalamic neurons. Physiol. Rev., *57*, 574–645, 1977.

205. *Henzl, M.:* Hormonal treatment of the dysfunctional uterine bleeding. (Summary in English.) Praha, Spofa, 1966.

206. *Henzl, M., Jirásek, J., Horský, J., Presl, J.:* Die Proliferationswirkung des 17α-Äthinyl-19- -Nor-Testosterons. Arch. Gynäk., *199*, 335–339, 1963.

207. *Hess, D. L., Wilkins, R. H., Moossy, J., Chang, J. L., Plant, T. M., McCormack, J. T., Nakai, Y., Knobil, E.:* Oestrogen-induced gonadotropin surges in decerebrated female Rhesus monkeys with medial basal hypothalamic peninsulae. Endocrinology, *101*, 1264–1270, 1977.

208. *Hienz, H. A.:* Chromosomen-Fibel. Stuttgart, Thieme Verlag, 1971.

209. *Hilgers, T. W., Abraham, G. E., Cavanagh, D.:* Natural family planning. I. The peak symptom and estimated time of ovulation. Obstet. and Gynec., *52*, 575–582, 1978.

210. *Hinz, W.:* Zur Abstossung der Gebärmutterschleimhaut bei anovulatorischen Blutungen. Geburtsh. u. Frauenheilk., *17*, 835–844, 1957.

211. *Hobson, W., Gosselin, R., Fuller, G. B.:* Inhibition of gonadotropin release in chimpanzees by the LH-RH antagonist (D-Phe[2], D-Trp[3], D-Phe[6]) LH-RH. Program of the 60th Ann. Mtg. Endocrine Soc., Miami Beach, Fla. Abst. No 765, 1978.

212. *Hoff, J. D., Kundell, S., Hopper, B., Yen, S. S. C.:* The development of rhythmic patterns of gonadotropin and oestrogen excretion before, during and after puberty. Gynaec. Invest., *8*, 91, 1977.

213. *Hoff, J. D., Lasley, B. L., Wang, C. F., Yen, S. S. C.:* The two pools of pituitary gonadotropin: Regulation during the menstrual cycle. J. clin. Endocr., *44*, 302–312, 1977.

214. *Hoffman, F., Kayser, W., Bergk, K. H.:* Untersuchungen über die hormonale Steuerung der Ovulation bei der Frau. Geburtsh. u. Frauenheilk., *30*, 347–355, 1970.

215. *Holmdahl, T. H., Johansson, E. D. B.:* Peripheral plasma levels of 17α-hydroxyprogesterone, progesterone and oestradiol during normal menstrual cycles in women. Acta endocr. (Kbh.), *171*, 743–754, 1972.

216. *Horský, J., Jouja, V., Štroufová, A., Presl, J.:* Day and night variations of LH excretion in urine and of oestradiol-17 β in plasma in the course of a normal menstrual cycle in human. In: Endocrinology of Sex. Dörner, G. (ed.). Proceedings of the Int. Symposium. Berlin (GDR) 20.–23. 9. 1972. Leipzig, Johann Ambrosius Barth, 1974, p. 384–387.

216a. *Horský, J., Štroufová, A., Kozlová, J., Divila, F., Presl, J.:* LH-RH test in anovulatory cycles unsuccessfully treated by clomiphene citrate. (Summary in English.) Čs. Gynek., *40*, 180–183, 1975.

389

217. *Horský, J., Herzmann, J., Presl, J.:* Correlation between the progesterone withdrawal bleeding test and the level of plasmatic oestradiol. (Summary in English.) Čs. Gynek., *40*, 587 to 590, 1975.

218. *Horský, J., Herzmann, J., Štroufová, A.:* Feedback effect of testosterone in the women. (Summary in English.) Čs. Gynek., *42*, 3–10, 1977.

219. *Horský, J., Herzmann, J., Štroufová, A.:* Biphasic action of oestrogens in the sensitivity of the anterior pituitary to LH-RH in amenorrhoeic woman. In: Research on Steroids. Vol. VIII. Klopper, A., Lerner, L., Van der Molen, H. J., Sciarra, F. (eds.). London, Academic Press, 1979, p. 231–234.

219a. *Horský, J., Herzmann, J., Štroufová, A., Kozlová, J., Jouja, V.:* Gonadotropin and steroid levels in urine and blood of normal menstrual cycles. (Summary in English.) Čs. Gynek., *42*, 83–88, and 779, 1977.

220. *Horský, J., Štroufová, A., Herzmann, J.:* A new modification of LH-RH test with a double-response for preciseness of the diagnostics in gynaecological endocrinology. (Summary in English.) Čs. Gynek., *43*, 583–588, 1978.

221. *Horský, J., Herzmann, J., Štroufová, A.:* The effect of a superactive LH-RH analogue (D-Leu[6], desGly-NH$_2$[10]) LH-RH ethylamid triacetate upon the plasma oestradiol level in women with normal cycle. (Summary in English.) Čs. Gynek., *44*, 24–26, 1979.

222. *Huber, S. C., Piotrow, P. T., Orlans, F. B., Kommer, G.:* IUDs reassessed. A decade of experience. Popul. Rep., Ser. B, 21–48, 1975.

223. *Huggins, G. R., Preti, G.:* Volatile constituents of human vaginal secretions. Amer. J. Obstet. Gynec., *126*, 129–136, 1976.

224. *Huppert, L. C.:* Induction of ovulation with clomiphene citrate. Fertil. and Steril., *31*, 1–8, 1979.

225. *Husslein, H.:* Zur Frage des Blutungsfaktors bei der Menstruation. Zbl. Gynäk., *75*, 963 to 968, 1953.

226. *Husslein, H., Stöger, H.:* Klinik und Therapie des Sheehan-Syndroms. Wien. klin. Wschr., *86*, 489–494, 1974.

227. *Hyyppä, M., Motta, M., Martini, L.:* Ultrashort feedback control of follicle-stimulation hormone-releasing factor secretion. Neuroendocrinology, *7*, 227–235, 1971.

228. *Insler, V., Melmed, H., Eden, E., Serr, D., Lunenfeld, B.:* Comparison of various methods used in monitoring gonadotropic therapy. In: Clinical Application of Human Gonadotropins. Bettendorf, G., Insler, V. (eds.). Stuttgart, G. Thieme, 1970, p. 87–100.

229. *Isojima, S., Koyama, K., Tsuchiya, K.:* The effect on fertility in women of circulating antibodies against human spermatozoa. J. Reprod. Fertil., Suppl. 21: 125, 1974.

230. *Israel, R., Mishell, D. R., Jr., Stone, S. C., Thorneycroft, I. H., Moyer, D. L.:* Single luteal phase serum progesterone assay as an indicator of ovulation. Amer. J. Obstet. Gynec., *112*, 1043–1046, 1972.

231. *Israel, R.:* Current concepts in female sterilization. Clin. Obstet. Gynec., *17*, 139–155, 1974.

232. *Jacobson, A., Marshall, J. R., Ross, G. T., Cargille, Ch. M.:* Plasma gonadotropins during clomiphene induced ovulatory cycles. Amer. J. Obstet. Gynec., *102*, 284–290, 1968.

233. *Jaramillo, C. J., Salgado, A. Ch., Perez-Infante, V., Puente-Cueva, M., Botella-Llusia, J., Coy, D. H., Schally, A. V.:* Levels of luteinizing hormone, follicle-stimulating hormone and 17β-oestradiol in response to D-Trp[6] LH-RH during different phases of the menstrual cycle in normal women. Fertil. and Steril., *29*, 153–158, 1978.

234. *Jaramillo-Jaramillo, C., Charro-Salgado, A., Perez-Infante, V., Lopez del Campo, G., Botella-Llusia, J., Coy, D. H., Schally, A. V.:* Clinical studies with D-Trp[6]-luteinizing hormone-releasing hormone in anovulatory women. Fertil. and Steril., *29*, 418–423, 1978.

235. *Jayle, M. F., Palmer, R.:* The concept of ovarian thecal insufficiency. Diagnosis, clinical and therapeutic incidences. Int. J. Fertil., *18*, 33–43, 1973.
236. *Jeffcoate, S. L., Greenwood, R. H., Holland, D. T.:* Blood and urine clearance of LH-RH in man measured by RIA. J. Endocr., *60*, 305–314, 1974.
237. *Jenkins, M. E.:* Precocious menstruation in hypothyroidism. Amer. J. Dis. Child., *109*, 252–254, 1965.
238. *Jenner, M. R., Kelch, R. P., Kaplan, S. L., Grumbach, M. M.:* Hormonal changes in puberty. IV. Plasma oestradiol, LH, and FSH in prepubertal children. J. clin. Endocr., *34*, 521–530, 1972.
239. *Jirásek, J. E.:* Disorders of somatosexual development. (In Czech.) Praha, Avicenum, 1974.
240. *Jirásek, J. E.:* Principles of reproductive embryology. In: Disorders of Sexual Differentiation. Simpson, J. L. (ed.). New York/San Francisco/London, Academic Press, 1976, p. 51–110.
241. *Jirásek, J. E.:* Morphogenesis of the genital system in the human. In: Morphogenesis and Malformation of the Genital System. Blandau, R. J., Bergsma, D. (eds.). New York, Alan R. Liss, 1977, p. 13–39.
242. *Johanson, A., Guyda, H., Light, C., Migeon, C. J., Blizzard, R. M.:* Serum luteinizing hormone by radioimmunoassay in normal children. J. Pediat., *74*, 416–424, 1969.
243. *Johansson, E. D. B.:* Progesterone levels in peripheral plasma during the luteal phase of the normal human menstrual cycle measured by a rapid competitive protein binding technique. Acta endocr. (Kbh.), *61*, 592–606, 1969.
244. *Johansson, E. D. B., Larsson-Cohn, U., Gemzell, C.:* Monophasic basal body temperature in anovulatory menstrual cycles. Amer. J. Obstet. Gynec., *113*, 933–937, 1972.
245. *Jones, G. S.:* The luteal phase defect. Fertil. and Steril., *27*, 351–356, 1976.
246. *Jones, G. S., Aksel. S., Wentz, A. C.:* Serum progesterone values in the luteal phase defects: effect of chorionic gonadotropin. Obstet. and Gynec., *44*, 26–34, 1974.
247. *Jones, J. R., Kemmann, E.:* Olfacto-genital dysplasia in the female. In: Obstetrics and Gynecology Annual, Vol. 5. Wynn, R. M. (ed.). New York, Appleton-Century-Crofts, 1976, p. 443–466.
248. *Judd, H. L.:* Endocrinology of polycystic ovarian disease. Clin. Obstet. Gynec., *21*, 99–114, 1978.
249. *Judd, H. L., Lucas, W. E., Anderson, D. C., Yen, S. S. C.:* The postmenopausal ovary. A continuing source of testosterone in women. Gynec. Invest., *5*, 12, 1974.
250. *Jürgensen, O., Hildebrandt, H., Fritz, I., Kronauer, J., Taubert, H.-D.:* Plasma LH und Progesteron in normalen und gestörten Cyclen. Arch. Gynäk., *214*, 418–420, 1973.
251. *Jutisz, M., Bérault, A., Kerdelhué, B., Théoleyre M.:* Some aspects of the cellular mechanism of action of gonadotrophin releasing hormones. Symp. med. Hoechst, 7, 33–46, 1975.
252. *Kaiser, R., Daume, E.:* Über eine einheitliche Nomenklatur für das Klimakterium und seine Begleitsymptome. Geburtsh. u. Frauenheilk., *25*, 974–986, 1965.
253. *Kaiser, R., Geiger, W., Künzig, H.-J., Weymar, P.:* Hormonal pattern in premenopausal cycles. Arch. Gynäk., *223*, 213–220, 1977.
254. *Kaplan, S. L., Grumbach, M. M., Aubert, M. L.:* The ontogenesis of pituitary hormones and hypothalamic factors in the human fetus. Recent Progr. Hormone Res., *32*, 161–243, 1976.
255. *Kappers, J. A.:* The pineal organ: An introduction. In: The Pineal Gland. Wolstenholme, G. E. W., Knight, J. (eds.). London and Edinburgh, Churchill Livingstone, 1971, p. 3–25.
256. *Karsch, F. J., Dierschke, D. J., Knobil, E.:* Sexual differentiation of pituitary function: apparent difference between primates and rodents. Science, *179*, 484–486, 1973.
257. *Karsch, F. J., Dierschke, D. J., Weick, R. F., Yamaji, T., Hotchkiss, J., Knobil, E.:* Positive

and negative feedback control by oestrogen of luteinizing hormone secretion in the Rhesus monkey. Endocrinology, *92*, 799–804, 1973.

258. *Kawakami, M., Yoshioka, E., Konda, N., Arita, J., Visessuvan, S.:* Data on sites of stimulatory feedback action of gonadal steroids indispensable for LH release in rat. Endocrinology, *102*, 791–798, 1978.

259. *Kelch, R. P., Kaplan, S. L., Grumbach, M. M.:* Suppression of urinary and plasma gonadotropins by exogenous oestrogens in prepubertal children. Pediat. Res., *6*, 354, 1972.

259a. *Keller, D. W., Wiest, W. G., Askin, F. B., Johnson, L. W., Strickler, R. C.:* Pseudocorpus luteum insufficiency: A local defect of progesterone action on endometrial stroma. J. clin. Endocr., *48*, 127–132, 1979

260. *Kemmann, E., Jones, J. R., Orti, E., Tricomi, V.:* 45,X ovarian karyotype in ovulating female patient with Turner phenotype. Amer. J. Obstet. Gynec., *129*, 341–342, 1977.

261. *Kendle, K. E., Paterson, S. R., Wilson, C. A.:* Effects of RMI 12,936, a synthetic antiprogestational steroid on the oestrous cycle and ovulation in the rat. J. Reprod. Fertil., *53*, 363–368, 1978.

262. *Kestelman, P.:* Contraception in Europe. IPPF Europ. region. Inform. Bull., *8*, 1–2, 1979.

263. *Kirschner, M. A., Jacobs, J. B.:* Combined ovarian and adrenal vein catheterization to determine the site(s) of androgen overproduction in hirsute women. J. clin. Endocr., *33*, 199–209, 1971.

263a. *Kirschner, M. A., Bardin, C. W.:* Androgen production and metabolism in normal and virilized women. Metabolism, *21*, 667–688, 1972.

264. *Kistner, R. W.:* The menopause. Clin. Obstet. Gynec., *16*, 106–129, 1973.

265. *Kistner, R. W.:* Endometriosis and infertility. Clin. Obstet. Gynec., *22*, 101–119, 1979.

266. *Kletzky, O. A., Davajan, V., Nakamura, R. M., Mishell, D. R. Jr.:* Classification of secondary amenorrhoea based on distinct hormonal patterns. J. clin. Endocr., *41*, 660–668, 1975.

267. *Kletzky, O. A., Nakamura, R. M., Thorneycroft, S. H., Mishell, D. R. Jr.:* Log normal distribution of gonadotropins and ovarian steroid values in the normal menstrual cycle. Amer. J. Obstet. Gynec., *121*, 688–694, 1975.

268. *Kletzky, O. A., Nicoloff, J., Davajan, V., Mims, R., Mishell, D. R. Jr.:* Idiopathic hypogonadotrophic hypogonadal primary amenorrhoea. J. clin. Endocr., *46*, 808–815, 1978.

269. *Klink, R.:* Epidemiologische Untersuchungen über die Coronarsklerose nach der Menopause. Gynäkologe, *2*, 139–145, 1970.

270. *Knobil, E.:* On the regulation of the primate corpus luteum. Biol. Reprod., *8*, 246–258, 1973.

271. *Knobil, E.:* On the control of gonadotropin secretion in the Rhesus monkey. Recent Progr. Hormone Res., *30*, 1–36, 1974.

271a. *Knobil, E., Plant, T. M., Wildt, L., Belchetz, P. E., Marshall, G.:* Control of the Rhesus monkey menstrual cycle: Permissive role of hypothalamic gonadotropin-releasing hormone. Science, *207*, 1371–1373, 1980.

272. *Knörr, K.:* Regelähnliche Blutungen in der Schwangerschaft und ihre forensische Bedeutung. Zbl. Gynäk., *75*, 1809–1814, 1953.

273. *Koester, H.:* Ovum transport. In: Mammalian Reproduction. Gibian, H., Plotz, E. J. (eds.). Berlin/Heidelberg/New York, Springer Verlag, 1970, p. 189–228.

274. *König, M. P., Cornu, F., Blaser, A., Zingg, E., Stirnemann, A., Trost, B.:* Transsexualismus. Schweiz. med. Wschr., *108*, 437–444, 1978.

275. *Koninckx, P. R., Goddeeris, P. G., Lauweryns, J. M., de Hertogh, R. C., Brosens, I. A.:* Accuracy of endometrial biopsy dating in relation to the midcycle luteinizing hormone peak. Fertil. and Steril., *28*, 443–445, 1977.

276. *Korenman, S. G., Sherman, B. M.:* Hormonal regulation in normal and abnormal menstrual

cycles. In: The Endocrine Function of the Human Ovary. James, J. H. T., Serio, M., Giusti, G. (eds.). London [N.Y.]/San Francisco, Academic Press, 1976, p. 359–372.

277. *Kosasa, T. S., Levesque, L. A., Goldstein, D. P., Taymor, M. L.:* Clinical use of a solid phase radioimmunoassay specific for human chorionic gonadotropin. Amer. J. Obstet. Gynec., *119,* 784–791, 1974.

278. *Kotz, H. L., Herrmann, W.:* A review of the endocrine induction of human ovulation. II. Thyroid. Fertil. and Steril., *12,* 102–107, 1961.

279. *Krey, L. C., Butler, W. R., Knobil, E.:* Surgical disconnection of the medial basal hypothalamus and pituitary function in the Rhesus monkey. I. Gonadotropin secretion. Endocrinology, *96,* 1073–1087, 1975.

280. *Krieg, R. J., Sawyer, Ch. H.:* Effects of intraventricular catecholamines on luteinizing hormone release in ovariectomized steroid-primed rats. Endocrinology, *99,* 411–419, 1976.

281. *Kuhl, H., Rosniatowski, Ch., Taubert, H.-D.:* The regulatory function of a pituitary LH-RH-degrading enzyme system in the feedback control of gonadotrophins. Acta endocr. (Kbh.), *86,* 60–70, 1977.

282. *Kulin, H. E., Grumbach, M. M., Kaplan, S. L.:* Changing sensitivity of the pubertal gonadal hypothalamic feedback mechanism in man. Science, *166,* 1012–1013, 1969.

283. *Kulin, H. E., Reiter, E. O.:* Gonadotropins during childhood and adolescence: A review. Pediatrics, *51,* 260–271, 1973.

284. *Kulin, H. E., Reiter, E. O.:* Gonadotropin and testosterone measurements after oestrogen administration to adult men, prepubertal and pubertal boys, and men with hypogonadotropism: Evidence for maturation of positive feedback in the male. Pediat. Res. *10,* 46–51, 1976.

285. *Kurcin, I. T.:* Teoretičeskije osnovy psichosomatičeskoj mediciny. Leningrad, Nauka, 1973. (Principles of the psychosomatic medicine – in Russian.)

286. *Labhart, A.:* Clinical Endocrinology. Theory and Practice. Berlin/Heidelberg/New York, Springer, 1974.

287. *Lachelin, G. C. L., Yen, S. S. C.:* Hypothalamic chronic anovulation. Amer. J. Obstet. Gynec., *130,* 825–831, 1978.

288. *Langreder, W., Zimmerer, G.:* Zur Cyclusdiagnostik vermittels Vaginalabstrich und Cytometrie insbesondere bei körpereigener und künstlicher Androgenwirkung. Arch. Gynäk., *184,* 1–31, 1953.

289. *Lasley, B. L., Judd, H. L.:* Pathophysiology of anovulation. Clin. Obstet. Gynec., *21,* 87–97, 1978.

290. *Lauritzen, Ch.:* The management of the pre-menopausal and the post-menopausal patient. In: Aging and Oestrogens. Front. Horm. Res. Vol. 2. Van Keep, P. A., Lauritzen, Ch. (eds.). Basel, S. Karger, 1973, p. 2–21.

291. *Lauritzen, Ch.:* The female climacteric syndrome: significance, problems, treatment. Acta obstet. gynec. scand., Suppl. 51: 47–62, 1975.

292. *Leblanc, H., Lachelin, G. C. L., Abu-Fadil, S., Yen, S. S. C.:* Effects of dopamine infusion on pituitary hormone secretion in humans. J. clin. Endocr., *43,* 668–674, 1976.

293. *Lee, C. Y.:* Human chorionic gonadotropin (hCG) binding and stimulation of adenyl cyclase (AC) of porcine granulosa cells during follicle development. In Vitro, *10,* 343–344, 1975.

294. *Leleux, P., Robyn, C.:* Immunohistochemistry of individual adenohypophyseal cells. Acta endocr. (Kbh.), *67,* Suppl. 153: 168–189, 1971.

294a. *Leridon, H.:* Contraceptive practice in France in 1978. Family Plan. Perspectives, *11,* 153–154, 1979.

295. *Lev-Ran, A.:* Secondary amenorrhoea resulting from uncontrolled weight-reducing diets. Fertil. and Steril., *25*, 459–462, 1974.

296. *Leyendecker, G., Wardlaw, S., Nocke, W.:* Experimental studies on the endocrine regulations during the periovulatory phase of the human menstrual cycle. Acta endocr. (Kbh.), *71*, 160–178, 1972.

297. *L'Hermite, M., Delogne-Desnoeck, J., Michaux-Duchene, A., Robyn, C.:* Alteration of feedback mechanism of oestrogen on gonadotropin by sulpiride-induced hyperprolactinemia. J. clin. Endocr., *47*, 1132–1136, 1978.

298. *Li, T. S.:* Sperm immunology, infertility, and fertility control. Obstet. and Gynec., *44*, 607–623, 1974.

299. *Liang, T., Tymoczko, J. L., Chan, K. M. B., Hung, S. C., Shutsung, L.:* Androgen action: Receptors and rapid responses. In: Androgens and Antiandrogens. Martini, L., Motta, M. (eds.). New York, Raven Press, 1977, p. 77–89.

300. *Liao, S., Fang, S.:* Receptor proteins for androgens and the mode of action of androgens on gene transcription in ventral prostate. Vitam. and Horm., *27*, 17–90, 1969.

301. *Libertun, C., McCann, S. M.:* The possible role of histamine in the control of prolactin and gonadotropin release. Neuroendocrinology, *20*, 110–120, 1976.

301a. *Lin, T. J., Billiar, R. B., Little, B.:* Metabolic clearance of progesterone in the menstrual cycle. J. clin. Endocr., *35*, 879–886, 1972.

302. *Lipner, H.:* Mechanism of mammalian ovulation. In: Handbook of Physiology. Sect. 7. Endocrinology Vol. II. Part I. Greep. R. O. (ed.). Washington, Amer. physiol. Soc., 1973, p. 409–437.

303. *Lipsett, M. B.:* Oestrogen use and cancer risk. J. Amer. med. Ass., *237*, 1112–1115, 1977.

304. *Little, B., Billiar, R. B., Rahman, S. S., Johnson, W. A., Takaoka, Y., White, R. J.:* In vivo aspects of progesterone distribution and metabolism. Amer. J. Obstet. Gynec., *123*, 527 to 534, 1975.

305. *Liu, W.:* Correlation between vaginal cytology and endometrial histology. Amer. J. Obstet. Gynec., *80*, 321–324, 1960.

306. *Liu, N., Grumbach, M., Napoli, R. A., de, Morishima, A.:* Prevalence of EEG abnormalities in idiopathic precocious puberty and premature pubarche: bearing on pathogenesis and neuroendocrine regulation of puberty. J. clin. Endocr., *25*, 1296–1308, 1965.

307. *Lloyd, Ch. W., Lobotsky, J., Baird, D. T., McCracken, J. A., Weisz, J., Pupkin, M., Zanartu, J., Puga, J.:* Concentration of unconjugated oestrogens, androgens and gestagens in ovarian and peripheral venous plasma of women. The normal menstrual cycle. J. clin. Endocr., *32*, 155–166, 1971.

308. *Loeber, J. G.:* Human luteinizing hormone. Structure and function of some preparations. Acta endocr. (Kbh.), *85*, Suppl. 210: 11–130, 1977.

309. *Longcope, C.:* Metabolic clearance and blood production rates of oestrogens in postmenopausal women. Amer. J. Obstet. Gynec., *111*, 778–781, 1971.

309a. *Loraine, J. A., Bell, E. T.,* eds.: Hormone Assays and their Clinical Application. 4th ed. London, Churchill, 1976.

310. *Louvet, J. P., Vaislic, M., Boulard, C.:* Glucocorticoid receptor in ovaries from oestrogen-stimulated immature female rats. Europ. J. Obstet. Gynec., *9*, 210, 1979.

310a. *Lucisano, A., Dell'Acqua, S., Montemurro, A., Rossetti, A., Cinque, B., Lafuenti. G., Arno, E., Bompiani, A.:* Peripheral and ovarian vein plasma levels of 20α-dihydroprogesterone in women with normal menstrual cycles. J. Steroid. Biochem., *9*, 643–648, 1978.

311. *Luksch, F., Reisenauer, R.:* Clinical evaluation of female puberty (in Czech). Praha, SZdN, 1966.

311a. *Lunan, C. B., Klopper, A.:* Antioestrogens: A review. Clin. Endocr., *4*, 551–572, 1975.

312. *Lundström, V.:* Treatment of primary dysmenorrhoea with prostaglandin synthetase inhibitors. — A promising therapeutic alternative. Acta obstet. gynec. scand., *57*, 421–428, 1978.

313. *Lundy, L. E., Lee, S. G., Levy, W., Woodruff, J. D., Wu, Ch.-H., Abdalla, M.:* The ovulatory cycle. A histologic, thermal, steroid and gonadotropin correlation. Obstet. and Gynec., *44*, 14–25, 1975.

314. *Lunenfeld, B., Insler, V.:* Diagnosis and Treatment of Functional Infertility. Berlin, Grosse Verlag, 1978.

315. *Luukkainen, T., Nielsen, N.-Ch., Nygren, K.-G., Pyörälä, T., Kosonen, A.:* Randomized comparison of clinical performance of two copper-releasing IUDs, Nova-T and Copper-T-200 in Denmark, Finland and Sweden. Contraception, *19*, 1–9, 1979.

316. *MacDonald, P. C.:* Determinants of the rate of oestrogen formation in postmenopausal women. Europ. J. Obstet. Gynec. Reprod. Biol., *9*, 187–189, 1979.

317. *MacLeod, J., Gold, R. Z.:* The male factor in fertility and infertility. Fertil. and Steril., *4*, 194–209, 1953.

318. *Makris, A., Ryan, K. J.:* Cyclic AMP and cyclic GMP accumulation in hamster pre-ovulatory follicles stimulated with LH and FSH. Acta endocr. (Kbh.), *87*, 158–163, 1978.

319. *Marshall, J. R.:* Induction of ovulation. Clin. Obstet. Gynec., *21*, 147–162, 1978.

320. *Martin, J. B., Renaud, L. P., Brazeau, P.:* Hypothalamic peptides: new evidence for peptidergic pathways in the CNS. Lancet, *2*, 393–394, 1975.

321. *Martin, J. B., Reichlin, S., Brown, G. M.:* Clinical Neuroendocrinology. Philadelphia, F.A. Davis Company, 1977.

322. *Martini, L.:* Recent views on the control of anterior pituitary function. Acta endocr. (Kbh.), *85*, Suppl. 214: 19–32, 1977.

323. *Martini, L.:* Future developments in the sphere of steroid hormones. Triangl, *17*, 75–80, 1978.

324. *Maruyama, T.:* A fluorescence-histochemical study of monoaminergic neurons in the hypothalamus in relation to sexual differentiation. Acta obstet. gynaec. Jap., *20*, 131, 1973.

325. *Matsumoto, S., Hosaka, H., Igarashi, M., et al.:* Evaluation of clinical and laboratory tests for menstrual disorders. Gunma J. med. Sci., *11*, 95–149, 1962.

326. *Matsumoto, S.:* Use of cyclofenil (sexovid) to induce ovulation. Int. J. Fertil., *18*, 209–214, 1973.

327. *McCormack, J .T., Plant, T. M., Hess, D. L., Knobil, E.:* The effect of luteinizing hormone releasing hormone (LH-RH) antiserum administration on gonadotropin secretion in the Rhesus monkey. Endocrinology, *100*, 663–667, 1977.

327a. *McEwen, B. S.:* Sexual maturation and differentiation: The role of the gonadal steroids. In: Progress in Brain Research. Vol. 48. Corner, M. A. et al. (eds.). Elsevier, North Holland Biomedical Press, 1978, p. 291–307.

328. *McNatty, K. P., Sawers, R., McNeilly, A. S.:* A possible role for prolactin in control of steroid secretion by the human Graafian follicle. Nature, *250*, 653–655, 1974.

329. *Menge, A. C., Behrman, S. J.:* Immunologic infertility. Clin. Obstet. Gynec., *22*, 231–244, 1979.

330. *Merrill, J. A.:* The morphology of the prepubertal ovary. Sth. med. J. (Birmingham, Ala.), *56*, 225–231, 1963.

331. *Mettler, L., Shirwani, D.:* The blood count during the ovarian cycle. Amer. J. Obstet. Gynec., *119*, 1038–1043, 1974.

332. *Michael, R. P., Bonsall, R. W., Kutner, M.:* Volatile fatty acids, "copulins", in human vaginal secretions. Psychoneuroendocrinology, *1*, 153–163, 1975.

333. *Midgley, A. R., Jr., Jaffé, R. B.:* Regulation of human gonadotropins. IV. Correlation of

serum concentrations of follicle stimulating and luteinizing hormones during the menstrual cycle. J. clin. Endocr., *28*, 1699–1703, 1968.

334. *Midgley, A. R. Jr., Gay, V. L., Keyes, P. L., Hunter, J. S.:* Human reproductive endocrinology. In: Human Reproduction. Conception and Contraception. Hafez, E. S. E., Evans, T. N. (eds.). Hagerstown, Harper & Row, 1973, p. 201–236.

335. *Mishell, D. R. Jr., Moore, D. E., Roy, S., Brenner, P. F., Page, M. A.:* Clinical performance and endocrine profiles with contraceptive vaginal rings containing a combination of estradiol and α-norgestrel, Amer. J. Obstet. Gynec., *130*, 55–62, 1978.

336. *Miyake, A., Tanizawa, O., Aono, T., Kurachi, K.:* Pituitary responses in LH secretion to LH-RH during pregnancy. Obstet. and Gynec., *49*, 549–551, 1977.

337. *Moghissi, K. S.:* Accuracy of basal body temperature for ovulation detection. Fertil. and Steril., *27*, 1415–1421, 1976.

338. *Moghissi, K. S.:* The cervix in infertility. Clin. Obstet. Gynec., 22, 27–42, 1979.

339. *Moghissi, K. S., Syner, F. N., Evans, T. N.:* A composite picture of the menstrual cycle. Amer. J. Obstet. Gynec., *114*, 405–418, 1972.

340. *Morgan, F. J., Birken, S., Canfield, R. E.:* Human chorionic gonadotropin: A proposal for the amino acid sequence. Mol. cell. Biochem., *2*, 97–102, 1973.

341. *Mori, T., Suzuki, A., Nishimura, T., Kambegawa, A.:* Inhibition of ovulation in immature rats by antiprogesterone antiserum. J. Endocr., *73*, 185–186, 1977.

342. *Mori, T., Fujita, Y., Suzuki, A., Kinoshita, Y., Nishimura, T., Kambegawa, A.:* Functional and structural relationships in steroidogenesis in vitro by human ovarian follicles during maturation and ovulation. J. clin. Endocr., *47*, 955–966, 1978.

343. *Morris, I. D., Kurl, R. D.:* A selective action of clomiphene upon central and peripheral oestrogen cytoplasmic receptors. J. Endocr., *68*, 29P, 1976.

344. *Morris, N. M., Underwood, L. E., Easterling, W. Jr.:* Temporal relationship between basal body temperature nadir and LH surge in normal women. Fertil. and Steril., *27*, 780–783, 1976.

345. *Mortimer, R. H., Fleischer, N., Lev-Gur, M., Freeman, R. G.:* Correlation between integrated LH and FSH levels and the response to luteinizing hormone releasing factor (LRF). J. clin. Endocr., *43*, 1240–1249, 1976.

346. *Motlik, K.:* Ovarian neoplasms. Morphology and classification. Acta Univ. Carol. med., Monographia XLIV. Praha, Universita Karlova, 1970.

346a. *Mozley, P. D.:* Psychophysiologic infertility: An overview. Clin. Obstet. Gynec., *19*, 407–417, 1976.

347. *Motta, M., Piva, F., Martini, L.:* The hypothalamus as the center of endocrine feedback mechanism. In: The Hypothalamus. Martini, L., Motta, M., Fraschini, F. (eds.). New York, Academic Press, 1970, p. 463–489.

348. *Mougdal, R. N., Mukku, V. R., Prahalade, S., Murty, G. S. R., Li, C. H.:* Passive immunization with an antibody to β-subunit of ovine LH as a method of early abortion. Feasibility study in monkeys (Macaca radiata). Fertil. and Steril., *30*, 223–229, 1978.

349. *Mühlenstedt, D., Wuttke, W., Schneider, H. P. G.:* Short luteal phase and prolactin. Fertil. and Steril., *28*, 373–374, 1977.

350. *Murray, D. S.:* Statistical method for determination of ovulation time in women. J. Amer. med. Ass., *170*, 42–43, 1959.

351. *Murray, J. L., Abraham, G. E.:* Pseudocyesis: A review. Obstet. and Gynec., *51*, 627–631, 1978.

352. *Murthy, Y. S., Arronet, G. H., Parekh, M. C.:* Luteal phase inadequacy. Its significance in infertility. Obstet. and Gynec., *36*, 758–761, 1970.

353. *Naftolin, F., Judd, H. L.:* Testicular feminization. In: Obstetrics and Gynecology Annual, Vol. 2, 1973. Wynn, R. M. (ed.). New York, Appleton Century Crofts, 1973, p. 25–53.

354. *Nakai, Y., Plant, T. M., Hess, D. L., Keogh, E. J., Knobil, E.:* Site of negative and positive feedback actions of oestradiol in control of gonadotropin secretion in Rhesus monkey. Endocrinology, *102*, 1008–1014, 1978.

355. *Nakano, R., Katayama, K., Mizuno, T., Tojo, S.:* Induction of ovulation with synthetic luteinizing hormone-releasing hormone. Fertil. and Steril., *25*, 471–477, 1974.

356. *Nakano, R., Kotsuji, F., Tojo, S.:* Pituitary responsiveness to synthetic luteinizing hormone- -releasing hormone (LH-RH) during the menstrual cycle and in female hypogonadism. Brit. J. Obstet. Gynaec., *82*, 805–811, 1975.

357. *Nakashima, I., Robinson, A.:* Fertility in a 45,X female. Pediatrics, *47*, 770–772, 1971.

358. *Nelboeck, M.:* Cyclisches Adenosinphosphat in der Kausalkette hormoneller Wirkungen. Naturwissenschaften, *59*, 209–313, 1972.

359. *Neumann, F.:* Physiological action of progesterone and pharmacological effects of pro- gestogens. Short review. Postgrad. med. J., *54*, Suppl. 2: 11–24, 1978.

360. *Neumann, F., Schenck, B.:* New antiandrogens and their mode of action. J. Reprod. Fertil., Suppl. 24: 129–145, 1976.

361. *Nieminieva, K.:* Observations on the development of the hypophyseal-portal system. Acta paediat. (Uppsala), *39*, 366–377, 1950.

362. *Nillius, S. J.:* Amenorrhoea after oral contraceptives. In: Hormonal Contraception. Haspels, A. A., Kay, C. R. (eds.).: Proc. of Int. Symposium on Hormonal Contraception, Utrecht 1977. Amsterdam, Exc. med., 1978, p. 39–49.

363. *Nillius, S. J., Johansson, E. D. B.:* Plasma levels of progesterone after vaginal, rectal or intramuscular administration of progesterone. Amer. J. Obstet. Gynec., *110*, 470–477, 1971.

364. *Nillius, S. J., Wide, L.:* Variation in LH and FSH response to LH-releasing hormone during the menstrual cycle. J. Obstet. Gynaec. Brit. Cwlth., *79*, 865–873, 1972.

365. *Nillius, S. J., Wide, L.:* Progesterone-induced augmentation of pituitary gonadotrophin responses to luteinizing hormone-releasing hormone in oestrogen-pre-treated amenorrhoeic women. Acta endocr. (Kbh.), *83*, 684–691, 1976.

366. *Nillius, S. J., Wide, L.:* Acute and chronic effects of the stimulatory luteinizing hormone- -releasing hormone analogue D-Ser(TBU[6])-EA[10]-LRH on the gonadotrophin and gonadal steroid secretion in women with amenorrhoea. Acta endocr. (Kbh.), *85*, Suppl. 212: 138, 1977.

367. *Nocke, W., Leyendecker, G.:* Neue Erkenntnisse über die endokrine Physiologie des men- struellen Cyklus. Gynäkologe, 5, 39–72, 1972.

368. *Nogales-Ortiz, F., Puerta, S., Nogales, F. F. Jr.:* The normal menstrual cycle: Chronology and mechanism of endometrial desquamation. Obstet. and Gynec., *51*, 259–264, 1978.

369. *Norman, R. L., Resko, J. A., Spies, H. G.:* Anterior hypothalamus. How it affects gonado- tropin secretion in Rhesus monkey. Endocrinology, *99*, 59–71, 1976.

370. *Nouza, K., John, C.:* Immunology and medicine (in Czech). 2nd ed. Praha, Avicenum, 1976.

371. *Noyes, R. W.:* Uniformity of secretory endometrium. Study of multiple sections from 100 uteri removed at operation. Fertil. and Steril., *7*, 103–109, 1956.

372. *Noyes, R. W., Hertig, A. T., Rock, J.:* Dating the endometrial biopsy. Fertil. and Steril., *1*, 1–25, 1950.

373. *Odell, W. D., Swerdloff, R. S.:* Progesterone induced luteinizing and follicle stimulating hormone surge in postmenopausal women: A simulated ovulation peak. Proc. nat. Acad. Sci. (Wash.), *61*, 529–536, 1968.

397

374. *Odell, W. D., Swerdloff, R. S., Wollesen, F.:* Selected aspects of control of LH and FSH secretion in women. In: The Endocrine Function of the Human Ovary. James, V. H. T., Serio, M., Guisti, G. (eds.). London, New York, San Francisco, Academic Press, 1976, p. 89–108.

375. *Ohno, S.:* Sex chromosomes and sex-linked genes. Berlin/Heidelberg/New York, Springer, 1967.

376. *Ohno, S.:* Simplicity of mammalian regulatory systems referred by single gene determination of sex phenotypes. Nature (London), *234*, 134–137, 1971.

377. *Ojeda, S. R., McCann, S. M.:* Control of LH and FSH release by LH-RH: Influence of putative neurotransmitters. Clin. Obstet. Gyneac., *5*, 283–303, 1978.

378. *Okon, E., Koch, Y.:* Localisation of gonadotropin-releasing and thyrotropin-releasing hormones in human brain by radioimmunoassay. Nature (London), *263*, 345–347, 1976.

379. *Ondo, J. G.:* Gamma-aminobutyric acid effects on pituitary gonadotropin secretion. Science, *186*, 738–739, 1974.

380. *Orcel, L., Smadja, A., Roland, J., Minh, H. N.:* Nouvelle hypothèse sur le mécanisme intime de la menstruation. Rev. franç. gynéc., *68*, 477–482, 1973.

381. *Osler, D. C., Crawford, J. D.:* Examination of the hypothesis of a critical weight at menarche in ambulatory and bedridden mentally retarded girls. Pediatrics, *51*, 675–679, 1974.

382. *Overzier, C.:* Intersexualität. Stuttgart, Georg Thieme Verlag, 1961.

383. *Paeschke, K.-D.:* Ovulationsvorbereitung und Ovulation. Bibl. Gynec. 56. Basel, S. Karger, 1970.

384. *Palkovits, M., Brownstein, M., Saavedra, J. M., Axelrod, J.:* Norepinephrine and dopamine content of hypothalamic nuclei in the rat. Brain Res., *77*, 137–149, 1974.

385. *Palkovits, M., Arimura, A., Brownstein, M., Schally, A. V., Saavedra, J. M.:* Luteinizing hormone-releasing hormone (LH-RH) content of the hypothalamic nuclei in rat. Endocrinology, *95*, 554–558, 1974.

386. *Palmer, J. P., Kneer, W. F., Eccleston, H. H.:* Endometrial biopsy. Comparison of aspiration curettage with conventional dilatation and curettage. Amer. J. Obstet. Gynec., *60*, 671–674, 1960.

387. *Palmer, R. L., Crisp, A., McKinnon, P. C. B., Franklin, M., Akand, E. O., Bonnar, J.:* Gonadotrophin response to LH/FSH-RH during weight gain in patients with anorexia nervosa. J. Endocr., *63*, 32P, 1974.

388. *Paola, G. R. di, Mendez Ribas, J. M., Arrighi, L. A.:* Critical study of the retarded progestational phase. Int. J. Fertil., *16*, 189–194, 1971.

389. *Pauerstein, C. J., Eddy, C. A., Croxatto, H. D., Hess, R., Siler-Khodr, T. M., Croxatto, H. B.:* Temporal relationships of oestrogen, progesterone and luteinizing hormone levels to ovulation in women and infrahuman primates. Amer. J. Obstet. Gynec., *130*, 876–886, 1978.

390. *Paulsen, R. P., Sobel, E. H., Shafran, M. S.:* Urinary steroid metabolites in children. I. Individual 17-ketosteroids in children with normal sexual development. J. clin. Endocr., *26*, 329–339, 1966.

391. *Penny, R., Olambiwonnu, N. O., Frasier, S. D.:* Serum gonadotropin concentrations during the first four years of life. J. clin. Endocr., *38*, 320–321, 1974.

391a. *Peretz, A., Sharf, M.:* Culdoscopy in gynecologic diagnosis. Amer. J. Obstet. Gynec., *82*, 582–587, 1961.

392. *Pepperell, R. J., deKretser, D. M., Burger, H. G.:* Studies on the metabolic clearance rate and production rate of human luteinizing hormone and on the initial half time of its subunits in man. J. clin. Invest., *56*, 118–126, 1975.

398

393. *Perez-Lopez, F. R., L'Hermite, M., Robyn, C.:* Gonadotrophin hormone releasing tests in women receiving hormonal contraception. Clin. Endocr., *4*, 477–485, 1975.

394. *Pernoll, M. L.:* Diagnosis and treatment of galactorrhoea. Postgrad. Med., *49*, 76–82, 1971.

395. *Peter, R., Veselý, K.:* Kindergynäkologie. Jena, VEB Georg Thieme, 1966.

396. *Peters, F., Richter, D.:* Psychosomatic conflicts and gonadotropin secretion. Acta endocr. (Kbh.), Suppl. 225: 471–472, 1979.

397. *Peters, H., Himelstein-Braw, R., Faber, M.:* The normal development of the ovary in childhood. Acta endocr. (Kbh.), *82*, 617–630, 1976.

398. *Petrusz, P., Sar, M.:* Light microscopic localization of gonadotropin binding sites in ovarian target cells. In: Cell Membrane Receptors for Drugs and Hormones: A Multidisciplinary Approach. Straub, R. W., Bolis, L. (eds.). New York, Raven Press, 1978, p. 167–182.

399. *Pimstone, B., Epstein, S., Hamilton, S. M., Lervith, D., Hendricks, S.:* Metabolic clearance and plasma half disappearance time of exogenous gonadotropin releasing hormone in normal subjects and in patients with liver disease and chronic renal failure. J. clin. Endocr., *44*, 356–360, 1977.

400. *Piotrow, P. T., Rinehart, W., Schmidt, J. C.:* IUDs — Update on safety, effectiveness, and research. Popul. Rep., Ser. B, 49–98, 1979.

401. *Pizzaro, E., Gomez-Rogers, C., Rowe, P. J., Lucero, S.:* Comparative study of the progesterone T (65 μg/d) and Copper 7 IUD. Contraception, 16, 313–323, 1977.

402. *Plant, T. M., Krey, L. C., Moossy, J., McCormack, J. T., Hess, D. L., Knobil, E.:* Arcuate nucleus and control of gonadotropin and prolactin secretion in female Rhesus monkey (Macaca mulatta). Endocrinology, 102, 58–62, 1978.

403. *Prasad, M. R. N., Sarkaran, M. S.:* Mode of action of non-steroidal antioestrogens. Acta endocr. (Kbh.), *71*, Suppl. 166: 448–456, 1972.

404. *Presl, J.:* Development of the oestrogen-feedback. (Summary in English.) Praha, Avicenum, 1974.

405. *Presl, J.:* Menstrual cycle disorders starting at menarche. (Summary in English.) Čs. Gynek., *39*, 356–359, 1974.

406. *Presl, J., Hrozek, D., Horský, J.:* Die Parotitis epidemica in der Anamnese von Frauen mit Störungen des Menstruationszyklus. Zbl. Gynäk., *90*, 1184–1189, 1968.

407. *Presl, J., Horský, J.:* Uterine bleeding as a placebo effect. (Summary in English.) Čs. Gynek., *35*, 413–415, 1970

408. *Presl, J., Bechinie, K., Horský, J.:* The possibility of placebo effect in the progesterone test. (Summary in English.) Čs. Gynek., *35*, 409–412, 1970.

409. *Presl, J., Herzmann, J., Horský, J.:* Developmental changes in urinary oestrogen secretion in girls. (Summary in English.) Čs. Gynek., *36*, 174–178, 1971.

410. *Presl, J., Pospíšil, J., Figarová, V., Wagner, V.:* Developmental changes in uptake of radio-activity by the ovaries, pituitary and uterus after $^{125}$I-labelled hCG administration in rats. J. Endocr., *52*, 585-586, 1972.

411. *Presl, J., Pospíšil, J., Figarová, V., Krabec, Z.:* Stage-dependent changes in binding of iodinated FSH during ovarian follicle maturation in rats. Endocr. exp., *8*, 291–298, 1974.

412. *Presl, J., Hořejší, J., Štroufová, A., Herzmann, J.:* Sexual maturation in girls and the development of oestrogen-induced gonadotropic hormone release. Ann. Biol. anim. Biochim. Biophys., *16*, 377–383, 1976.

413. *Preslock, J. P.:* Gonadal steroid regulation of pineal malatonin synthesis. Life Sci., *20*, 1299–1304, 1977.

414. *Procopé, B. J., Adlercreutz, H.:* Studies on the influence of age on oestrogens in post--menopausal women with atrophic endometrium and normal liver function. Acta endocr. (Kbh.), *62*, 461–467, 1969.

414a. *Pundel, J. P.:* Les frottis vaginaux endocriniens. Paris, Masson & Cie, 1952, p. 102.
415. *Purandare, T., Sar, M., Stumpf, W. E.:* Immunohistochemical localization of FSH and LH in rat pituitary. Mol. cell. Endocr., *10,* 57–62, 1978.
416. *Raacke, I. D.:* Protein hormones and the eucaryotic genome: A general theory of hormone action. Perspect. Biol. Med., *21,* 139–157, 1977.
417. *Raj, S. G., Thompson, I. E., Berger, M. J., Taymor, M. L.:* Clinical aspects of the polycystic ovary syndrome. Obstet. and Gynec., *49,* 552–556, 1977.
418. *Rakoff, J., Vandenberg, G., Siler, T. M., Yen, S. S. C.:* An integrated direct functional test of the adenohypophysis. Amer. J. Obstet. Gynec., *119,* 358–368, 1974.
419. *Rauscher, H.:* Die Ermittlung der präovulatorischen Phase durch die Simultanuntersuchung von Vaginalabstrich (Smear) und Zervix. Geburtsh. u. Frauenheilk., *16,* 890–906, 1956.
420. *Rawlings, N. C., Kennedy, S. W., Henricks, D. M.:* Effect of active immunization of the cyclic ewe against oestradiol-17β. J. Endocr., *76,* 11–19, 1978.
421. *Rebar, R., Judd, H. L., Yen, S. S. C., Rakoff, J., Vandenberg, G., Naftolin, F.:* Characterization of the inappropriate gonadotropin secretion in polycystic ovary syndrome. J. clin. Invest., *57,* 1320–1329, 1976.
422. *Rebar, R., Lucky, A., Rakoff, J., Johnsonbaugh, E., Vaitukaitis, J., Yen, S.:* Hypothalamic-gonadotropin maturation in the absence of gonadal feedback: Chronologic studies in gonadal dysgenesis. Gynec. Invest., *8,* 92, 1977.
423. *Reilly, W. A.:* Thyrotoxicosis. Amer. J. Dis. Child., *60,* 79–86, 1940.
424. *Reiter, R. J., Vaughan, M. K.:* Pineal antigonadotrophic substances: polypeptides and indoles. Life Sci., *21,* 159–172, 1977.
425. The Pineal and Reproduction. (Progress in Reproductive Biology. Vol. 4.) Reiter, R. J. (ed.). Basel, Karger, 1978.
426. *Reuter, L. A., Lisk, R. D.:* Progesterone may act at hypothalamus and pituitary by way of enhancement of oestrogen retention. Nature, *262,* 790–791, 1976.
427. *Reuter, A. M., Ketelslegers, J. M., Hendrick, J. C., Franchimont, P.:* Radioimmunoassay of protein hormones: Principles and methodology. Hormone Res., *9,* 404–421, 1978.
428. *Reyes, F. I., Boroditsky, R. S., Winter, J. S. D., Faiman, C.:* Studies on human sexual development. II. Fetal and maternal serum gonadotropin and sex steroid concentration. J. clin. Endocr., *38,* 612–617, 1974.
429. *Reyes, F. I., Winter, J. S. D., Faiman, C.:* Gonadotropin–gonadal interrelationships in the fetus. In: Diabetes and Other Endocrine Disorders during Pregnancy and in the Newborn. New York, Alan R. Liss, 1976, p. 83–106.
430. *Reyes, F. I., Winter, J. S. D., Faiman, C.:* Pituitary-ovarian relationship preceeding menopause. 1. Cross-sectional study of serum FSH, LH, prolactin, estradiol and progesterone levels. Amer. J. Obstet. Gynec., *129,* 557–564, 1977.
431. *Rigler, G. L., Peake, G. T., Ratner, A.:* Effect of luteinizing hormone releasing hormone on accumulation of pituitary cyclic AMP and GMP in vitro. J. Endocr., *76,* 367–368, 1978.
432. *Rinehart, W., Piotrow, P. T.:* Oral contraceptives. Update on usage, safety, and side effects. Popul. Rep., Ser. A, 133–186, 1979.
433. *Rockenschaub, A.:* Der menstruelle Zyklus. Z. Geburtsh. Gynäk., *155,* 105–156, 1960.
434. *Roemer, H.:* Das Sexualleben der Frau und seine Störungen. In: Gynäkologie und Geburtshilfe, Bd. 1. Käser, O. et al. (eds.). Stuttgart, Thieme, 1969, p. 487–544.
435. *Römmler, A., Baumgarten, S., Hammerstein, J.:* Doppelstimulierung der Hypophyse mit synthetischem LH-Releasinghormon an drei aufeinanderfolgenden Tagen bei Männern sowie menstruierenden und amenorrhoischen Frauen. Geburtsh. u. Frauenheilk., *34,* 842–850, 1974.
436. *Rosemberg, E.:* A comparison of treatment schedules for ovulation induction with HMG

400

and HCG. In: Gonadotropin Therapy in Female Infertility. Rosenberg, E. (ed.). Amsterdam, Exc. Medica, 1973, p. 103–108.

437. *Rosenfield, A.:* Oral and intrauterine contraception: A 1978 risk assessment. Amer. J. Obstet. Gynec., *132*, 92–106, 1978.

438. *Rosenfield, R. L.:* Studies of the relation of plasma androgen levels to androgen action in women. J. Steroid Biochem., *6*, 695–702, 1975.

439. *Ross, C., Piotrow, P. T.:* Birth control without contraceptives. Popul. Rep., Ser. I, 1–19, 1974.

440. *Ross, G. T.:* Clinical relevance of research on the structure of human chorionic gonadotropin. Amer. J. Obstet. Gynec., *129*, 795–808, 1977.

441. *Ross, G. T.:* Morphologic correlates of hormone profiles in blood and antral fluid during ovulatory cycles in women. Uppsala J. med. Sci., Suppl. 22: 7–15, 1978.

442. *Ruf, K. B.:* How does the brain control the process of puberty? Z. Neurol., *204*, 96–105, 1973.

443. *Ryan, R. J., Lee, C. T.:* The role of membrane bound receptors. Biol. Reprod., *14*, 16–29, 1976.

444. *Rybo, G.:* Clinical and experimental studies on menstrual blood loss. Acta obstet. gynaec. scand., *45*, Suppl. 7: 1–23, 1966.

445. *Sadeghi-Nejad, A., Senior, B.:* Sexual precocity: an unusual complication of propylthiouracil therapy. J. Pediat., *79*, 833–837, 1971.

446. *Sandow, J., von Rechenberg, W., Jerzabek, G., Stoll, W.:* Pituitary gonadotropin inhibition by a highly active analog of luteinizing hormone-releasing hormone. Fertil. and Steril., *30*, 205–209, 1978.

447. *Sawyer, C. H., Hilliard, J., Kanematsu, S., Scaramuzzi, R., Blake, C. A.:* Effects of intraventricular infusions of norepinephrine and dopamine on LH release and ovulation in the rabbit. Neuroendocrinology, *15*, 328–337, 1974.

448. *Saxena, B. B., Rathnam, P., Römmler, A.:* Human pituitary follicle stimulating and luteinizing hormones: Current status. Endocr. exp., 7, 19–36, 1973.

449. *Saxena, B. B., Landesman, R.:* Does implantation occur in the presence of an IUD? Res. in Reprod., *10*, 1–3, 1978.

450. *Schally, A. V., Kastin, A. J., Arimura, A.:* The hypothalamus and reproduction. Amer. J. Obstet. Gynec., *114*, 423–442, 1972.

451. *Schally, A. V., Kastin, A. J., Coy, D. H.:* LH-releasing hormone and its analogues: Recent basis and clinical investigations. Int. J. Fertil., *21*, 1–30, 1976.

452. *Schmidt-Elmendorff, H.:* Klinische und experimentelle Ergebnisse mit dem Ovulationsauslöser Fertodur (Cyclofenil). Geburtsh. u. Frauenheilk., *31*, 693, 1971. (Ref.)

452a. *Schmidt-Elmendorff, H., Kämmering, R.:* Vergleichende klinische Untersuchungen von Clomiphen, Cyclofenil und Epimestrol. Geburtsh. u. Frauenheilk., *37*, 531–541, 1977.

453. *Schmidt-Gollwitzer, K., Schmidt-Gollwitzer, M., Sackmann, U., Eiletz, J.:* Ovulation timing by radioreceptor assay for human luteinizing hormone. Int. J. Fertil., *22*, 232–237, 1977.

454. *Schneider, P. B.:* Laboratory examination of the thyroid. 1., 2. Postgraduate Med., *56*, 91–106, 1974.

455. *Schneider, W.:* Dysfunktionelle Blutung. Zbl. Gynäk., *92*, 1062–1067, 1970.

456. *Schomberg, D. W., Williams, R. F., Tyrey, L., Ulberg, L. C.:* Reduction of granulosa cell progesterone secretion in vitro by intraovarian implants of antiandrogen. Endocrinology, *102*, 984–987, 1978.

457. *Schröder, R.:* Die Klinik des normalen und gestörten menstruellen Cyclus. Arch. Gynäk., *183*, 204–236, 1953.

458. *Schulster, D.:* Radioreceptor assays: plasma membrane receptors and assays for polypeptide and glycoprotein hormones. J. Reprod. Fertil., *51*, 295–301, 1977.

459.  *Schulz, K. D., Geiger, W., Del Pozo, E., Kunzig, H. J.:* Pattern of sexual steroids, prolactin and gonadotropic hormones during prolactin inhibition in normally cycling women. Amer. J. Obstet. Gynec., *132,* 561–566, 1978.
460.  *Schumacher, G. F. B.:* Biochemistry of cervical mucus. Fertil. and Steril., *21,* 697–705, 1970.
461.  *Schwartz, N. B., Channing, C. P.:* Evidence for "inhibin": Suppression of the secondary rise in serum follicle stimulating hormone levels in proestrous rats by injection of porcine follicular fluid. Proc. nat. Acad. Sci. (Wash.), *74,* 5721–5724, 1977.
462.  *Seif, S. M., Robinson, A. G.:* Localization and release of neurophysins. Ann. Rev. Physiol., *40,* 345–376, 1978.
463.  *Selmanoff, M. K., Pramik-Holdaway, M. J., Weiner, R. I.:* Concentrations of dopamine and norepinephrine in discrete hypothalamic nuclei during the rat oestrous cycle. Endocrinology *99,* 326–329, 1976.
464.  *Sen, K. K., Menon, K. M. J.:* Oestradiol receptors in the rat anterior pituitary gland during the oestrous cycle: Quantitation of receptor activity in relation to gonadotrophin releasing hormone-mediated luteinizing hormone release. J. Endocr., *76,* 211–218, 1978.
465.  *Serra* (discussion) — In: Recent Progress in Reproductive Endocrinology. Crosignani, P. G., James, V. H. T. (eds.). London/New York, Academic Press, 1974, p. 569–570.
466.  *Shanklin, D. R.:* Symposium on histologic dating of the endometrium. J. reprod. Med., *3,* 179–200, 1969.
467.  *Shaw, R. W.:* Differential response to LH-RH following oestrogen therapy in women with amenorrhoea. Brit. J. Obstet. Gynaec., *86,* 69–75, 1979.
468.  *Shaw, R. W., Butt, W. R., London, D. R., Marshall, J. C.:* The oestrogen provocation test: A method of assessing the hypothalamic-pituitary axis in patients with amenorrhoea. Clin. Endocr., *4,* 267–276, 1975.
469.  *Shaw, R. W., Butt, W. R., London, D. R.:* The effect of oestrogen pretreatment on subsequent response to luteinizing hormone releasing hormone in normal women. Clin. Endocr., *4,* 297–304, 1975.
470.  *Shaw, R. W., Butt, W. R., London, D. R.:* The effect of progesterone on FSH and LH response to LH-RH in normal women. Clin. Endocr., *4,* 543–550, 1975.
471.  *Shearman, R. P.:* Post-coital contraception. A review. Contraception, *7,* 459–476, 1973.
472.  *Sheehan, H. L.:* The frequency of post-partum hypopituitarism. J. Obstet. Gynaec. Brit. Cwlth, *72,* 103–111, 1965.
473.  *Shepard, M. K., Senturia, Y. D.:* Comparison of serum progesterone and endometrial biopsy for confirmation of ovulation and evaluation of luteal function. Fertil. and Steril., *28,* 541–548, 1977.
474.  *Sherman, B. M., Korenman, S. G.:* Measurement of serum LH, FSH, oestradiol and progesterone in disorders of the human menstrual cycle: The inadequate luteal phase. J. clin. Endocr., *39,* 145–149, 1974.
475.  *Sherman, B. M., West, J. H., Korenman, S. G.:* The menopausal transition: Analysis of LH, FSH, oestradiol and progesterone concentrations during menstrual cycles of older women. J. clin. Endocr., *42,* 629–636, 1976.
476.  *Shippel, S.:* The ovarian theca cell. Part IV — The hyperthecosis syndrome. J. Obstet. Gynaec. Brit. Emp., *62,* 321–353, 1955.
477.  *Shoemaker, E. S., Forney, J. P., MacDonald, P. C.:* Oestrogen treatment of postmenopausal women. Benefits and risks. J. Amer. med. Ass., *238,* 1524–1530, 1977.
478.  *Shome, B., Parlow, A. F.:* The primary structure of the hormone-specific, β-subunit of human luteinizing hormone (hLH). J. clin. Endocr., *36,* 618–621, 1973.
479.  *Shome, B., Parlow, A. F.:* Human follicle stimulating hormone: First proposal for the amino

acid sequence of the α-subunit (hFSHα) and first demonstration of its identity with the α-subunit of human luteinizing hormone (hLHα). First proposal for the amino acid sequence of the hormone-specific β-subunit (hFSHβ). J. clin. Endocr., *39*, 199–202; 203–205, 1974.

480. *Shome, B., Parlow, A. F.:* Human pituitary prolactin (hPRL): The entire linear amino acid sequence. J. clin. Endocr., *45*, 1112–1115, 1977.

481. *Shulman, S., Friedman, M. R.,:* Antibodies to spermatozoa. 5. Antibody activity in human cervical mucus. Amer. J. Obstet. Gynec., *122*, 101–105, 1975.

482. *Slaunwhite, W. R., Jr., Kirdani, R. Y., Sandberg, A. A.:* Metabolic aspects of oestrogens in man. In: Handbook of Physiology. Sec. 7. Endocrinology Vol. II. Greep, R. O. (ed.). Washington, Amer. Physiol. Soc., 1973, p. 485–523.

483. *Smith, R. G.:* Hormone-receptor interactions – Basic mechanisms. Int. J. Fertil., *21*, 159–162, 1976.

484. *Smith, R. P., Ross, B.:* Post-coital contraception using dl-norgestrel/ethinyl oestradiol combination. Contraception, *17*, 247–252, 1978.

485. *Soria, J., Zarate, A., Canales, E. S., Ayala, A., Schally, A. V., Coy, D. H., Coy, E. J., Kastin, A. J.:* Increased and prolonged LH-RH/FSH-RH activity of synthetic (D-Ala[6], desGly-NH2[10]) LH-RH ethylamide in normal women. Amer. J. Obstet. Gynec., *123*, 145–146, 1975.

486. *Southam, A. L., Richart, R. M.:* The prognosis for adolescents with menstrual abnormalities. Amer. J. Obstet. Gynec., *94*, 637–645, 1966.

487. *Spona, J.:* Rapid timing of imminent ovulation in sterility patients. Endocr. exp., *7*, 125 to 128, 1973.

488. *Spona, J., Schneider, W. H. F., Wacheck, W.:* Rascher Radioimmunoassay für die Bestimmung von Progesteronserumspiegeln. Wien. klin. Wschr., *90*, 654–658, 1978.

489. *Staemmler, H. J.:* Die gestörte Regelung der Ovarialfunktion. Berlin, Springer, 1964.

490. *Stange, H. H.:* Zur Morphologie, Klinik und Genese der hochgradig unterentwickelten „Eierstöcke". Z. Geburtsh. Gynäk., *147*, 261–332, 1956.

491. *Starup, J., Sele, V.:* Premature ovarian failure. Acta obstet. gynaec. scand., *52*, 259–268, 1973.

492. *Stein, I. R., Leventhal, M. L.:* Amenorrhoea associated with bilateral polycystic ovaries. Amer. J. Obstet. Gynec., *29*, 181–191, 1935.

493. *Stein-Werblowsky, R.:* Penetration of spermatozoa into the uterine mucosa: a possible cause of infertility in the human. Int. J. Fertil., *18*, 74–80, 1973.

494. *Steiner, R. A., Clifton, D. K., Spies, H. G., Resko, J. A.:* Sexual differentiation and feedback control of luteinizing hormone secretion in the Rhesus monkey. Biol. Reprod., *15*, 206–212, 1976.

495. *Steiner, R. A., Schiller, H. S., Barber, J., Gale, C. C.:* Luteinizing hormone regulation in the monkey (Macaca nemestrina): Failure of testosterone and dihydrotestosterone to block the oestrogen-induced gonadotropic surge. Biol. Reprod., *19*, 51–56, 1978.

496. *Stevens, V. C.:* Research on the development of antifertility vaccines. Acta obstet. gynaec. jap., *29*, 1203, 1977.

497. *Stieve, H.:* Der Einfluss des Nervensystems auf Bau und Tätigkeit der Geschlechtsorgane des Menschen. Stuttgart, Thieme, 1952.

498. *Stone, S. C., Mickal, A., Rye, P. H., Dickey, R. P.:* Postmenopausal symptomatology, maturation index, plasma oestrogen levels. Obstet. and Gynec. (ref.), *43*, 622, 1974.

499. *Strott, C. A., Cargille, C. M., Ross, G. T., Lipsett, M. B.:* The short luteal phase. J. clin. Endocr. *30*, 246–251, 1970.

500. *Sykes, D. W., Einsburg, J.:* The use of laparoscopic ovarian biopsy to assess gonadal function. Amer. J. Obstet. Gynec., *112*, 408–413, 1972.

501. *Szontagh, F. E.:* Short-loop (internal) pituitary-hypothalamus gonadotropin feedback in the human. Endocr. exp., *7,* 65–67, 1973.

502. *Talbot, N. R., Jubel, E. H., McArthur, J. W., Crawford, J. D.:* Functional endocrinology, from birth through adolescence. Cambridge (Massachusetts), Harvard University Press, 1952.

503. *Talwar, G. P.:* The present and future of immunologic approaches to contraception. Int. J. Gynaec. Obstet., *15,* 410–414, 1978.

504. *Tamaya, T., Furuta, N., Motoyama, T., Boku, S., Ohono, Y., Okada, H.:* Mechanism of antiprogestational action of synthetic steroids. Acta endocr. (Kbh.), *88,* 190–198, 1978.

505. *Tamura, T., Minaguchi, H., Sakamoto, S.:* Responsiveness of human fetal pituitary to hypothalamic hormones in vitro. Endocr. jap., *20,* 545–553, 1973.

506. *Tatum, H. J.:* Clinical aspects of intrauterine contraception: Circumspection 1976. Fertil. and Steril., *28,* 3–28, 1977.

507. *Taubert, H.-D., Jürgensen, O.:* The treatment of monophasic cycles with the retroprogesterone Ro4-8347. Bull. schweiz. Akad. med. Wiss., *25,* 503–511, 1969.

508. *Taymor, M. L.:* The use of luteinizing hormone-releasing hormone in gynecologic endocrinology. Fertil. and Steril., *25,* 992–1005, 1974.

509. *Tietze, Ch.:* The pill and mortality from cardiovascular disease: Another look. Fam. Plan. Perspectives, *11,* 80–84, 1979.

510. *Tillson, S. A., Marian, M., Hudson, R., Wong, P., Pharriss, B., Aznar, R., Martinez--Manautou, J.:* The effect of intrauterine progesterone on the hypothalamo-hypophyseal--ovarian axis in humans. Contraception, *11,* 179–192, 1975.

511. *Tima, L., Flerkó, B.:* Ovulation induced by norepinephrine in rats made anovulatory by various experimental procedures. Neuroendocrinology, *15,* 346–354, 1974.

512. *Timonen, S., Procopé, B.-J.:* The premenstrual syndrome; frequency and association of symptoms. Ann. Chir. Gynaec. Fenn., *62,* 108–116, 1973.

513. *Treloar, A. E., Boynton, R. E., Behn, B. G., Brown, B. W.:* Variation of the human menstrual cycle through reproductive life. Int. J. Fertil., *12,* 77–126, 1967.

514. *Trygstad, O., Foss, I., Edminson, P. D., Johansen, J. H., Reichelt, K. L.:* Humoral control of appetite: An urinary anorexigenic peptide. Chromatographic patterns of urinary peptides in anorexia nervosa. Acta endocr. (Kbh.), *89,* 196–208, 1978.

515. *Tsafriri, A., Pomerantz, S. H., Channing, C. P.:* Inhibition of oocyte maturation by porcine follicular fluid. Partial characterization of the inhibitor. Biol. Reprod., *14,* 511–516, 1976.

516. *Tseng, L., Gurpide, E.:* Competition of oestetrol and ethinyloestradiol with oestradiol for nuclear binding in human endometrium. J. Steroid Biochim., *7,* 817–822, 1976.

517. *Valcke, J. Cl., Mahoudeau, J. A., Thieblot, P., Pique, L., Luton, J. P., Franchimont, P.:* Critères d'interprétation du test utilisant l'hormone de libération de la lutéostimuline (LH--RH). Ann. Endocr. (Paris), *35,* 423–443, 1974.

518. *Vale, W., Rivier, C., Brown, M.:* Regulatory peptides of the hypothalamus. Ann. Rev. Physiol., *39,* 473–527, 1977.

519. *Vandalem, J. L., Pirens, G., Hennen, G., Gaspard, U.:* Thyroliberin and gonadoliberin tests during pregnancy and the puerperium. Acta endocr. (Kbh.), *86,* 695–703, 1977.

520. *Van Orden, D. E., Swanson, J. A., Clancey, C. J., Farley, D. B.:* Plasma prostaglandins in the normal menstrual cycle. Obstet. and Gynec., *50,* 639–643, 1977.

521. *Van Look, P. F. A., Hunter, W. M., Fraser, I. S., Baird, D. T.:* Impaired oestrogen-induced luteinizing hormone release in young women with anovulatory dysfunctional uterine bleeding. J. clin. Endocr., *46,* 816–823, 1978.

522. *Van Wyk, J. J., Grumbach, M.:* Syndrome of precocious menstruation and galactorrhoea in

404

juvenile hypothyroidism: an example of hormonal overlap in pituitary feedback. J. Pediat., 57, 416–435, 1960.

523. *Vermeulen, A.:* The hormonal activity of the postmenopausal ovary. J. clin. Endocr., 42, 247–253, 1976.

524. *Vessey, M. P.:* Contraceptive methods: risks and benefits. Brit. med. J., 2, 721–722, 1978.

525. *Villa de, G. O., Roberts, K., Wiest, W. G., Flickinger, G.:* A specific radioimmunoassay of plasma progesterone. J. clin. Endocr., 35, 458–460, 1972.

526. *Volkova, O. V.:* Struktura i reguljacija funkcij jaičnikov. Moskva, Medicina, 1970, p. 34–51. Structure and regulation of the ovarian function (in Russian).

526a. *Vorherr, H.:* The Breast. New York/San Francisco/London, Academic Press, 1974.

527. *Wallach, E. E.:* Dysfunctional uterine bleeding. Clin. Obstet. Gynec., 13, 363–385, 1970.

528. *Wallach, E. E.:* Evaluation and management of uterine causes of infertility. Clin. Obstet. Gynec., 22, 43–60, 1979.

529. *Wan, L. S., Weiss, G., Ganguly, M.:* Pituitary response to LH-RH stimulation in women on oral contraceptives. Contraception, 17, 1–7, 1978.

530. *Wasada, T., Akamine, Y., Kato, K., Ibayashi, H., Nomura, Y.:* Adrenal contribution to circulating oestrogens in woman. Endocr. jap., 25, 123–128, 1978.

531. *Weiser, P.:* Zur Funktionsdiagnose im weiblichen Zyklus. Geburtsh. u. Frauenheilk., 25, 550–552, 1965.

532. *Weiss, G., Nachtigall, L. E., Ganguly, M.:* Induction of an LH surge with estradiol benzoate: a clinical test of pituitary-hypothalamic axis competence. Obstet. and Gynec., 47, 415–418, 1976.

533. *Werder, K. von, Rjosk, H. K.:* Menschliches Prolaktin. Klin. Wschr., 57, 1–12, 1979.

534. *Whitelaw, M. J.:* Statistical examination of female fertility. Fertil. and Steril., 11, 428–436, 1960.

535. WHO expert committee on biological standardization. Twenty-sixth Report. Technical Report Series 565. Geneva, World Health Organization, 1975.

535a. *Wide, L.:* In: Hormone assays and their clinical application. Loraine, J. A., Bell, E. T. (eds.). 4th ed., London, Churchill, 1976, p. 87.

536. *Wide, L., Roos, P., Gemzell, C.:* Immunological determination of human pituitary luteinizing hormone (LH). Acta endocr. (Kbh.), 37, 445–449, 1961.

537. *Wildschut, J.:* Das limbische System und die Ovulation. Organorama, 10, 3–8, 1973.

537a. *Williams, R. H.. (ed.):* Textbook of Endocrinology. 5th ed. Philadelphia /London/Toronto, W. B. Saunders, 1974.

537b. *Wilson, E. A., Erickson, G. F., Zarutski, P., Finn, A. E., Tulchinsky, D., Ryan, K. J.:* Endocrine studies of normal and polycystic ovarian tissues in vitro. Amer. J. Obstet. Gynec., 134, 56–63, 1979.

538. *Winter, J. S. D., Faiman, C.:* Serum gonadotropin concentrations in agonadal children and adults. J. clin. Endocr., 35, 561–564, 1972.

539. *Winter, J. S. D., Faiman, C.:* Pituitary-gonadal relations in female children and adolescents. Pediat. Res., 7, 948–953, 1973.

540. *Winter, J. S. D., Faiman, C., Reyes, F. I.:* Normal and abnormal pubertal development. Clin. Obstet. Gynec., 21, 67–86, 1978.

540a. *Wood, L. C., Olichney, M., Locke, H., Crispell, K. R., Thornton, W. N., Kitay, J. I.:* Syndrome of juvenile hypothyroidism associated with advanced sexual development: Report of two new cases and comment on the management of an associated ovarian mass. J. clin. Endocr., 25, 1289–1295, 1965.

541. *Worm, M.:* Menstruation und Fertilität bei Diabetes mellitus. Zbl. Gynäk., 77, 886–893, 1955.

542. *Wu, Ch., Motohashi, T., Abdel-Rahman, H. A., Flickinger, G. L., Mikhail, G.:* Free and protein-bound plasma oestradiol-17β during the menstrual cycle. J. clin. Endocr., *43*, 436–445, 1976.

543. *Wurtman, J., Axelrod, J., Kelly, D. E.:* The pineal. New York, Academic Press, 1968.

544. *Wurtman, R. J., Moskowitz, M. A.:* The pineal organ. New Engl. J. Med., *296*, 1329–1333, 1383–1386, 1977.

545. *Yen, S. S. C., Tsai, C. C., Naftolin, F., Vandenberg, G., Ajabor, L.:* Pulsatile patterns of gonadotropin release in subjects with and without ovarian function. J. clin. Endocr., *34*, 671–675, 1972.

546. *Yen, S. S. C., Vandenberg, G., Rebar, R., Ehara, Y.:* Variation of pituitary responsiveness to synthetic LRF during different phases of the menstrual cycle. J. clin. Endocr., *35*, 931 to 934, 1972.

547. *Yen, S. S. C., Lasley, B. L., Wang, C. F., Leblanc, H., Siler, T. M.:* The operating characteristics of the hypothalamic-pituitary system during the menstrual cycle and observations of biological action of somatostatin. Recent Progr. Hormone Res., *31*, 321–363, 1975.

548. *Ylikorkala, O., Dawood, M. Y.:* New concepts of dysmenorrhoea. Amer. J. Obstet. Gynec., *130*, 833–847, 1978.

549. *Zacur, H. A., Chapanis, N. P., Lake, C. R., Ziegler, M., Tyson, J. E.:* Galactorrhoea — amenorrhoea: Psychological interaction with neuroendocrine function. Amer. J. Obstet. Gynec., *125*, 859–862, 1976.

550. *Zander, J., Holzmann, K.:* Störungen des menstruellen Zyklus und ihre Behandlung. In: Gynäkologie und Geburtshilfe. Bd. I. Käser, O. et al. (eds.) Stuttgart, Thieme, 1969, p. 315–461.

551. *Zarate, A., Canales, E. S., Soria, J., Forsbach, G., Kastin, A. J., Schally, A. V.:* Therapeutic use of gonadoliberin (follicle-stimulating hormone) luteinizing hormone-releasing hormone in women. Fertil. and Steril., *27*, 1233–1239, 1976.

552. *Zuspan, F. P., Rao, P.:* Thermogenic alterations in the woman. I. Interaction of amines, ovulation and basal body temperature. Amer. J. Obstet. Gynec., *118*, 671–678, 1974.

# Subject Index

Basal body temperature (BBT), **203—208**, 215, 222, 223, 242, 243, 312, 339
  biphasic, 152, **155**, 157, 165, 205, 232, 244, 258, 259, **262**, 269, 302
  hyperthermic, 155, 156
  monophasic, 154, 155, 175, 221, 244, 258, 262, 266, 267
  pregnancy, 205, **207—208**
Basal metabolic rate (BM) 17, 189, 230, 284
Beling's method. *See* Method(s).
Biogenic amines. *See* Amines, biogenic, *also* Neurotransmitters.
Bleeding, dysfunctional uterine. *See* Dysfunctional uterine bleeding.
  physiological uterine. *See* Menstruation.
Body fat ratio, menarche, **17**
Brain,
  foetal, LH-RH occurrence, 32
  sexual maturation, **14—15**
Breakthrough bleeding. 264, 265, 311, 317, 367, 369, 372
Breast(s), development, 12, 88, 171
Breastfeeding, 76
Bromocriptine, 65, 258, 260, 277
  amenorrhoea-galactorrhoea, 274, **282**, 332
  anovulation, 332
  premenstrual tension, 164
Brown's method. *See* Method(s).

cAMP, 46, 113, 118, 375
  adenylate cyclase-cAMP system, 32, 46, 66, 67, 68, 69
  and gonadotropins, **66—69**
Castration, 46, 134, 135, 136, 140, **295—296**, 301. *See also* Ovariectomy.
  neurosis, 24
  postnatal/prepubertal, 296
Catecholamines, 17, 29, 43, 45, 67, 123, 140, 169, 178
Catechol oestrogens. *See* Hydroxyoestrogens.
Central nervous system. *See* CNS.
Cerebral cortex (neocortex), function of, **23—24**
Cervical cycle. *See* Cycle, cervical.
Cervical mucus, **124—126**, 152, **206**, 213, 214, 215, 223, 238, **239—241**, 329, 340, 341, 342, 370

  arborization, 125, 126, **210**, 215, 240
  enzymes in, 241
  ovulation tests, **239—241**
  sodium chloride in, 240
Cervix,
  sterility, cervical causes, **340—342**
Chlormadinone acetate, 361, 366, 367, 371
Cholesterol, 88, 123, 142, 284
  steroidogenesis, ovarian and, **80**, 81
Chorionepithelioma, 170, 292
Chromosomal (gonosomal) aberrations, **174—175, 198**, 201
  classification, pathogenic, **174**
Chromosome(s), sex determination, **1—2, 297**, 298
Chronic anovulation. *See* Anovulation.
Circadian rhythms, endocrine system, **46**
Climacteric, **131—148**. *See also* Menopause.
  anatomical changes, **138—139**
  clinical symptoms, **139—144**
  coronary disease in, **141—142**
  dysfunctional uterine bleeding, **139**
  endocrine regulatory mechanism, **132** to **138**
  hypothalamic neurohormones in, **137**
  osteoporosis, 138, **142—143**
  premature, 293
  steroids, **133—135, 137—138**
  therapy hormonal and non-hormonal, **143—148**
  vegetative disorders, **140**, 266, 305, 307
Clauberg test. *See* Test(s).
Clitoris, hypertrophy, 164, 297
Clomiphene citrate, 111, 223, 226, 253, 263, 276, 320, 322, **324—327**
  mechanism of action, 212
  therapy, 93, 207, 263, 274, 275, 277, 282, 322, 338, 366
Clonidine, 65
CNS, 24, 30, 152, 279, 280, 300
  foetal, 197, 198
  menstrual cycle, corticovisceral disorders, **177**
Coitus, frequency, 25, 333, 334, 341
Competitive protein binding (CPB). *See* Protein binding, competitive.
Conception, 253, 254, 340

Norethisterone acetate, 259, 268, 313, 366, 367, 369, 371

Norethynodrel, 313, 361

Norgestrel, 313, 366, 367, 369, 371, 372
Levo-norgestrel, 361, 372

Norsteroids, **95, 99**

Nuclei, hypothalamic. *See* Hypothalamic nuclei.

Nutrition disorders, menstrual dysfunction, **191—194, 202,** 261


Obesity, 272
menstrual dysfunction, **193—194,** 257, 269, 372

Oestradiol ($E_2$), 18, 22, 85, 86, 87, 91, 145, 206, 229
assessment, 91, **234**
benzoate, 34, 39, 44, 145, 146, 147
excretion, 217
metabolism, 85, 86, 87, 89, 133
physiological action, 39, 74, **87—88**
placental, 9
plasma, 12, 56, 90, 91, 133, 209, 221, 228, 257, 278, 295, 324
production, 85, 86, 309
secretion, 85, 86, 87
sexual maturation, 12
urinary, 87, 90
valerate, 145, 146, 147, 213, 259, 310, 339

Oestriol ($E_3$), 18, 82, 86, 87, 91
assessment, 90
plasma, 89
therapy, 88, 89, 310
climacteric syndrome, 144, 145, 146
premenopause, 144, 145
urinary, 87, 89, 90

Oestrogen(s), **84—91.** *See also* specific compounds.
assessment, **90—91,** 140, 234, **262**
basal body temperature, **206**
biosynthesis, 8, 82, 183, 215
climacteric/menopause, **144—148**
conjugated, 86, 87, 90, 91, 145, 146, 147, 257
contraception, **368,** 369
cytoplasmic oestrogen receptor protein, 14, **113,** 183, 324
endometrium, stimulation, 208
excretion, 18, 209, 215

feedback, inhibitory (negative), **14—15,** 29, **38,** 43, 182, 294, 328
stimulatory (positive), 9, **15,** 29, 36, **39,** 43, 44, 182, 229, 294, 328

MCR, 86

mechanism of action on target tissue, 113, 115, 314

menopause, **135—135,** 144, 145, 146 147, 148

natural, 83, **84—85**

ovarian, 18, 212, 213

physiological action, **87—89, 113—114**

placental, 9, 20

plasma, **89—90,** 134, **265,** 266, 310

provocation test, hypothalamic-hypophyseal axis, functional evaluation, **229**

secretion, circulation and metabolism, **85—87,** 194, 198

sexual maturation, 12, 14

sources and production, **88, 133**

Stein-Leventhal syndrome, **273**

structure, 83, 84

synthetic, 84, **85**

test, **212—213**

therapy, 87, 144, **145,** 146, 147, 148, 203, 212, 223, 229, 268, 279, **309—312, 315**

total oestrogen activity urinary, 19, **89—90,** 134, 208, 209, 213, 214, 226, **234,** 243, 249, 295, 301, 304

vaginal stimulation, **218**

Oestrone ($E_1$), 85, 86, 88, 206
excretion **213,** 214, 215
metabolism, 133
plasma, 12, 86, 90, 133, 135, 295
production, 85, 86, 309
sexual maturation, 12, 14
therapy, 134
urinary, 87, 90

Olfactory communication, 24, 25

Olfacto-genital dysplasia, 246, **279.** *See also* Kalmann-de Morcier syndrome.

Oligomenorrhoea, 24, **155—156,** 159, 180, 183, 187, 194, 195, 207, 212, 223, 257, 266
anovulatory, 260, 261
temporary, 294

Oocyte(s), 4, 5, 71, 72, 73, 74, 201

Oogenesis, **4—5**

Opsomenorrhoea, 155

Ossification age, X-ray examination, **236**

419